COAGULATION:
THE ESSENTIALS

COAGULATION:
THE ESSENTIALS

David P. Fischbach, M.D.
Assistant Professor
Stanford University School of Medicine
Stanford, California

Richard P. Fogdall, M.D.
Associate Professor
Stanford University School of Medicine
Stanford, California

with illustrations by Barbara Haynes

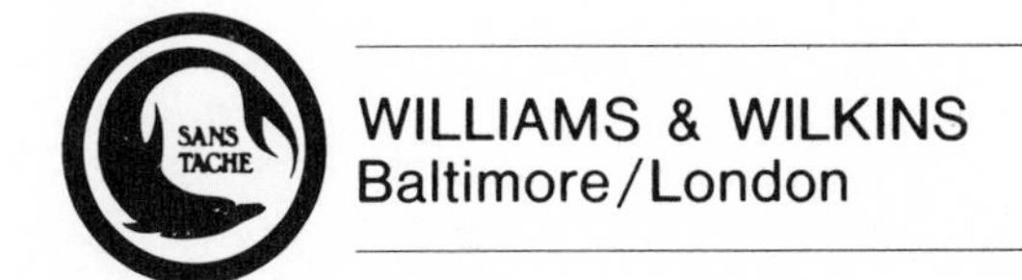

WILLIAMS & WILKINS
Baltimore/London

Made in the United States of America

Library of Congress Cataloging in Publication Data

Fischbach, David P.

Coagulation, the essentials.

Bibliography: p.
Includes index.
1. Blood—Coagulation, Disorders of. 2. Blood—Coagulation. I. Fogdall, Richard P. II. Title.
[DNLM: 1. Blood coagulation. WH 310 F528c]
RC647.C55F57 616.1'57 81-11623
ISBN 0-683-03312-3 AACR2

Composed and printed at
Waverly Press, Inc.
Mt. Royal and Guilford Aves.
Baltimore, MD 21202, U.S.A.

To Jon Kosek and Janet Solomon,
for their unwavering support.

DPF

To Lynne, for her patience and support.

RPF

PREFACE

This book is written primarily for anesthesiologists, surgeons, critical-care physicians and nurses, and medical students. Since an understanding of coagulation is becoming increasingly important in the management of the critically ill patient, we hope that our succinct account will be useful to all who care for these patients.

All books contain a bias from the authors. Ours is to provide the reader with an organized way of thinking, rather than to provide a compendium of facts. To achieve this goal several teaching aids have been used. First, each chapter is divided into the same four topics for organization and ease of comprehension. These same four areas are then used to organize the reader's thinking in analyzing and treating the bleeding patient. Second, illustrations are profuse, enabling the reader to visualize the concepts presented within these four areas.

A difficult aspect of writing such a brief text is that many fascinating areas of coagulation cannot be covered fully. Our major consolation is that busy professionals will appreciate the conciseness. As new information about coagulation is published, the reader should be able to assimilate this new information into the framework we have provided.

David P. Fischbach, M.D.
Richard P. Fogdall, M.D.
Stanford, California

ACKNOWLEDGMENTS

The authors are indebted to many individuals for assistance, suggestions, and comments throughout the preparation of this book. Many of our professional colleagues have spent hours in discussion and review, and we apologize if we have omitted any of them in the list to follow:

Robert T. Wall, MD
Michael Link, MD
Jon Kosek, MD
Willard Spiegelman, MD, PhD
William Dolan, MD
Gene Schmitt, MD
Norig Ellison, MD
Terry S. Vitez, MD
Ronald D. Kolkka, MD
David J. Ruderman, MD
Adele Nelson, RN
Linda Greco, RN
Virginia Duncan
Susan Ahlering
Barbara Ybarra

The illustrations in this text are the combined efforts of three illustrators. We are deeply indebted to our major illustrator, Barbara Haynes, for her work, commitment, patience, and for her being there when we needed her.

It is common in textbooks for the authors to thank such individuals for help, assistance, patience, inspiration, motivation, etc. Only after completion of such a task as a textbook do we fully understand what that means. We truly thank all who have aided us.

RPF/DPF

CONTENTS

INTRODUCTION

This book provides a framework to help the reader organize, catalogue, remember, and use the fundamental facts of hemostasis. The framework is easy to remember and apply because it follows the natural physiological sequence of hemostasis—namely, disruption of vascular integrity, platelet reaction, coagulation cascade, and clot lysis. These four areas are presented in the same order in each chapter, to facilitate comprehension and learning.

We have designed a unique page layout to encourage use of this framework. The four common themes: vascular integrity, platelets, coagulation cascade, and clot lysis are found in the upper right-hand corner of each page. The area under active discussion is in bold type for emphasis. The text and illustrations provide the fundamental knowledge of the topic, and the "questions" or key phrases at the bottom of each pge may be used for review or further emphasis. We have provided many illustrations and flow charts, each of which is designed specifically to reinforce the accompanying text. At the end of the book, we have provided some "Cut-out and use" sections which the reader may remove and keep at hand during daily work.

Let us begin with a brief overview of the coagulation and hemostatic processes.

Chapter 1
OVERVIEW OF HEMOSTASIS

1. VASCULAR INTEGRITY
2. PLATELETS
3. COAGULATION CASCADE
4. CLOT LYSIS

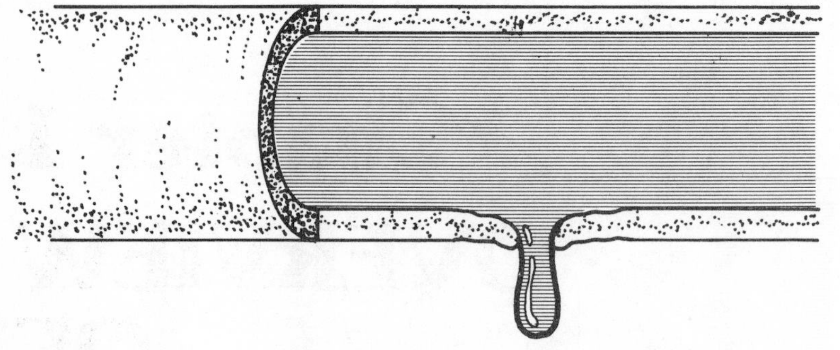

Injured Vessel

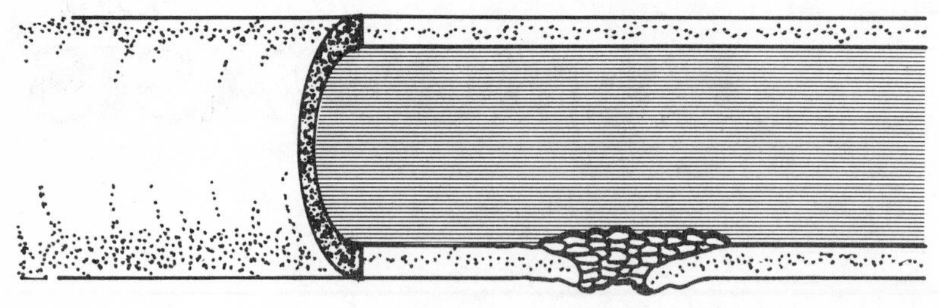

Platelet Plug

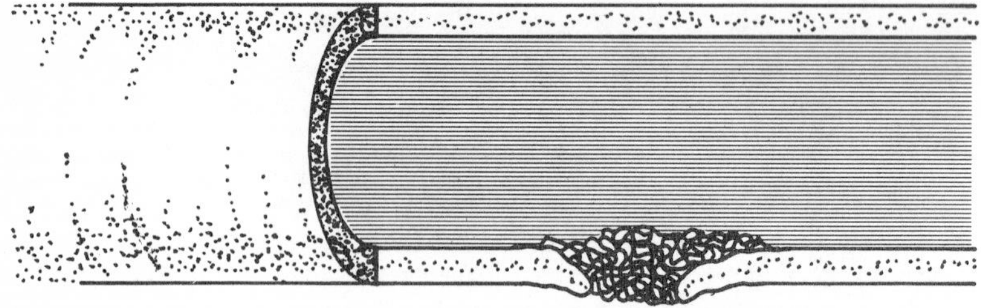

Fibrin Clot

The hemostatic mechanism is designed to maintain blood within injured vessels. Bleeding occurs when vascular integrity is lost. The arrest of that bleeding is accomplished by three sequential events: vascular reaction, formation of a platelet plug, and activation of the coagulation cascade.

---

1. *Bleeding implies loss of ____________.*	***vascular integrity***
2. *Arrest of bleeding is assisted by the formation of a ____________ plug.*	***platelet***
3. *During platelet plug formation, the ____________ is activated.*	***coagulation cascade***

1. VASCULAR INTEGRITY
2. PLATELETS
3. COAGULATION CASCADE
4. CLOT LYSIS

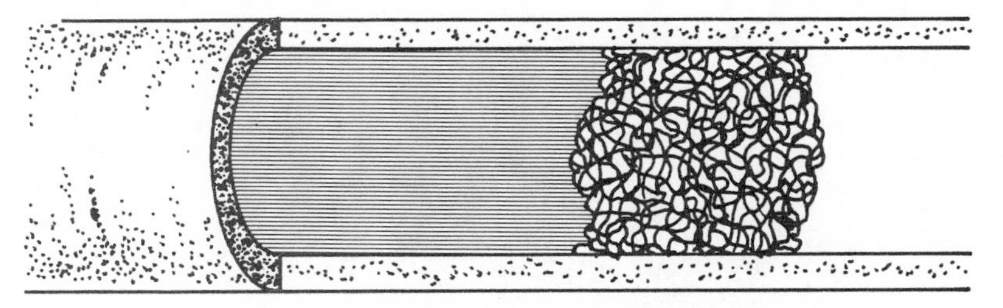

Thrombosis

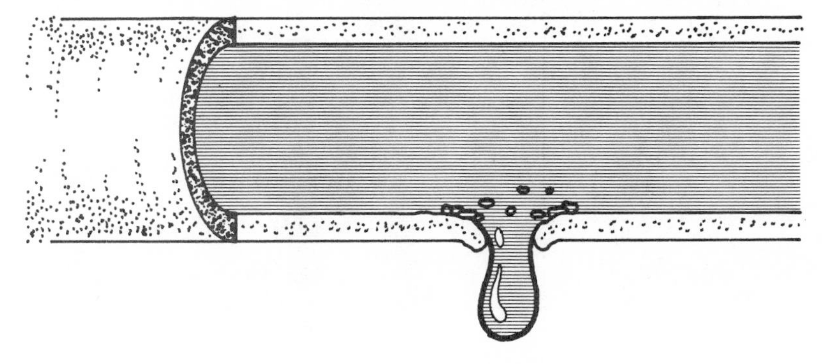

Inadequate Hemostasis

The basic hemostatic mechanism normally is rapid and localized. But the system is not without risk.

Too much hemostasis at the site of injury leads to excessive **thrombosis** (with vascular obstruction and ischemia).

Too little hemostasis at the site of injury leads to **persistent bleeding.**

---

1. *Persistent bleeding may occur with ______________ hemostasis.* — ***inadequate***
2. *Detrimental thrombosis may occur with ______________ hemostasis.* — ***excessive***
3. *This process is normally ______________ to the area of injury.* — ***localized***

1. VASCULAR INTEGRITY
2. PLATELETS
3. COAGULATION CASCADE
4. CLOT LYSIS

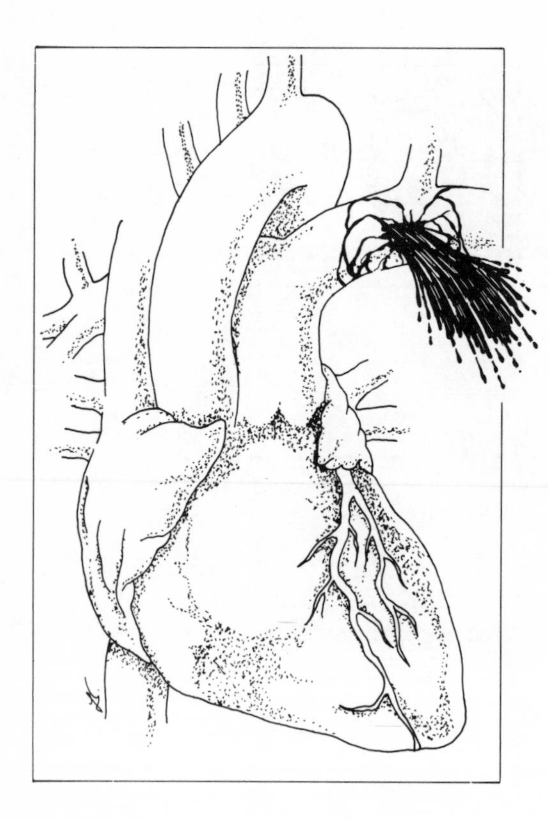

Large breaks cannot be sealed by platelets or fibrin clot.

Why is vascular integrity important?

Because large breaks in vessel walls, especially in vessels under pressure, cannot be sealed by platelets or fibrin meshwork. There are normal mechanisms by which the blood flow through an injured vessel can be reduced (vasoconstriction, shunting, tissue swelling, etc.).

---

1. *Platelet plugs and protein mesh are __________ to close large defects in broken blood vessels.* — ***inadequate***
2. *The body has normal mechanisms which serve to __________ blood flow in injured vessels.* — ***decrease***
3. *The first basic component of hemostasis is __________.* — ***vascular integrity***

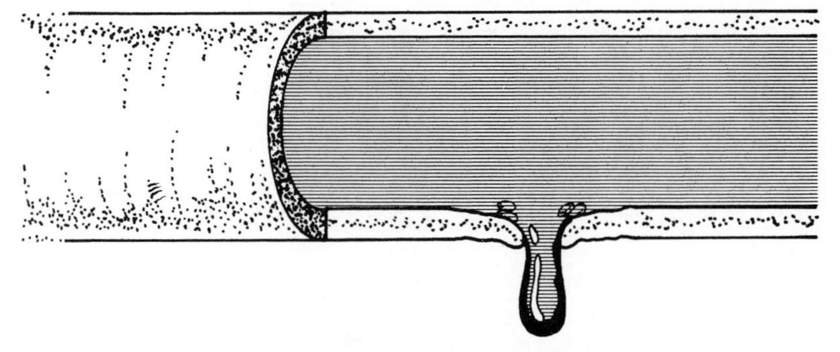

1-2 Seconds

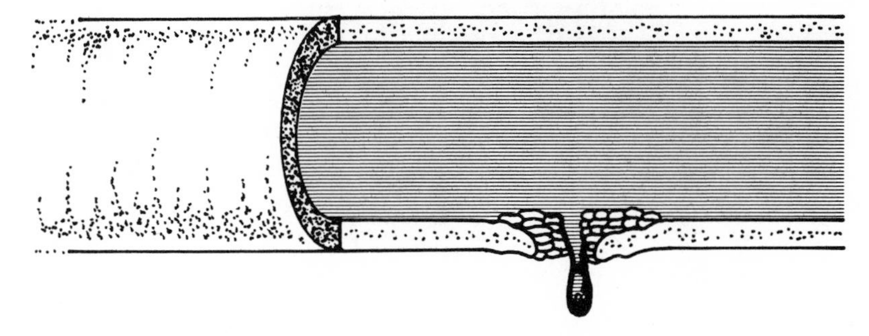

15-20 Seconds
Platelet Reaction

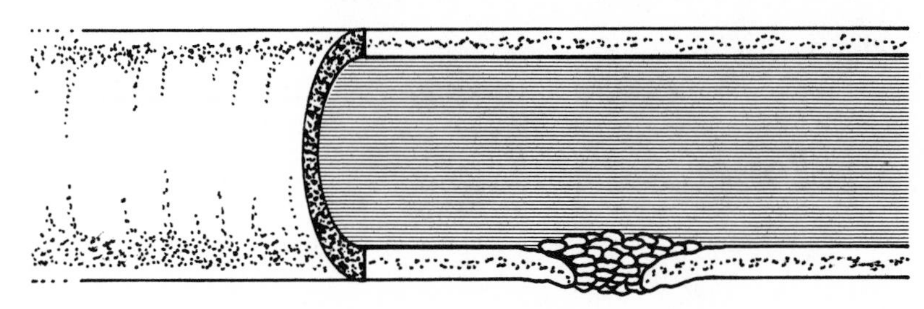

3-5 Minutes
Platelet Plug

Why are platelets important?

The initial plug is formed by platelets within five minutes of vascular injury. In addition, the platelet surface membrane is required to initiate and support the enzymatic reactions of the coagulation cascade.

---

1. *The initial plug is composed of _______________.* — ***platelets***
2. *The platelet surface also supports _______________ necessary for the coagulation cascade.* — ***enzyme reactions***
3. *The second basic component of hemostasis is the _______________ reaction.* — ***platelet***

1. VASCULAR INTEGRITY
2. PLATELETS
3. COAGULATION CASCADE
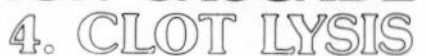

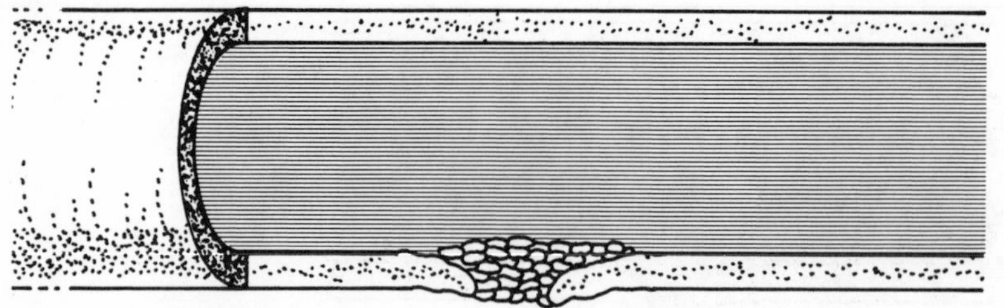

Platelet Plug

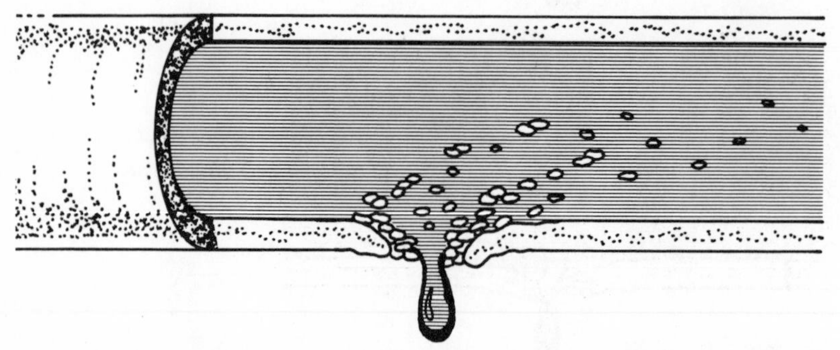

Platelet plug disintegration with time (re-bleeding occurs without fibrin)

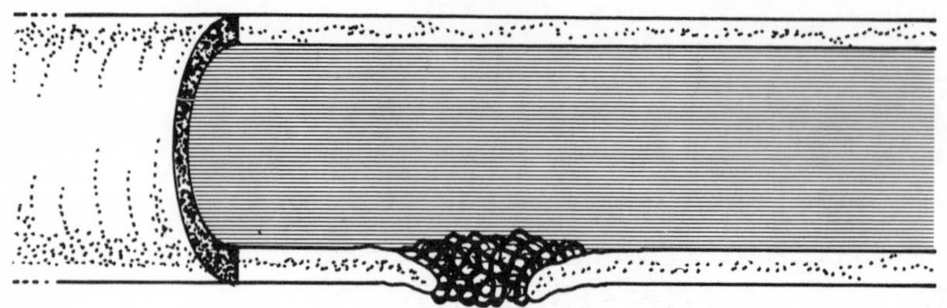

Platelet plug consolidated with fibrin meshwork

Why is the coagulation cascade important?

The platelet plug is only temporary. Without fibrin strands providing structural support to the platelet plug, the plug would soon fall apart. This fibrin meshwork is called a clot.

Fibrin deposition is localized to the site of injury by requiring an activated platelet surface upon which to interact.

---

1. *The platelet plug is only __________.* — ***temporary***
2. *__________ strands give structural support to the platelet plug.* — ***fibrin***
3. *The third basic component of hemostasis is the __________.* — ***coagulation cascade***

1. VASCULAR INTEGRITY
2. PLATELETS
3. COAGULATION CASCADE
4. CLOT LYSIS

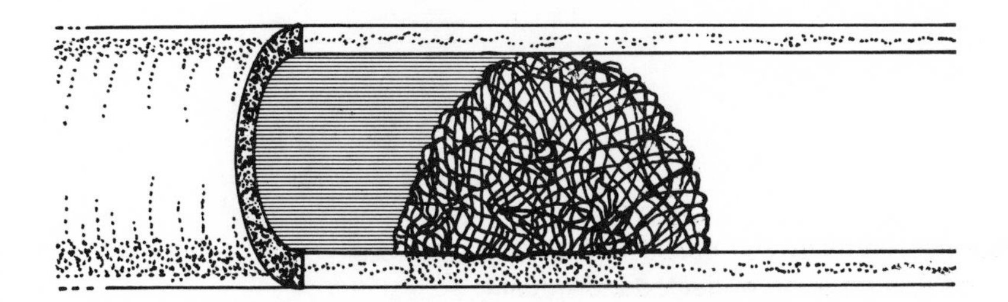

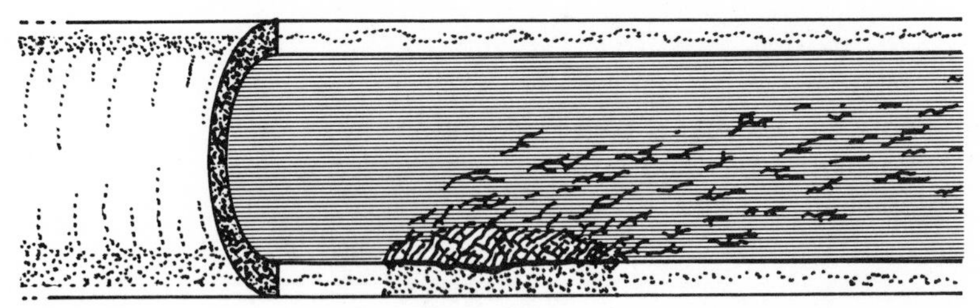

Clot Lysis

Why is clot lysis important?

Re-establishing normal blood flow in a vessel previously injured requires removal of the fibrin clot and any trapped platelets. This occurs by clot lysis. However, lysis must proceed with caution, for too much too soon might result in re-bleeding from early clot removal.

---

1. *Re-establishing flow in a clotted vessel occurs by* ______________. — ***clot lysis***
2. *Lysis occuring too early may produce* ______________. — ***bleeding***
3. *Without lysis, the vessel may remain* ______________. — ***occluded***

1. VASCULAR INTEGRITY
2. PLATELETS
3. COAGULATION CASCADE
4. CLOT LYSIS

In order to diagnose correctly the cause of bleeding, the four components of hemostasis must be evaluated individually:

Vascular integrity—is there a large hole in a vessel?	Inspect surgical sutures and injured vessels.
Platelets—Are there enough, and are they functioning properly?	Order a platelet count and bleeding time.
Coagulation cascade—Is the coagulation cascade functioning properly?	Order a prothrombin time (PT and a partial thrombo-plastin time (PTT).
Clot lysis—Is the lytic system functioning properly?	Order a fibrin split products level.

(Coagulation testing will be covered in detail later.)

---

1. *Inspection of the surgical field evaluates ____________.* — ***vascular integrity***
2. *The bleeding time tests ____________ function.* — ***platelet***
3. *The PT and PTT test the ____________.* — ***coagulation cascade***
4. *A fibrin split products level evaluates the effectiveness of ____________.* — ***clot lysis***

Chapter 2
BASICS OF CLOTTING AND LYSIS

This chapter presents the basics of the normally functioning hemostatic system. We have provided an organized way of thinking, which is easily visualized to facilitate recall. If the basics are comprehended, the following chapters will not need to be memorized, but rather will be derivable from the basics.

For our illustrations, we have given specific shapes to various surfaces and structures. These are representative only of the concepts we want the reader to remember.

1. VASCULAR INTEGRITY

2. PLATELETS
3. COAGULATION CASCADE
4. CLOT LYSIS

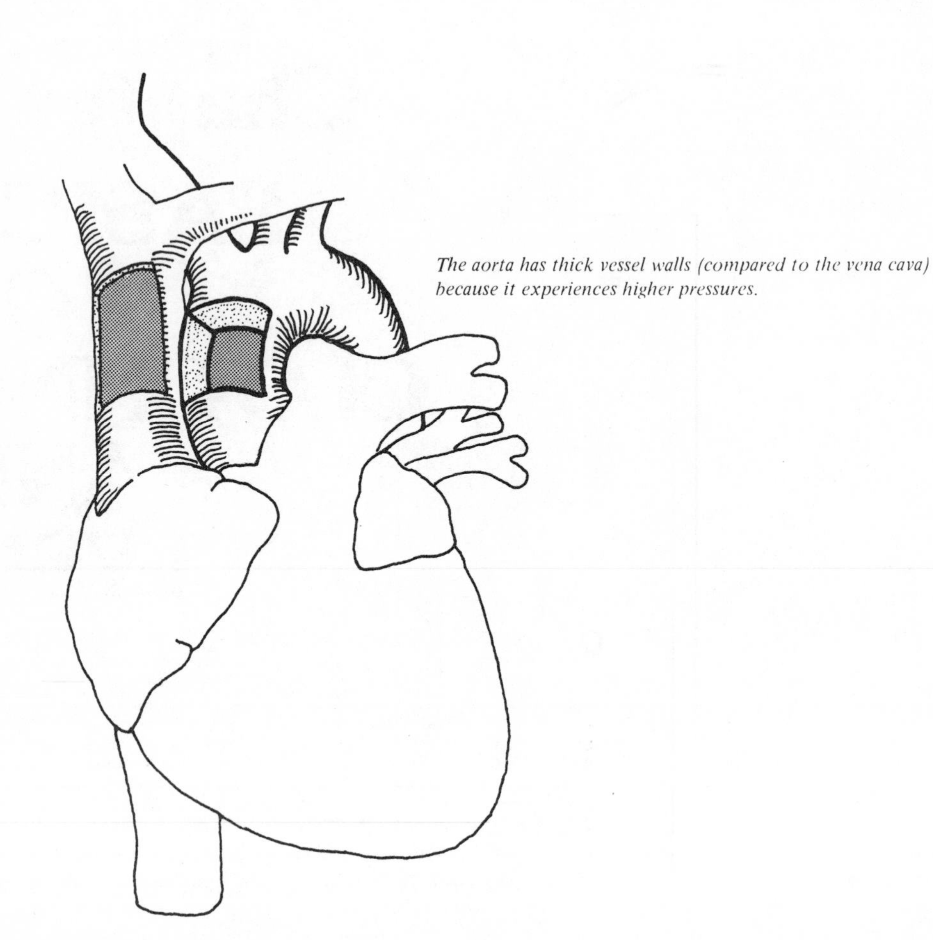

The aorta has thick vessel walls (compared to the vena cava) because it experiences higher pressures.

The structural integrity of vessels is necessary to prevent bleeding. Vessels experiencing high pressures or frequent trauma are structurally more sturdy than those experiencing low pressures and infrequent trauma.

---

1. The first component of hemostasis is ______________.	***vascular integrity***
2. Vascular integrity is most important in vessels under ______________ pressure.	***high***
3. Vascular integrity is disturbed by violent or surgical ______________.	***trauma***

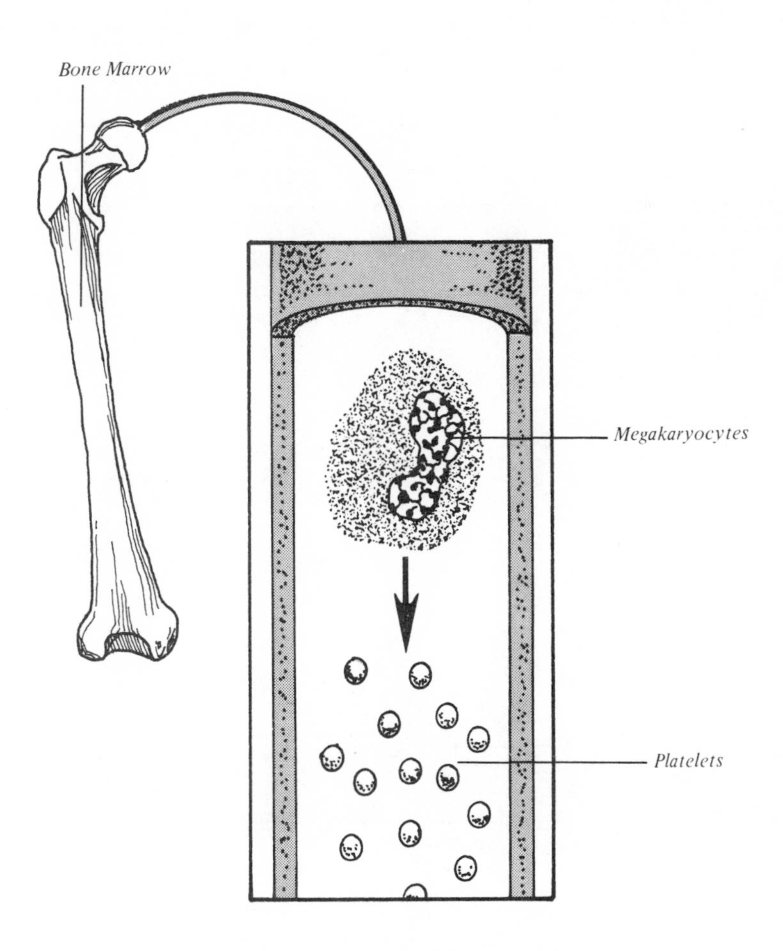

Platelets are the second component of hemostasis.

Platelets are blood elements that are approximately two microns in diameter. They are released from megakaryocytes produced in bone marrow. Platelet production takes approximately four days, and they have a half-life of 9-10 days in the normal human being.

---

1. Platelets have a size of approximately two ______.	***microns***
2. Megakaryocytes, which produce platelets, are made in ______.	***bone marrow***
3. The platelet half-life is normally ______ days.	***9-10***

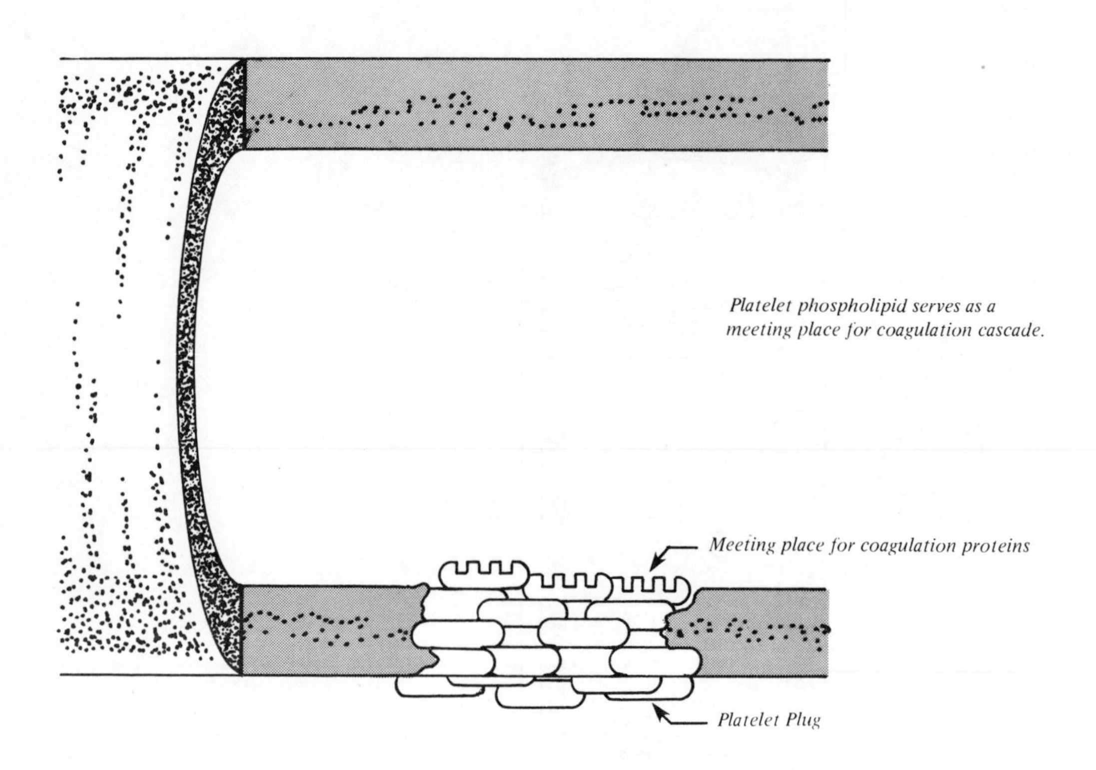

Platelets play a crucial role in initiating and localizing clot formation, once vascular integrity has been disturbed. Platelets serve two functions, the first is to form a temporary platelet plug, the second is to provide a meeting place for the proteins of the coagulation cascade. This meeting place is a platelet phospholipid, and is termed platelet factor 3 (PF-3).

---

1. Platelets aid in __________ and __________ clot formation.	***initiating*** ***localizing***
2. The platelet phospholipid is known as __________.	***Platelet Factor 3***
3. Platelets are recruited after __________ is disturbed.	***vascular integrity***

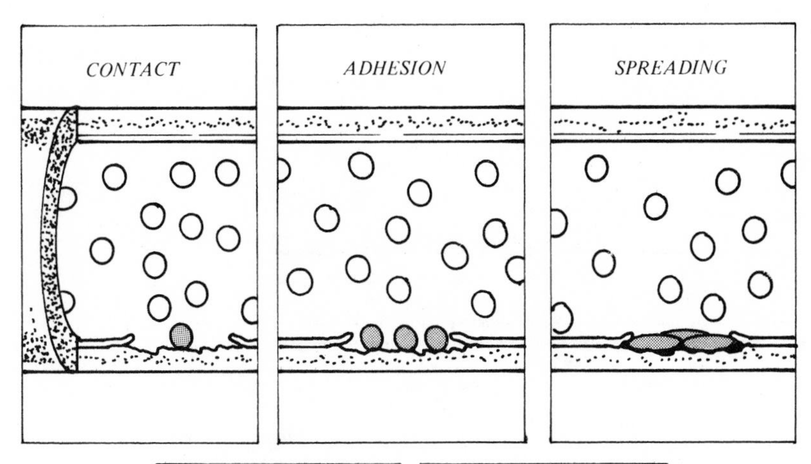

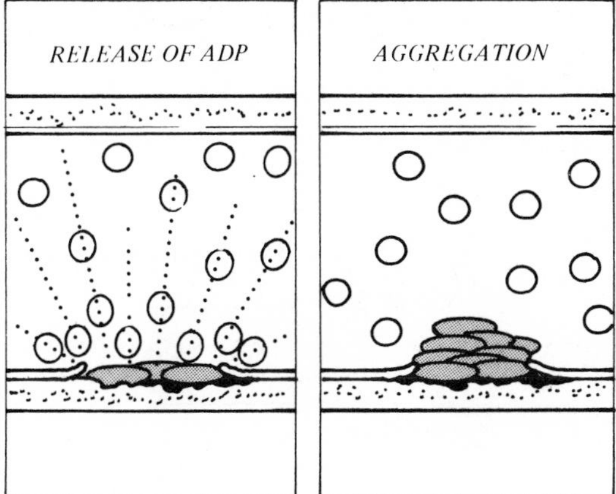

The sequential mechanics of the platelet interaction with a damaged vessel include:

contact — with a damaged vessel wall
adhesion — to subendothelial connective tissue
spreading — to cover the damaged surface
release — of multiple compounds
aggregation — of many platelets to form an effective barrier to further blood loss

---

1. *Platelets contact and adhere to ____________ vessel wall.* — ***damaged***
2. *When a platelet contacts, adheres, and spreads, the platelet ____________ multiple compounds.* — ***releases***
3. *The final step in platelet mechanics is ____________.* — ***aggregation***

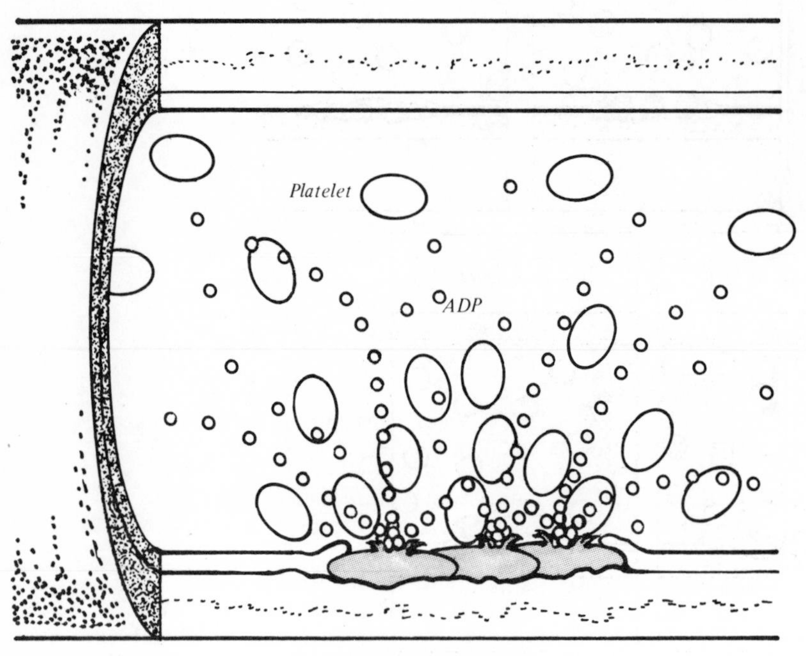

Aggregated platelets release ADP to recruit additional platelets.

Platelet contact, adhesion, and spreading results in **release** of multiple compounds. One of these compounds, adenosine diphosphate (ADP), is an **aggregating** signal to other platelets. Aggregation, the fifth and last step of platelet mechanics, is controlled by the amount of ADP released from a platelet.

---

1. *Platelets release multiple ______________.* — ***compounds***
2. *One of the released compounds is ______________.* — ***ADP***
3. *ADP release controls platelet ______________.* — ***aggregation***

1. VASCULAR INTEGRITY
2. PLATELETS
3. COAGULATION CASCADE
4. CLOT LYSIS

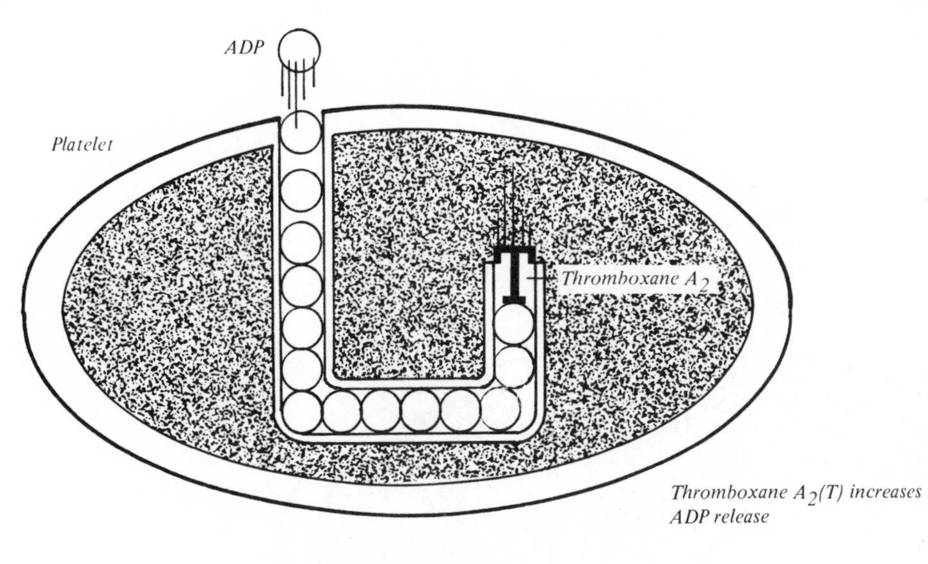

Thromboxane A_2(T) increases ADP release

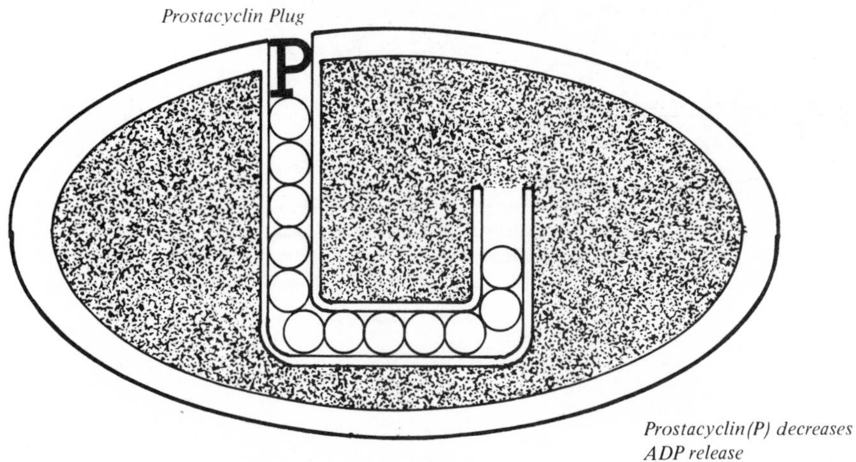

Prostacyclin(P) decreases ADP release

ADP release is regulated locally by the prostaglandins, thromboxane A2 and prostacyclin (PGI2). These two prostaglandins have opposite effects. Thromboxane A2 increases ADP release, while prostacyclin (PGI2) decreases ADP release.

---

1. *ADP release is regulated locally by ______________.*	***prostaglandins***
2. *Thromboxane A2 ______________ ADP release.*	***increases***
3. *Prostacyclin (PGI2) ______________ ADP release.*	***decreases***

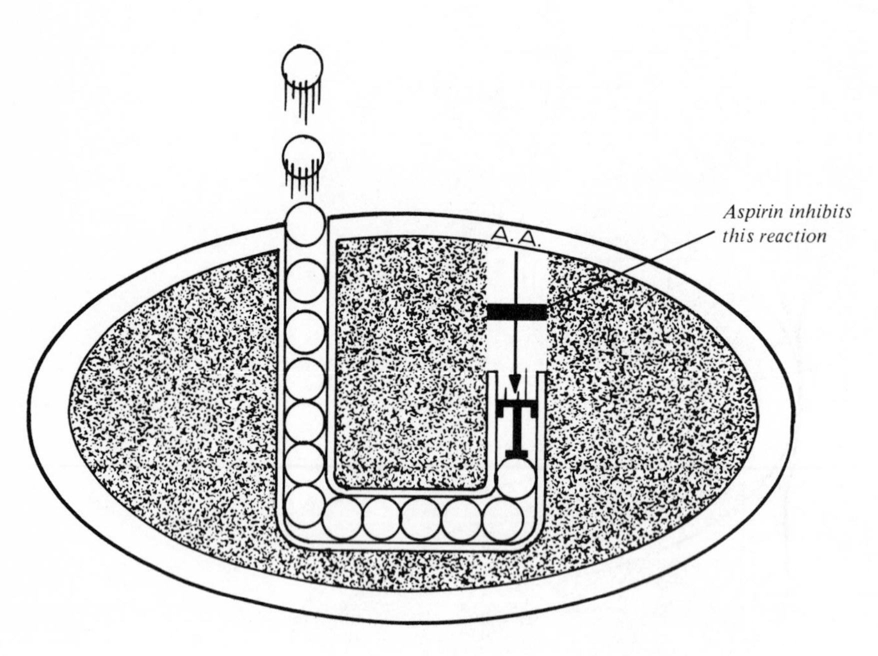

Thromboxane is synthesized by arachidonic acid(AA) in activated platelet cell membrane.

Thromboxane A_2, a prostaglandin, is synthesized by an activated platelet from arachidonic acid, a normal constituent of cell membranes. Thromboxane A_2 produces platelet aggregation by increasing the release of ADP. Inhibitors of thromboxane A_2 synthesis (such as aspirin) will inhibit platelet aggregation, by inhibiting ADP release.

---

1. *Thromboxane A_2 is produced by an activated ______________.* — ***platelet***
2. *By increasing the release of ADP, thromboxane A_2 causes platelet ______________.* — ***aggregation***
3. *Inhibitors of thromboxane A_2 synthesis will ______________ platelet aggregation.* — ***inhibit***

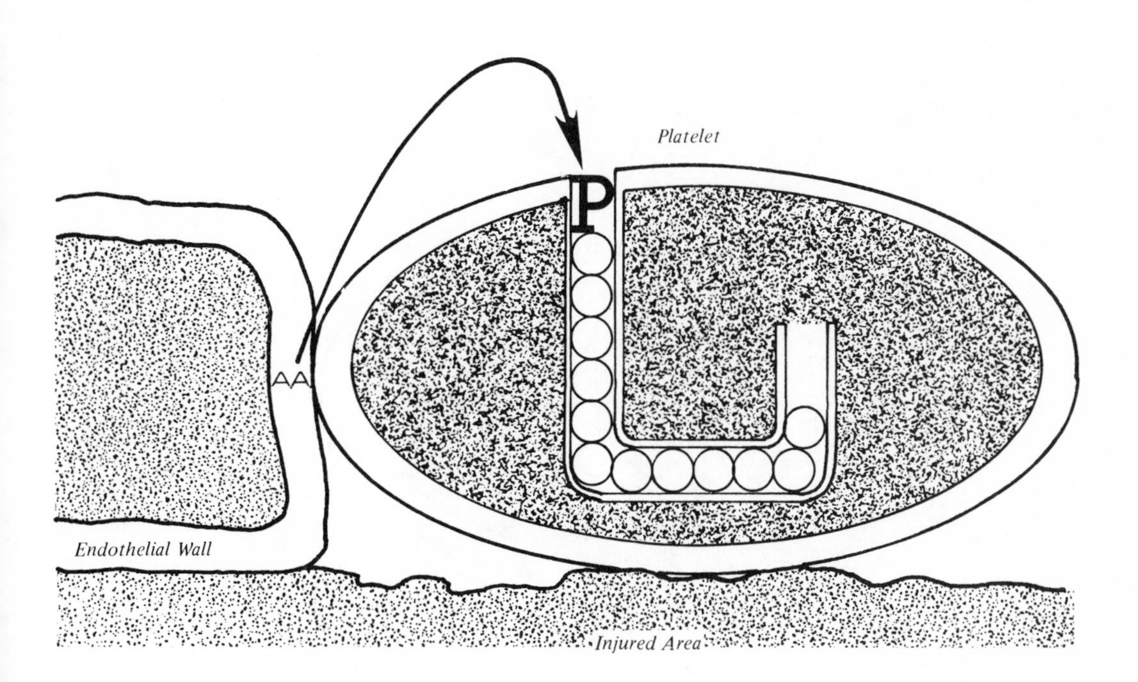

Prostacyclin (PGI_2) is synthesized by endothelial cells from arachidonic acid. It inhibits platelet aggregation by decreasing the release of ADP.

---

1. *Prostacyclin (PGI_2) is synthesized by blood vessel ______________.* — ***endothelium***
2. *Prostacyclin (PGI_2) ______________ platelet aggregation.* — ***inhibits***
3. *Prostacyclin (PGI_2) inhibits platelet aggregation by decreasing the release of ______________.* — ***ADP***

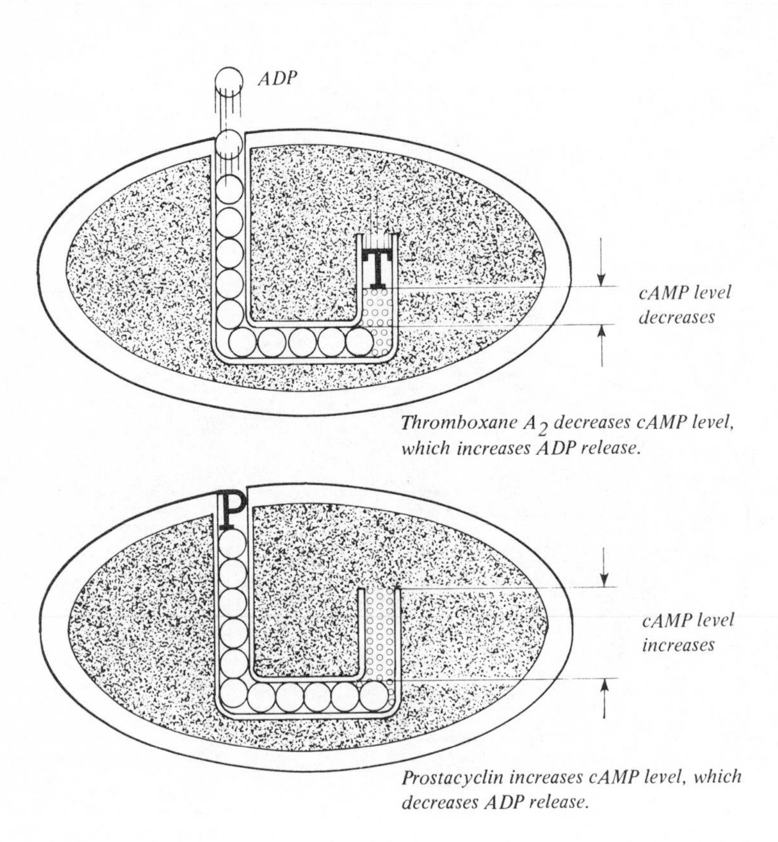

Thromboxane A_2 decreases cAMP level, which increases ADP release.

Prostacyclin increases cAMP level, which decreases ADP release.

Platelet ADP release is regulated by the prostaglandins [thromboxane A_2 and prostacyclin (PGI_2)], via the secondary messenger cyclic adenosine monophosphate (cAMP). By functioning via the secondary messenger cAMP, and separating the site of synthesis of the different prostaglandins, localization of platelet aggregation occurs naturally. Vascular endothelial cells prevent platelet aggregation from extending past the area of injury, by synthesizing prostacyclin. Simultaneously, platelets can continue to aggregate to plug areas of injury by releasing thromboxane A_2. The balance provided by synthesis of opposing prostaglandins results in adequate hemostasis without excessive thrombosis.

---

1. *ADP release is regulated via a secondary messenger ______________.* — ***cAMP***
2. *Platelet aggregation occurs after release of ADP which is increased by ______________.* — ***thromboxane A_2***
3. *Inhibition of platelet aggregation occurs after release of ______________.* — ***prostacyclin***

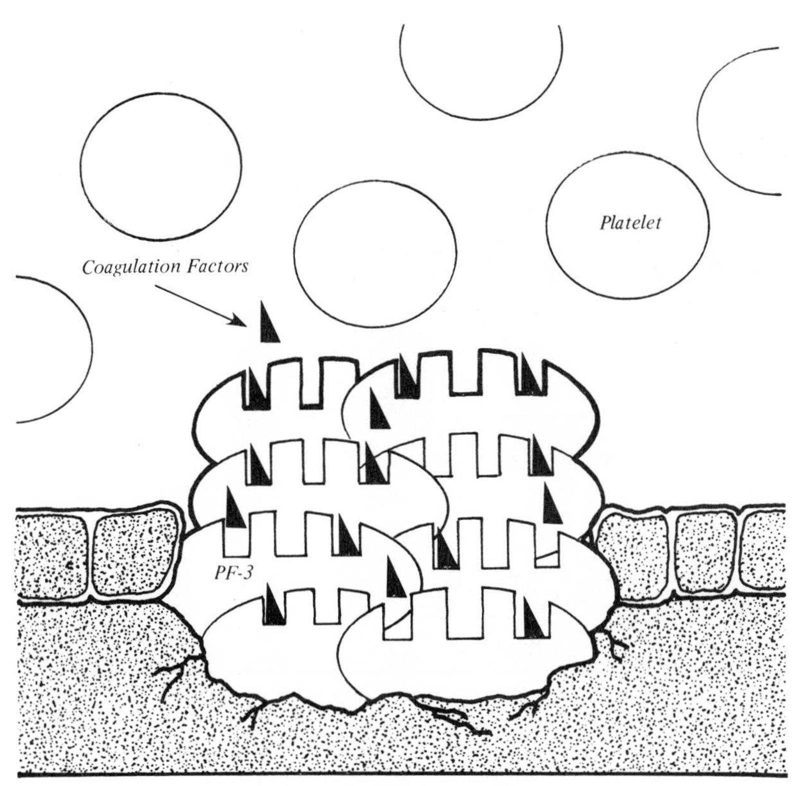

Aggregated platelets expose PF-3, which acts as congregating place for coagulation factors.

Platelet aggregation normally takes place within seconds of vessel injury. The formation of the unstable platelet plug results in exposure of a **phospholipid** (PF-3) on the platelet surface membrane. This phospholipid (PF-3) serves as a congregating place for the **coagulation proteins**. Fibrin, the end-product of the coagulation cascade, will stabilize the platelet plug.

---

1. *Platelet aggregation is a ______________ phenomenon after endothelial damage.*	***rapid***
2. *Platelet ______________ (PF-3) is exposed on the platelet surface.*	***phospholipid***
3. *The platelet plug is stabilized by ______________.*	***fibrin***

In order to avoid confusion, an international committee* established a standard nomenclature assigning Roman Numerals to the clotting factors. They were numbered in the order of discovery. Active factors were indicated by the subscript "a".

Roman Numeral	Protein Coagulation Factor
I	Fibrinogen
II	Prothrombin
III	Platelet Factor 3 (thromboplastin)
IV	Calcium
V	Labile Factor (proaccelerin)
VI	(Not Assigned)
VII	Stable Factor—Proconvertin
VIII	Antihemophiliac Factor A (AHF)
IX	Antihemophiliac Factor B , Christmas Factor
X	Stuart-Prower Factor
XI	Antihemophiliac Factor C
XII	Hageman Factor
XIII	Fibrin Stabilizing Factor

Note: Factor III is a phospholipid in the platelet surface membrane. Factor IV is the calcium ion.

(*Biggs—Second Edition, p. 15.)

---

1. *Factor VI is not presently assigned. The Roman Numerals were assigned in order of* ***discovery****, and subsequently factor ______________ was later shown* ***not*** *to be involved in the clotting system.* — ***VI***

2. *The Roman numerals assigned to the factors were assigned in the order of ______________, thus* ***the numeral implies nothing about the sequence of action.*** — ***discovery***

3. *The Roman Numerals, as seen above, refer to* ***non-****activated factors. The activated forms are indicated by the lower case "a". Thus after activation, for example, Factor XII would be indicated by ______________.* — ***XIIa***

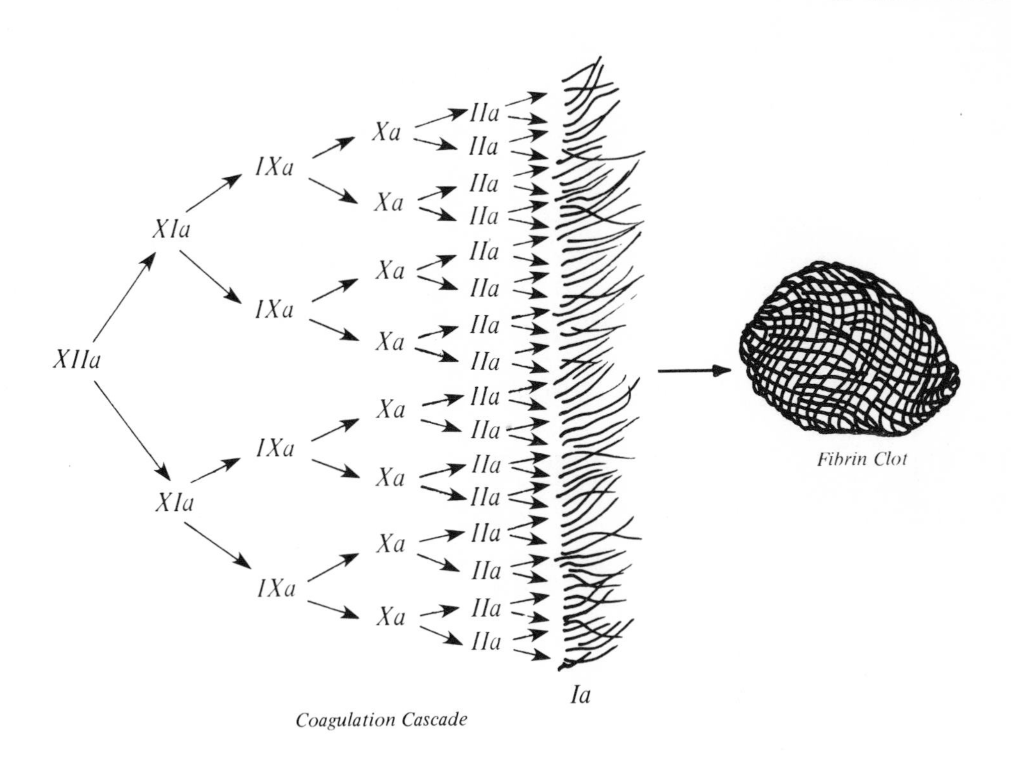

Coagulation Cascade

The coagulation proteins form an enzyme cascade analogous to a chain reaction. The coagulation process is a biologic amplification system, that enables relatively few molecules of initiator products to induce **sequential** activation of a series of inactive proteins. This culminates in the explosive production of **fibrin**.

Because knowledge of the specific properties of these proteins and enzymes is important to the understanding of their function, let us look at these properties in more detail.

---

1. *The coagulation proteins form an ____________ cascade.* — ***enzyme***
2. *The process of coagulation activation is a ____________ one.* — ***sequential***
3. *The end-product of the coagulation protein cascade is ____________.* — ***fibrin***

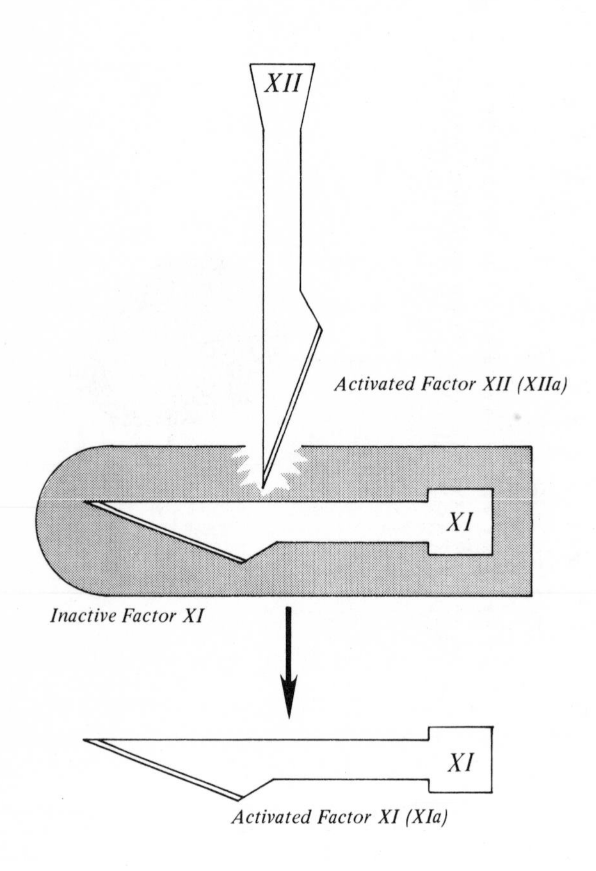

Most circulating coagulation factors are serine proteases. Serine proteases are cleavage enzymes. We can think of these cleavage enzymes as knives. The knife is sheathed (in an inactive form) until it is unsheathed (**activated**), by the serine protease one step back in the coagulation cascade. Activation of factors XII, XI, IX, X, VII and II is accomplished by a common **mechanism**, but with a high specificity for the factor immediately following it in the cascade.

(Only factors V, VIII and Fibrinogen are NOT cleavage enzymes.)

---

1. *Each protease (factor) circulates as an ____________ enzyme precursor.* — ***inactive***
2. *Each protease (factor) is ____________ by the preceding protease (cleavage enzyme).* — ***activated***
3. *Each activated factor only activates the factor ____________ following it in the coagulation cascade.* — ***immediately***

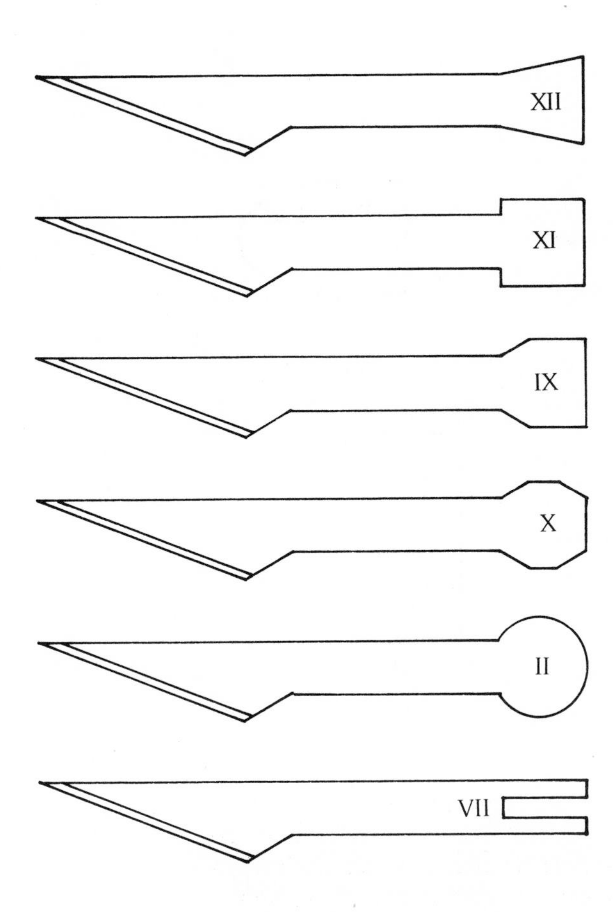

The serine proteases are similar to each other in that they are all cleavage enzymes. They are different from each other in that they cleave different substrates. We diagram their similarity by drawing all the cutting edges the same. We diagram their differences by drawing their "handles" with different shapes. The serine proteases all circulate in the inactive form.

---

1. *The serine proteases all have a basically ______________ structure.* — ***similar***
2. *However, there are specific ______________.* — ***differences***
3. *They circulate in the ______________ form.* — ***inactive***

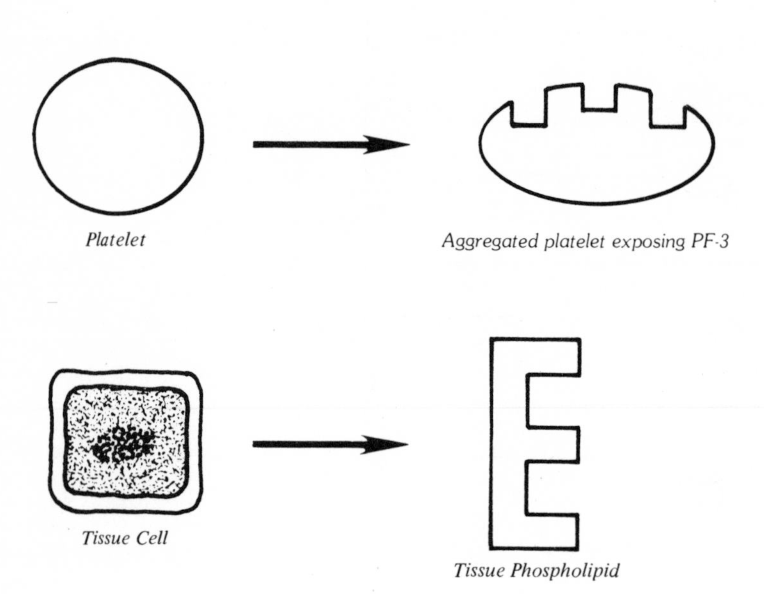

The coagulation factors which are serine proteases circulate in the inactive form and in high concentration. The rate-limiting step is the availability of an appropriate phospholipid surface for coagulation protein binding and activation. There are two types of biological lipid surfaces which become available at the time of injury:

• Platelet membrane phospholipid (PF-3) is made available on activated platelets at the site of injury. Non-activated platelets do not reveal this phospholipid.

• Tissue phospholipid is released from cell surface membranes of injured tissues.

---

1. *Activated platelets make available ____________.* — ***platelet phospholipid***

2. *Injured cellular membranes make available ____________.* — ***tissue phospholipids***

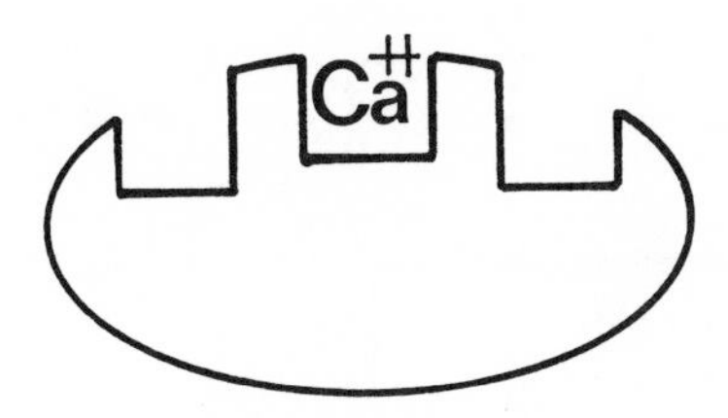

Platelet exposing PF-3

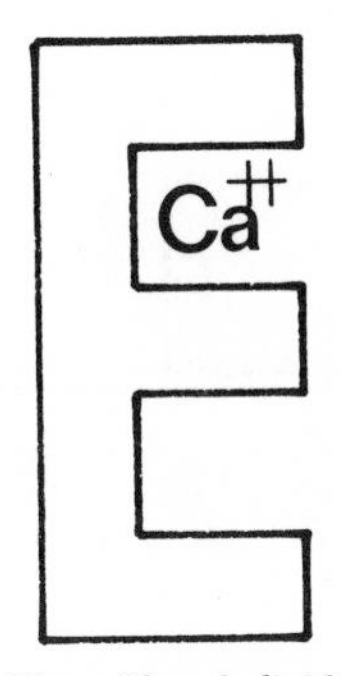

Tissue Phospholipid

The biochemical reactions of the coagulation cascade occur on the platelet phospholipid (PF-3) or, if it is available, on the tissue phospholipid. The phospholipids bind coagulation proteases via a Ca^{++} bridge.

---

1. *Platelets are an integral part of the coagulation pathway. By providing ______________, they provide a meeting place for the coagulation proteins.*	***PF-3***
2. *PF-3 is a membrane ______________ on the platelet surface.*	***phospholipid***
3. *Phospholipids bind coagulation proteases via a ______________ bridge.*	***calcium***

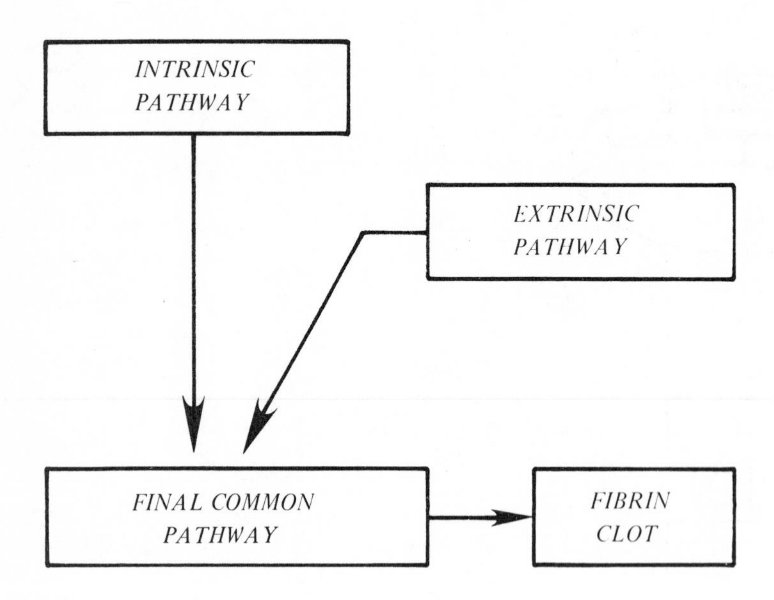

The reactions leading to fibrin formation can be divided into two major overlapping pathways, **intrinsic** and **extrinsic.** The final portion of both pathways is the final common pathway. The end product of both the intrinsic and the extrinsic pathways is a fibrin clot, which is generated from fribrinogen.

(Note: We reserve the term "clot" to refer to a fibrin meshwork. The term "plug" refers to an aggregation of platelets.)

---

1. *The end-product of the coagulation cascade, ______, is generated from ______.* — ***fibrin***, ***fibrinogen***
2. *Two pathways, the intrinsic and the ______, both result in the formation of a final common product ______.* — ***extrinsic***, ***fibrin***
3. *The intrinsic and extrinsic pathways share a ______.* — ***final common pathway***

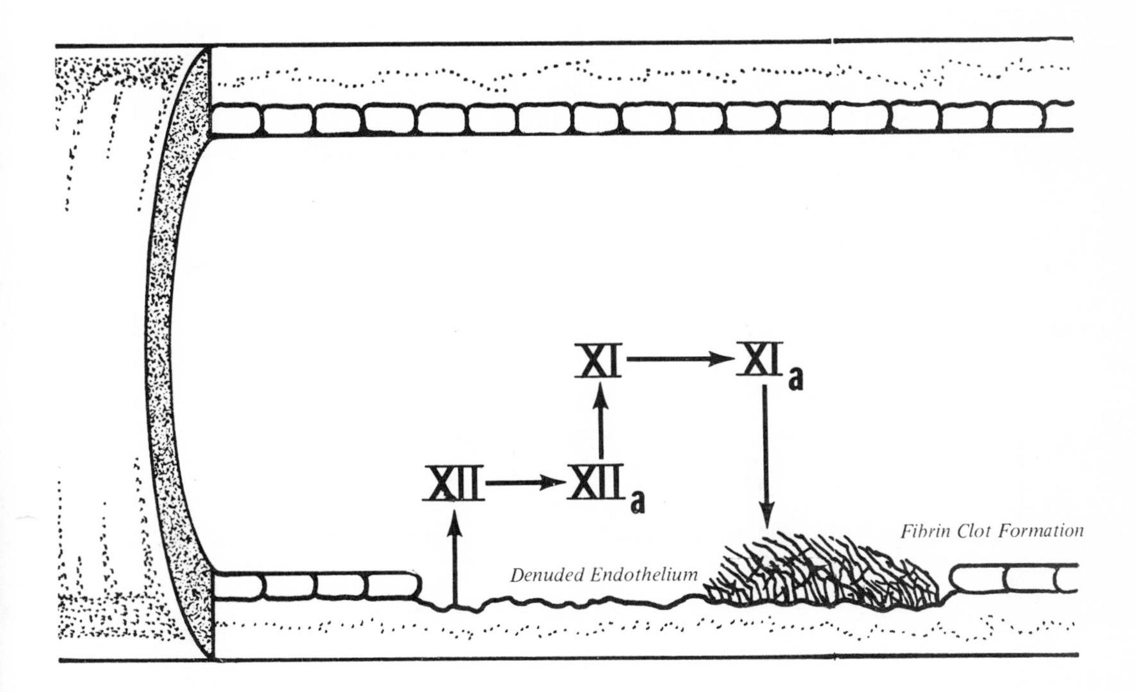

The intrinsic coagulation cascade begins intravascularly with activation of factor XII. Factor XII is activated by surface contact with a vessel denuded of endothelium. Factor XII becomes XIIa, and XIIa in turn, activates factor XI.

The platelet **surface** becomes involved at the next step in the cascade.

---

1. *The ______________ pathway functions intravascularly.* — ***intrinsic***
2. *Denuded vascular endolethium, in contact with factor ______________, initiates the intrinsic pathway.* — ***XII***
3. *Factor XII is activated, and in turn activates factor ______________.* — ***XI***

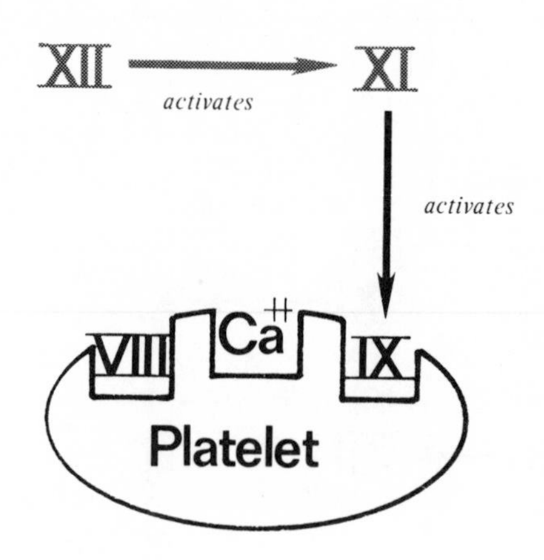

Platelet surfaces become involved because their phospholipids **bind**, and thereby facilitate the interaction of, the coagulation factors.

The **first** set of factors **bound** by the platelet phospholipid are the two factors deficient in the two types of hemophilia, factors VIII and IX. Factor IX is bound by PF-3. The binding site for Factor VIII has not been characterized completely.

---

1. *The "hemophiliac factors" VIII and IX interact on the portion of the surface of the platelet composed of the __________, or PF-3.* — ***phospholipid***
2. *The two "hemophiliac factors" bound on the platelet are __________ and __________.* — ***VIII and IX***
3. *Note that __________ is involved in the binding of factor IX.* — ***calcium***

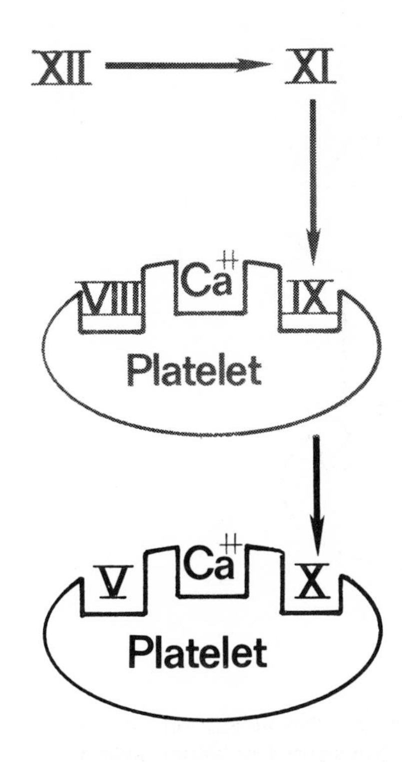

The **second** set of factors **bound** by the platelet phospholipid are the nickel and dime factors, V and X.

---

1. *Remember, the ______ pathway is initiated by activation of factor ______.*	***intrinsic XII***
2. *The first set of factors bound on the platelet are the ______ factors VIII, IX.*	***hemophiliac***
3. *The second set of factors bound on the platelet are factors ______ and ______.*	***V and X***

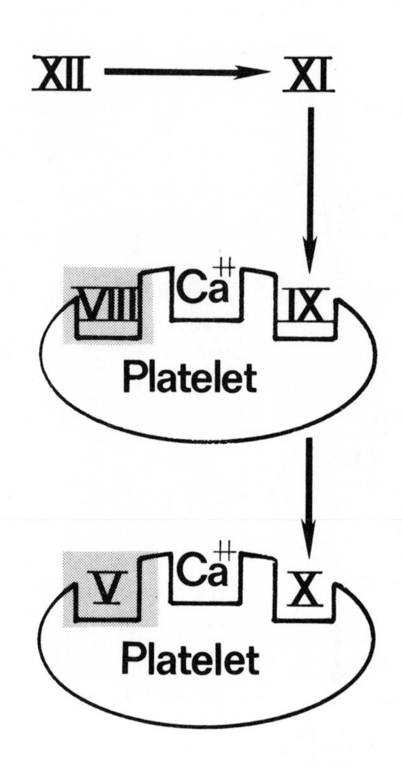

The **smaller** number of each of the first two sets bound to the platelet (VIII, and V, respectively), are the **coenzymes** or **helper** factors. They are **not** serine proteases. The cofactors VIII and V circulate only in the active form, and are very labile. (They are prone to destruction, and are deficient in stored bank blood, but are preserved in freshly frozen plasma.)

---

1. *Factor VIII is a coenzyme, and helps bind the serine protease, factor __________, to the platelet.*	***IX***
2. *Factor V is also a coenzyme, and helps bind the serine protease, factor __________, to the platelet.*	***X***
3. *Thus, the two coenzymes (helper factors) are __________ and __________.*	***VIII and V***
4. *These two cofactors circulate in the __________ form.*	***active***

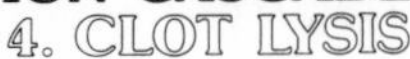

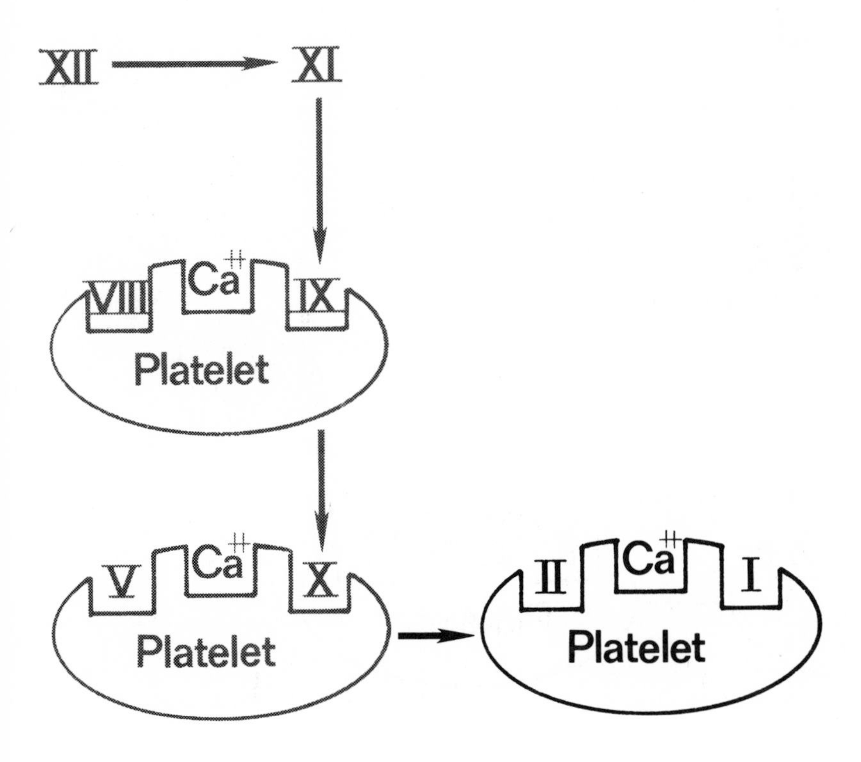

The **third** set of factors **bound** on the platelet surface are the factors that conclude the pathway, II and I. Factor II is prothrombin, Factor I is fibrinogen. Factor II is activated by the action of Xa, and Factor I by the action of IIa.

---

1. *Factor ______________, a serine protease, splits prothrombin (II), to form thrombin (IIa).*	***X***
2. *Factor IIa (______________) is the active form of prothrombin.*	***thrombin***
3. *Thrombin (IIa) converts fibrinogen (I) to ______________ (Ia).*	***fibrin***

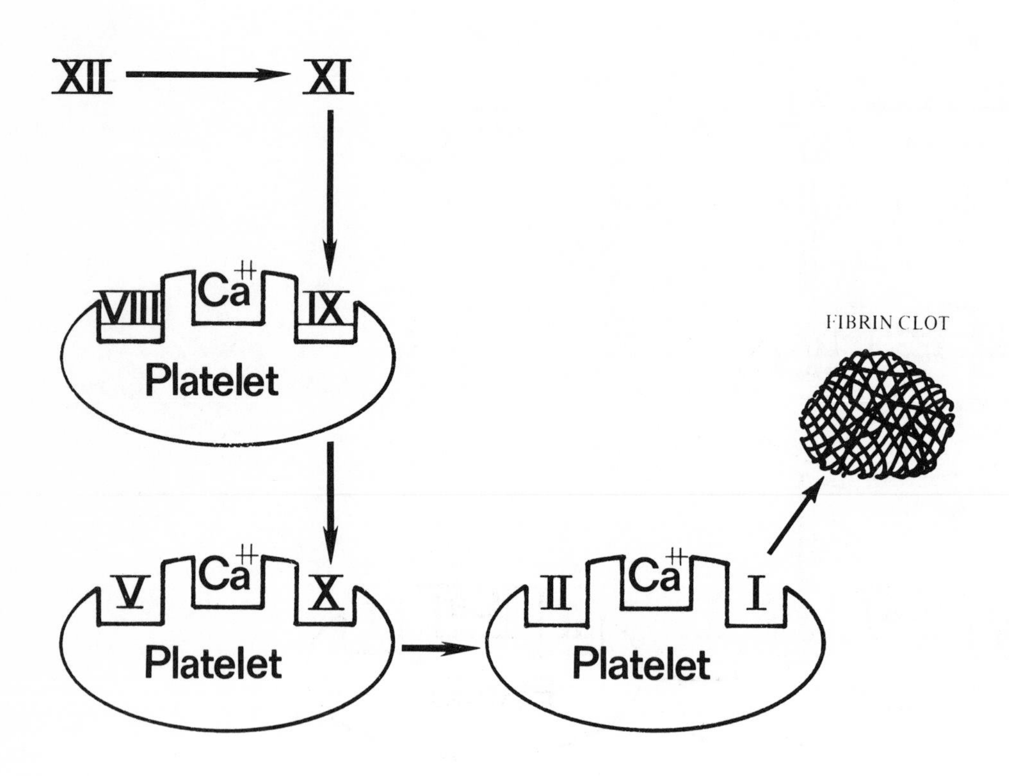

Fibrin (Ia) is the cross-linked end-product of the coagulation cascade. Its production from fibrinogen is the result of a **sequential** activation of inactive proteins, amplified at each stage. This results in an **explosive** production of fibrin, which polymerizes or cross-links to form the fibrin clot.

---

1. Fibrin is designated ______, and is the end-product of the ______.	***Ia*** ***coagulation cascade***
2. The stages of the cascade provide ______ amplification toward the end-product.	***sequential***
3. Activation at each step usually can be done only by the ______ preceding step in the cascade.	***immediately***

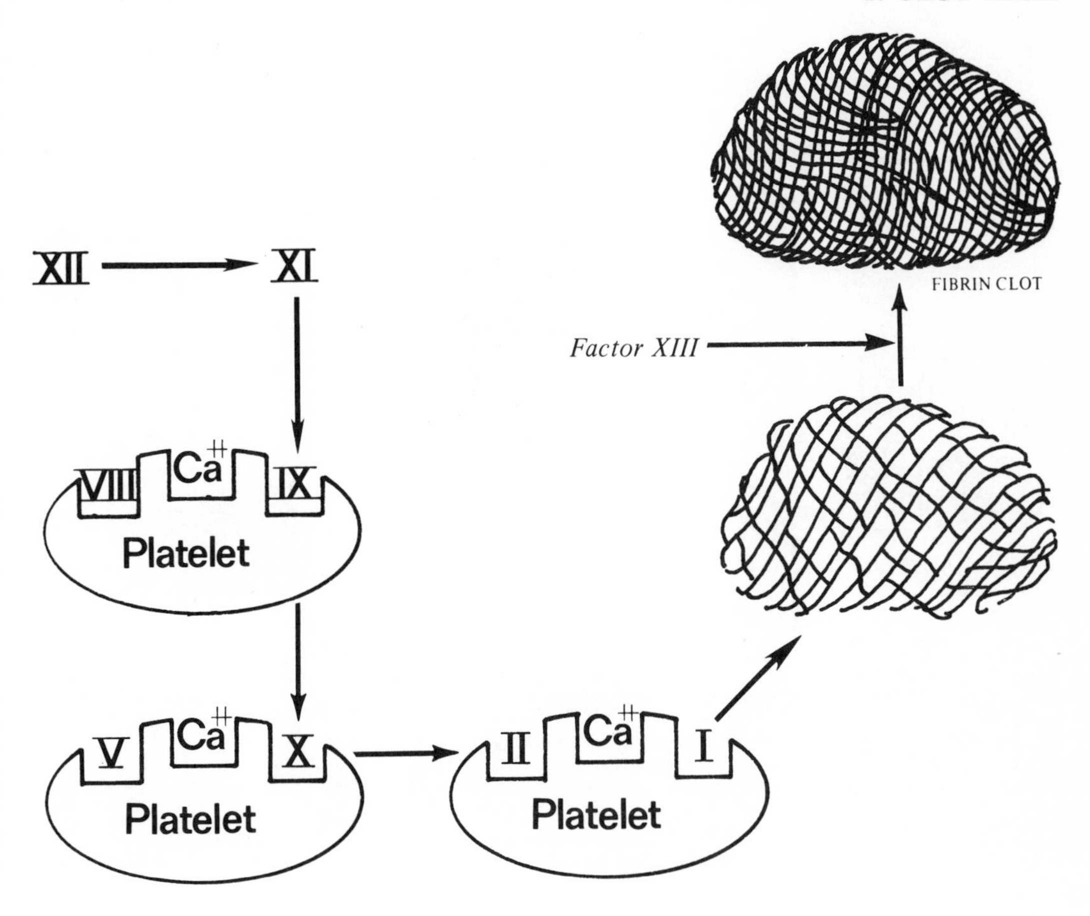

Factor XIII (fibrin stabilizing factor) enzymatically cross-links fibrin at additional sites. The testing of factor XIII is complicated by the fact that all laboratory tests are normal even with less than 5 percent factor XIII. Thus even a red cell transfusion will likely contain enough factor XIII to normalize the patient both clinically and in subsequent screening tests. Factor XIII deficiency is associated with wound dehiscence, late postoperative bleeding, and an increased incidence of abortions.

---

1. *Factor XIII is termed ______________.* — ***fibrin stabilizing factor***
2. *The level of factor XIII necessary for adequate clot formation is less than ______________.* — ***5 percent***
3. *A transfusion of red cells has enough plasma to correct a deficiency of factor ______________.* — ***XIII***

1. VASCULAR INTEGRITY
2. PLATELETS
3. COAGULATION CASCADE
4. CLOT LYSIS

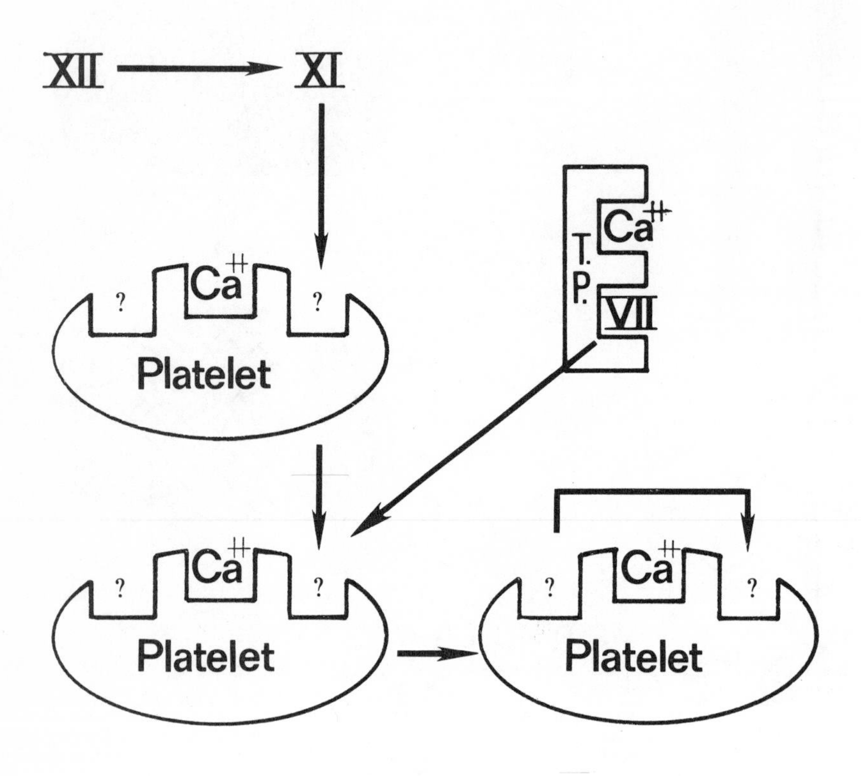

Before leaving the intrinsic pathway, see if you can recall the three sets of factors bound to the platelet surface. (The intrinsic pathway begins with the large numerals and concludes with the smallest numerals. In between, the numbers do not follow numerically.)

Let us now turn our attention to the **extrinsic pathway.** This pathway involves **tissue** activation, and is a much shorter path to fibrin formation.

---

1. *The first set is involved in hemophilia* ______, ______. — ***VIII, IX***
2. *The second set are the nickel and dime factors.* ______, ______. — ***V, X***
3. *The third set are the smallest numbered factors* ______, ______. — ***II, I***

1. VASCULAR INTEGRITY
2. PLATELETS
3. COAGULATION CASCADE
4. CLOT LYSIS

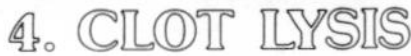

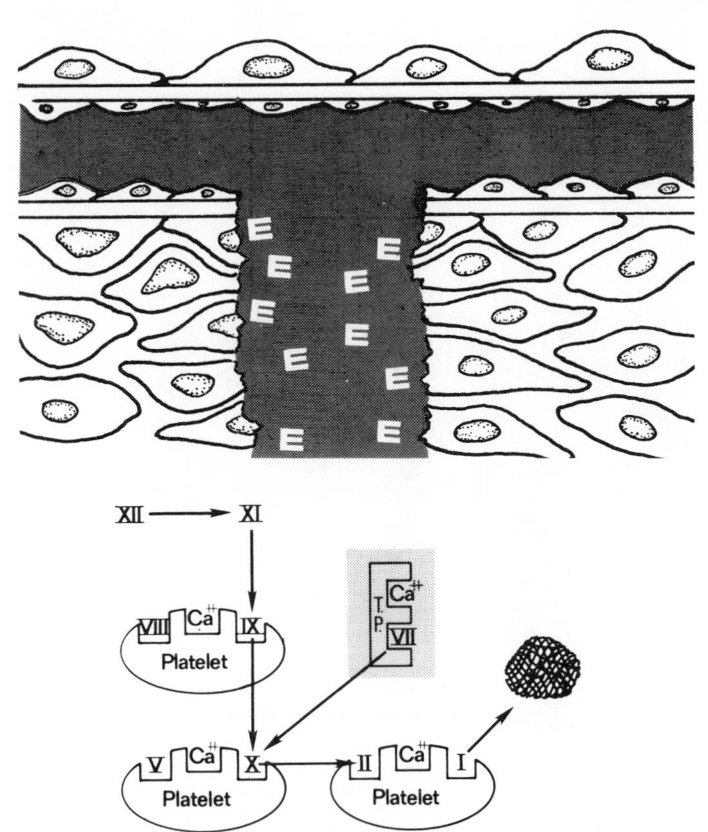

The Extrinsic Pathway serves as an alternate method to activate Factor X, and therefore an alternate method to produce fibrin.

A **tissue** phospholipid provides a suitably charged surface to bind both Ca^{++} and factor VII. The tissue phospholipid is not normally present in the blood, but is released upon **tissue** damage. Thus, the key to the extrinsic pathway is the extravascular **tissue phospholipid.**

(We have diagrammed this phospholipid as a "Big E" to remind the reader that this tissue phospholipid is in the Extrinsic Pathway. Also, an E binds two factors, Ca^{++} and VII, rather than three, as in the Intrinsic Pathway.)

---

1. *Tissue phospholipid, in the ________ pathway, is analogous to ________ phospholipid (PF-3) in the intrinsic pathway.*	***extrinsic*** ***platelet***
2. *The important difference between PF-3 and tissue phospholipid is ________.*	***location***
3. *Tissue phospholipid binds both factors ________ and ________.*	***calcium and VII***

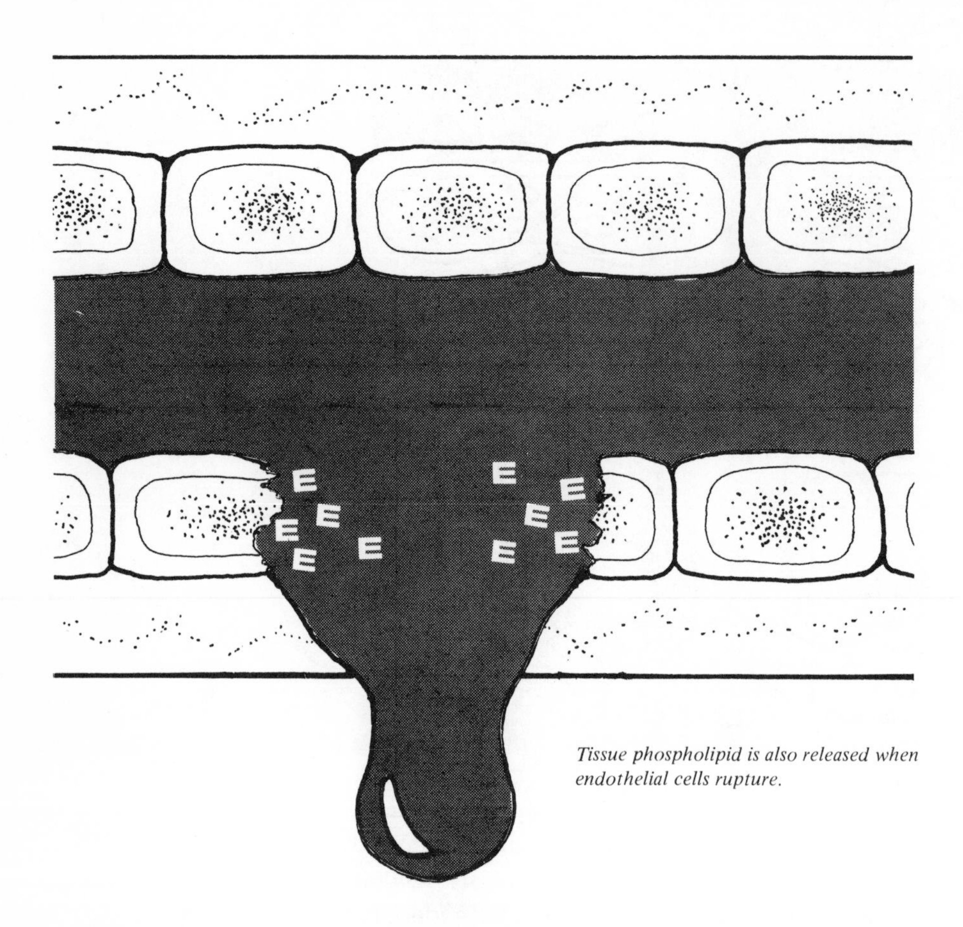

Tissue phospholipid is also released when endothelial cells rupture.

Tissue phospholipid, besides being present extravascularly, is also released when endothelial cells rupture. The amount of tissue phospholipid contributed by endothelial cells usually is small, but it is enough so that both the intrinsic and extrinsic pathways may be activated by relatively trivial vascular injury.

---

1. The only factor not in the intrinsic pathway is factor ______.	***VII***
2. Factor VII and ______ bind to tissue phospholipid.	**Ca^{++}**
3. Under normal conditions, tissue phospholipid is not found in the ______ space.	***intravascular***
4. The end-product of the extrinsic pathway is ______.	***fibrin***

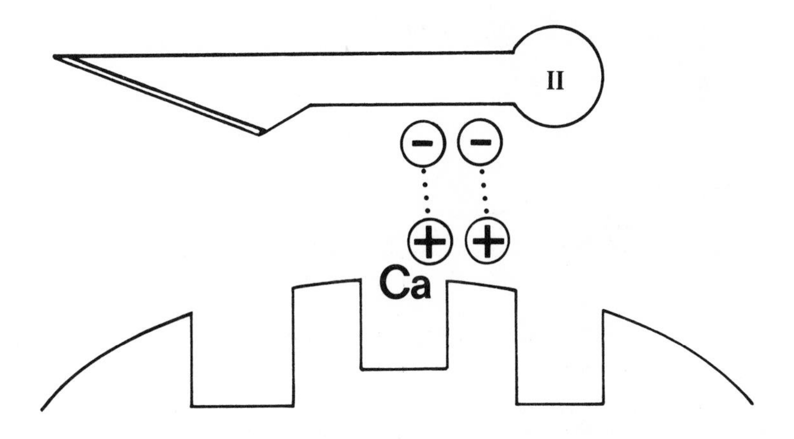

Before leaving the coagulation cascade, notice that the phospholipids always bind Ca^{++}. The reason for this is that Ca^{++} actually binds the **serine proteases** to the phospholipids by an electrostatic charge. This electrostatic charge is **double** positive to **double** negative.

---

1. *Ca^{++} acts as a ______ between the phospholipids and the ______.* — ***bridge***, ***serine proteases***
2. *Binding between Ca^{++} and the serine proteases is an ______ bond.* — ***electrostatic***
3. *Ca^{++} has a ______ charge.* — ***double positive***
4. *Serine proteases require a ______ charge for phospholipid binding.* — ***double negative***

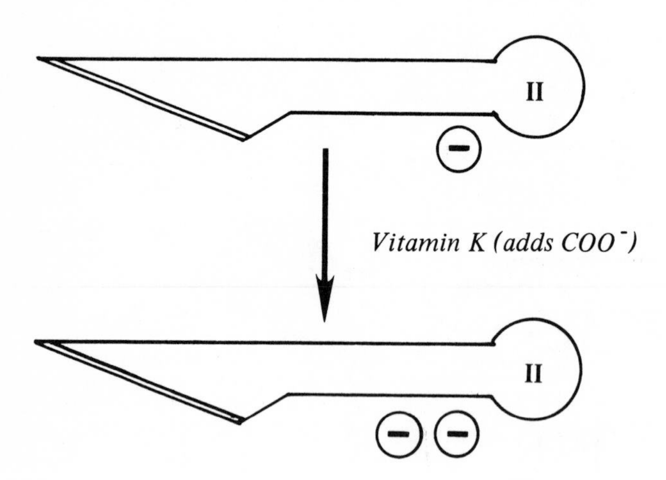

None of the serine protease amino acid side chains has the **double negative** charge necessary to bind to the platelet or tissue phospholipid by the double positive calcium bridge. Glutamic acid, an amino acid contained in the serine proteases, has a side chain with a single negative charge. Vitamin K enzymatically adds a carboxyl (COO^-) group to the glutamic acid side at the gamma carbon, to produce the double negative charge. Hence the term gamma carboxy glutamic acid.

Vitamin K enzymatically adds this carboxyl (COO^-) to each of four serine proteases which bind to platelet or tissue phospholipid. These serine proteases are appropriately termed vitamin K dependent factors.

---

1. A ________ charge is required by four proteases to bind to phospholipids.	***double negative***
2. This charge is added as a ________ group.	***carboxyl***
3. This group is enzymatically added by ________.	***Vitamin K***

1. VASCULAR INTEGRITY
2. PLATELETS
3. COAGULATION CASCADE
4. CLOT LYSIS

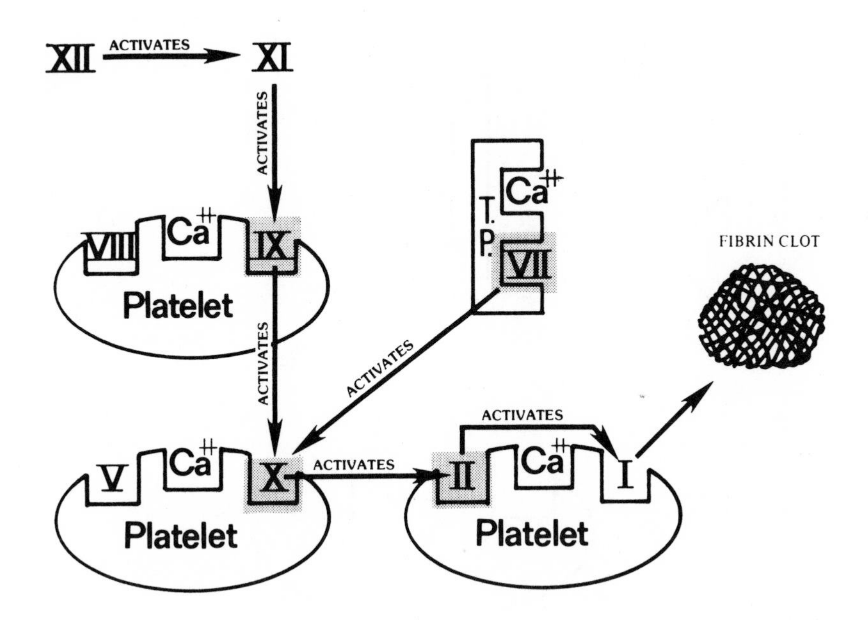

The four factors which bind to the platelet or tissue phospholipid are non-functional without the addition of the carboxyl group (COO^-). These four factors—II, VII, IX, and X—are all serine proteases. One can derive which serine proteases are vitamin K dependent by recalling the basic diagram, and noticing which serine proteases are bound to either the platelet or tissue phospholipid. (We will discuss the importance of this modification in the chapter on disorders.)

---

1. *An additional carboxyl group is enzymatically added to factors ______, ______, ______, and ______ by ______.* — ***II, VII, IX, X*** / ***vitamin K***
2. *The carboxyl group added to make a double negative charge, is a ______ of the serine protease, required for binding to a platelet or tissue phospholipid.* — ***modification***

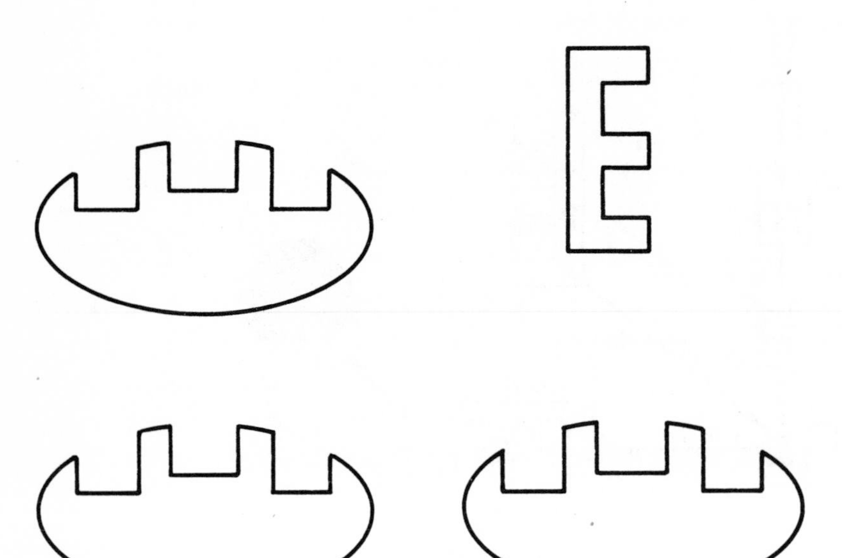

DRAW THE COMPLETE COAGULATION CASCADE ABOVE

(We'll have a totally filled in one on the next page, but give it a good try before you peek.) Draw the phospholipids first.

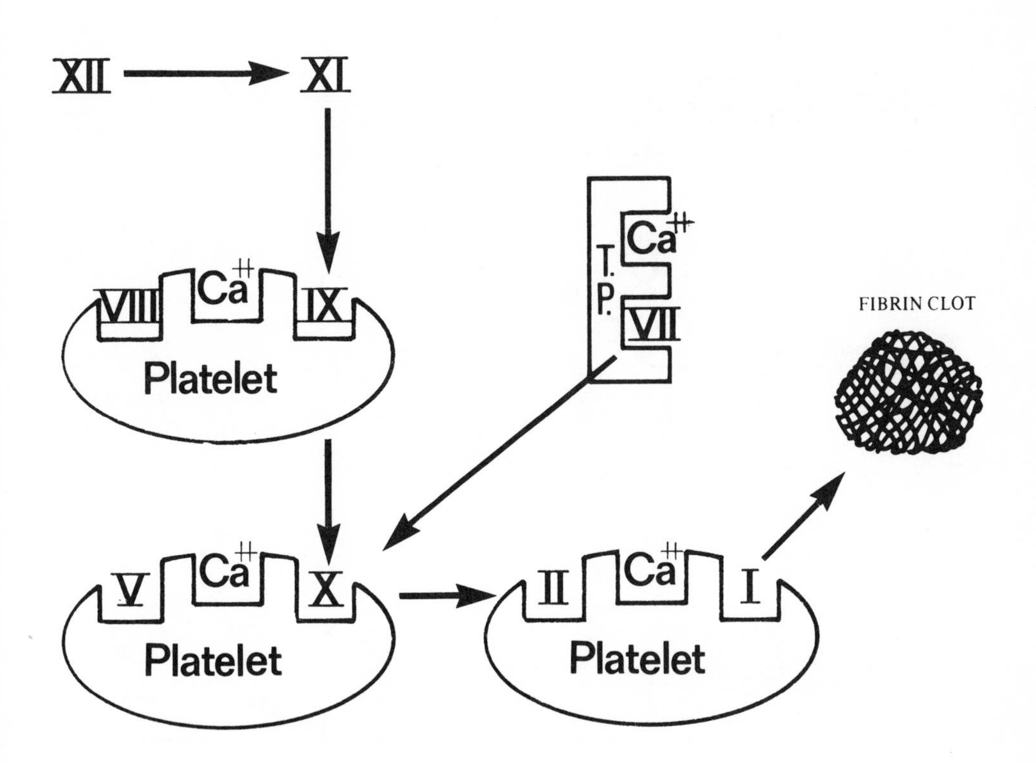

Helpful hints to re-derive the coagulation cascade anywhere, anytime:

1. Draw the platelet phospholipids and the tissue phospholipid in the forms we have illustrated, to have a "landing area" for each of the coagulation factors. Three slots on each "platelet", and an "E" for the extrinsic tissue phospholipid.
2. Add Ca^{++} to each phospholipid.
3. Platelet — 1st set add hemophiliac factors.
   2nd set add the nickel and dime factors.
   3rd set add smallest two numbers.
4. Tissue phospholipid—add the lucky number seven.

[Note that the two factors which are helpers are bound on the platelet and are diagramatically at the **outside** slot. This has helped us remember which factors are helpers (they are different from the proteases that dominate the rest of the diagram).]

1. VASCULAR INTEGRITY
2. PLATELETS
3. COAGULATION CASCADE
4. CLOT LYSIS

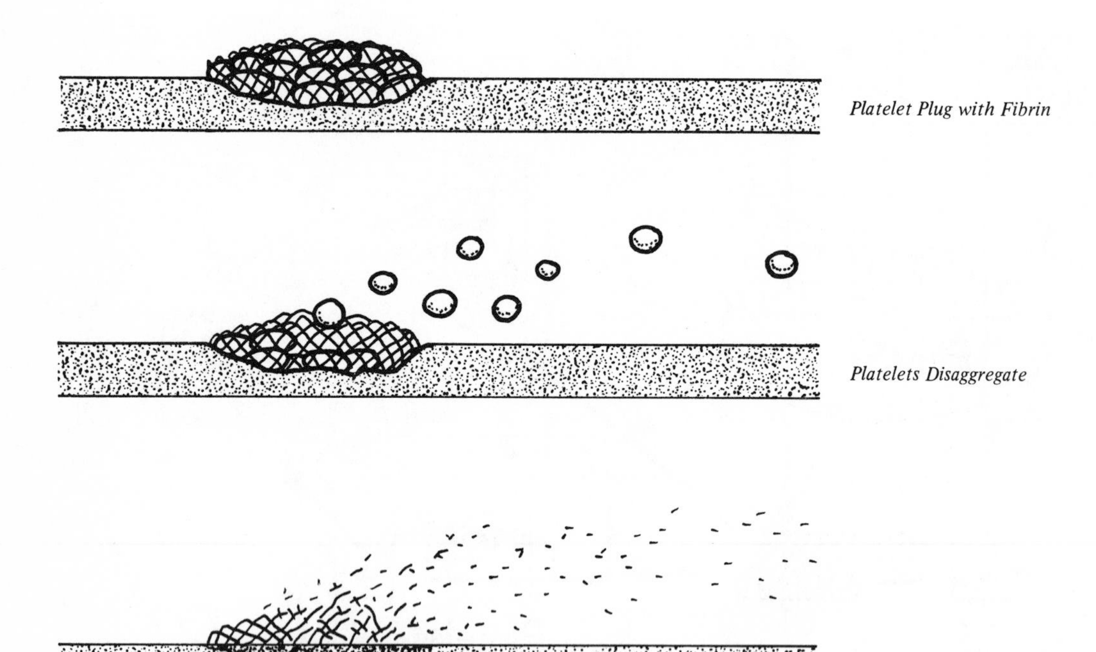

Platelet Plug with Fibrin

Platelets Disaggregate

Fibrin Clot Lysed

We are now ready to study the fourth component of the hemostatic system, clot lysis.

Re-establishing normal circulation requires that, over time, the injured vessel heals, and the fibrin clot is removed. Lysis must proceed slowly and with caution, since too much too soon will result in rebleeding from the injured and incompletely healed vessel.

(Note: Platelets disaggregate after 24-48 hours, leaving the fibrin clot to maintain hemostatis. Thus during clot lysis, there are normally no platelets involved.)

---

1. *Clot lysis thus serves to help ____________ normal circulation.* — **re-establish**
2. *The purpose of the lytic system is to remove the ____________.* — **fibrin clot**
3. *This lytic system must be coordinated with ____________ of the injured vessel.* — **healing**

1. VASCULAR INTEGRITY
2. PLATELETS
3. COAGULATION CASCADE
4. CLOT LYSIS

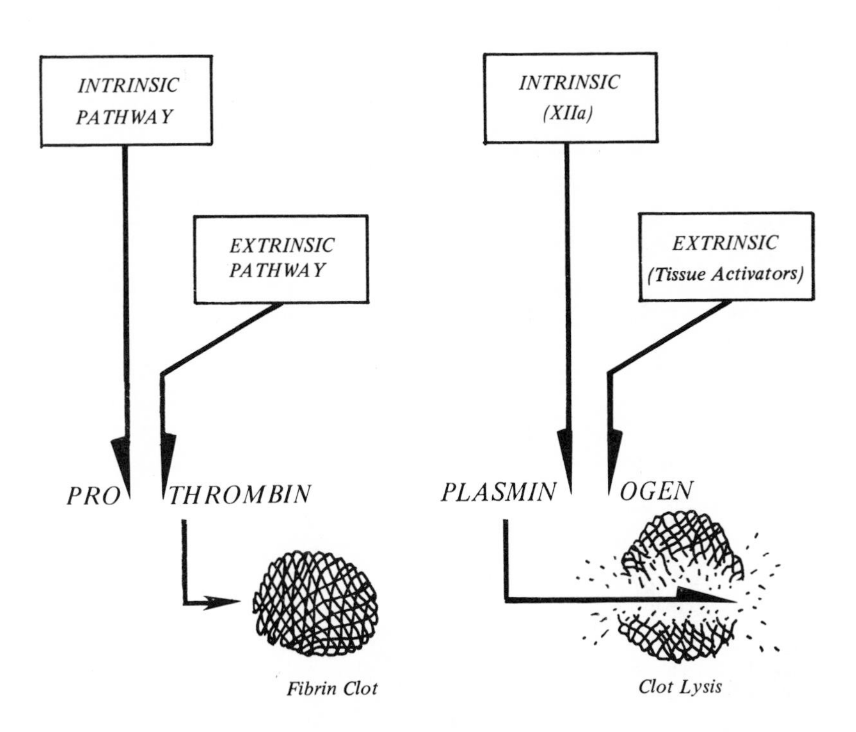

Fibrin Clot

Clot Lysis

The diagram above is the coagulation cascade with the **parallel** lytic system to the right.

The lytic system is simple compared to the coagulation cascade. In designing clot lysis, nature took the first and last steps of the coagulation cascade, and left out everything in-between. By having the first steps the same, the body initiates clot lysis simultaneously with clot formation. The last steps are also almost identical. The last cleavage enzymes, thrombin in coagulation and plasmin in lysis, are essentially the same enzyme (only a few amino acids are different). This difference is enough, however, for plasmin to cleave fibrinogen at additional sites (plasmin cleaves fibrinogen into much smaller pieces than does thrombin).

---

1. *The initial steps for both the coagulation cascade and the lytic system are ______________.* — ***identical***
2. *The lytic system is more ______________ than the coagulation cascade.* — ***simple***
3. *Clot formation and clot lysis may occur ______________.* — ***simultaneously***

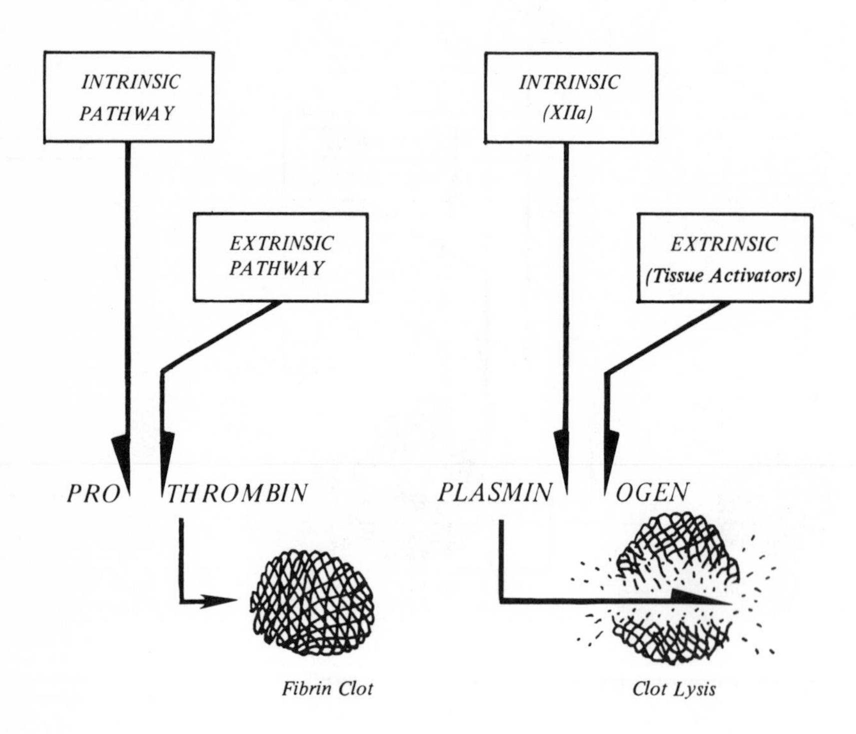

Fibrin Clot *Clot Lysis*

The first of the two steps in the lytic system is activation of plasminogen to plasmin via either of two pathways. Plasminogen is activated to plasmin intravascularly (intrinsic pathway) by Factor XIIa (the initiator of the coagulation cascade). Extravascularly (extrinsic pathway), plasminogen is activated by "tissue activators" in a manner similar to the tissue phospholipid activation of factor VII in the coagulation cascade.

Thus there are two ways of activating plasminogen to plasmin, just as there are two pathways for activating prothombin to thrombin.

---

1. *The intrinsic activator of plasmin formation is factor__________.* — **XIIa**
2. *The extrinsic activators of plasmin formation are__________.* — ***tissue activators***
3. *Intrinsic activation occurs__________, while extrinsic activation occurs__________.* — ***intravascularly*** / ***extravascularly***

4. CLOT LYSIS

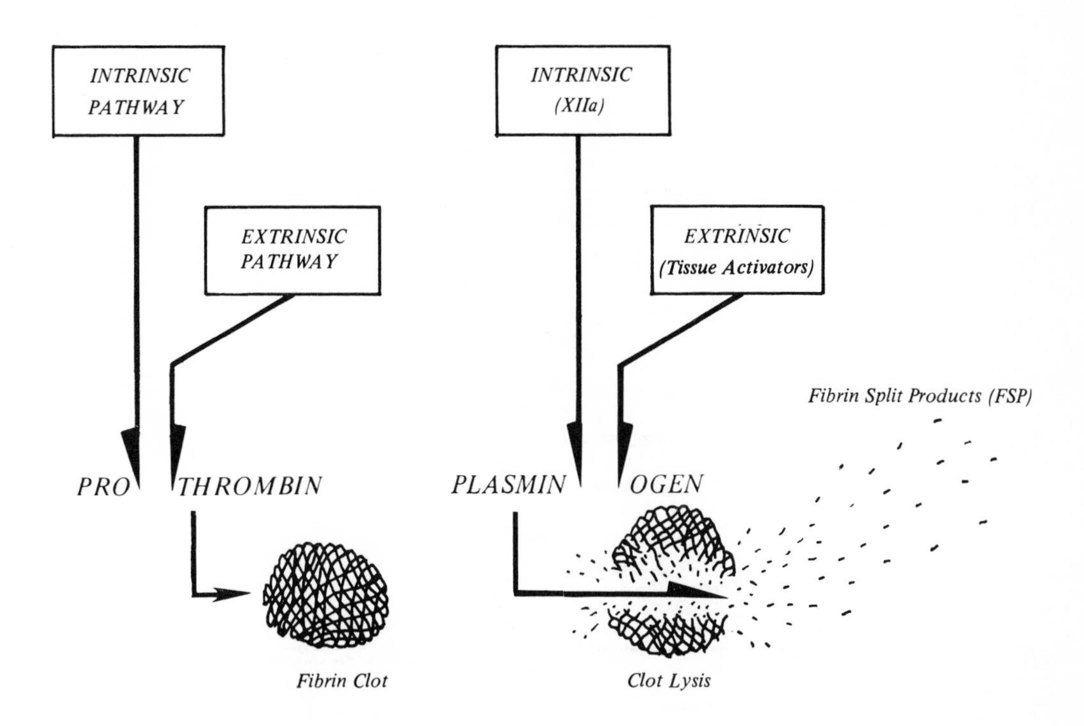

The second of the two steps in the lytic system is the cleavage action of plasmin. Plasmin, the activated form of plasminogen, slices fibrin into small pieces effectively lysing the fibrin clot. The activity of plasmin is almost identical to thrombin in the coagulation cascade. Thrombin, however, only cleaves fibrinogen, while plasmin cleaves both fibrinogen and fibrin. When plasmin cleaves fibrin or fibrinogen, the result is the formation of fibrin split products.

---

1. *Plasmin is a ______ enzyme almost identical in structure and function to the coagulation cascade enzyme ______.* — **cleavage**; **thrombin**
2. *The end-product of the lytic system is the formation of ______.* — **fibrin split products**
3. *Thrombin can only cleave ______.* — **fibrinogen**
4. *Plasmin can cleave ______ and ______.* — **fibrinogen**; **fibrin**

1. VASCULAR INTEGRITY
2. PLATELETS
3. COAGULATION CASCADE
4. CLOT LYSIS

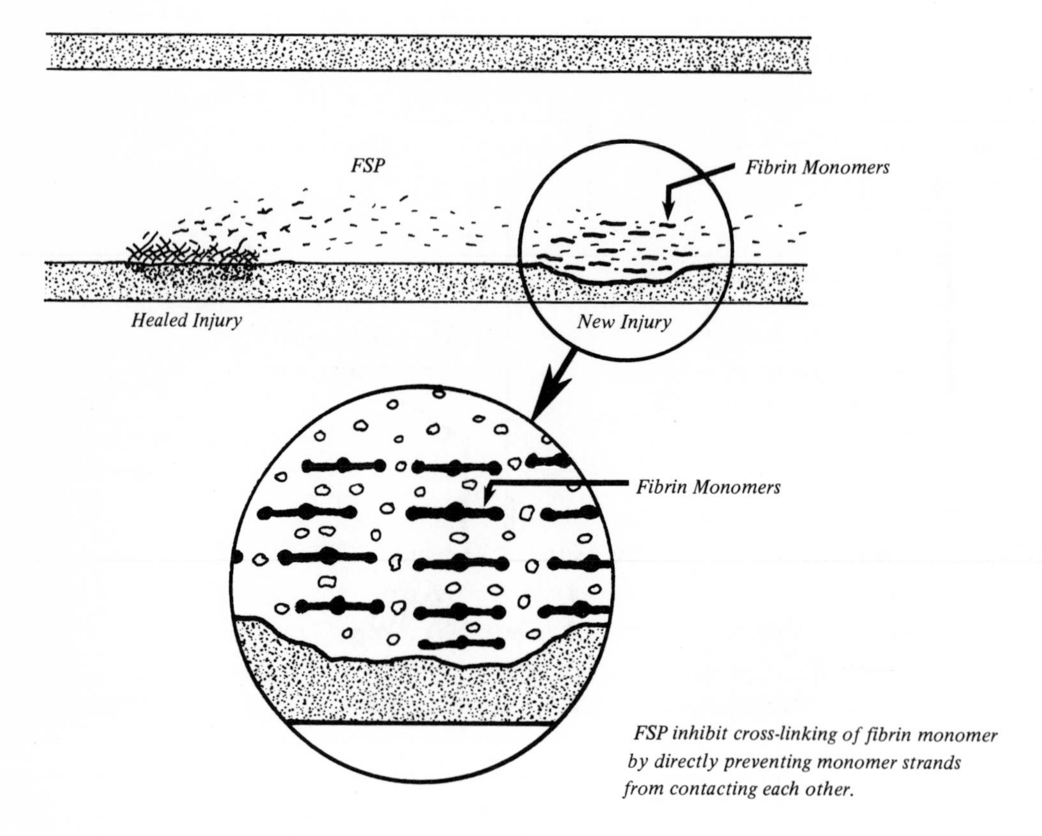

FSP inhibit cross-linking of fibrin monomer by directly preventing monomer strands from contacting each other.

The small peptides resulting from clot lysis are appropriately termed fibrin split products (FSP), or fibrin degradation products (FDP). They are normally removed by the reticuloendothelial system especially by the Kupffer cells in the liver. If they are not removed, they reach high concentrations and become potent inhibitors of clot formation. FSP inhibit cross-linking of fibrin monomer by directly preventing monomer strands from contacting each other. In high concentrations they also can produce platelet dysfunction.

---

1. *Breakdown products of fibrin are termed __________ or __________.* — **FSP, FDP**
2. *Fibrin split products are normally removed by the hepatic __________ cells.* — **Kupffer**
3. *High concentrations of FSP inhibit __________ of fibrin monomer.* — **cross-linking**
4. *High concentractions of FSP may produce __________ dysfunction.* — **platelet**

In summary:

Clot lysis closely resembles the coagulation cascade. In fact, by thinking of both processes in a parallel fashion, much information falls into place. Both systems involve:

Precursor Activation	Coagulation Cascade	Clot Lysis
Intrinsic	XIIa	XIIa
Extrinsic	Tissue activators	Tissue activators
Proenzyme	Prothrombin	Plasminogen
Active enzyme	Thrombin	Plasmin
"Substrate" for end-product	Fibrinogen	Fibrin
End-product	Fibrin	Fibrin Split Products
Natural Inhibitor*	Anti-thrombin	Anti-plasmin

(*We have not discussed this concept yet—but have just given you a peek at the next chapter. Read on!)

Chapter 3
LOCALIZATION OF CLOTTING AND LYSIS

This chapter contains many of the "pearls" we are presenting in the text. While some of the concepts previously presented are reexamined, the organization is such that we answer the question: "why doesn't blood clot everywhere?"

As we discuss each localizing mechanism, realize that if these mechanisms are prevented from operating, coagulation loses its localized nature and diffuse thrombosis may compromise vital organs. We will discuss this loss of localization in the chapter on DIC (disseminated intravascular coagulation).

1. VASCULAR INTEGRITY
2. PLATELETS
3. COAGULATION CASCADE
4. CLOT LYSIS

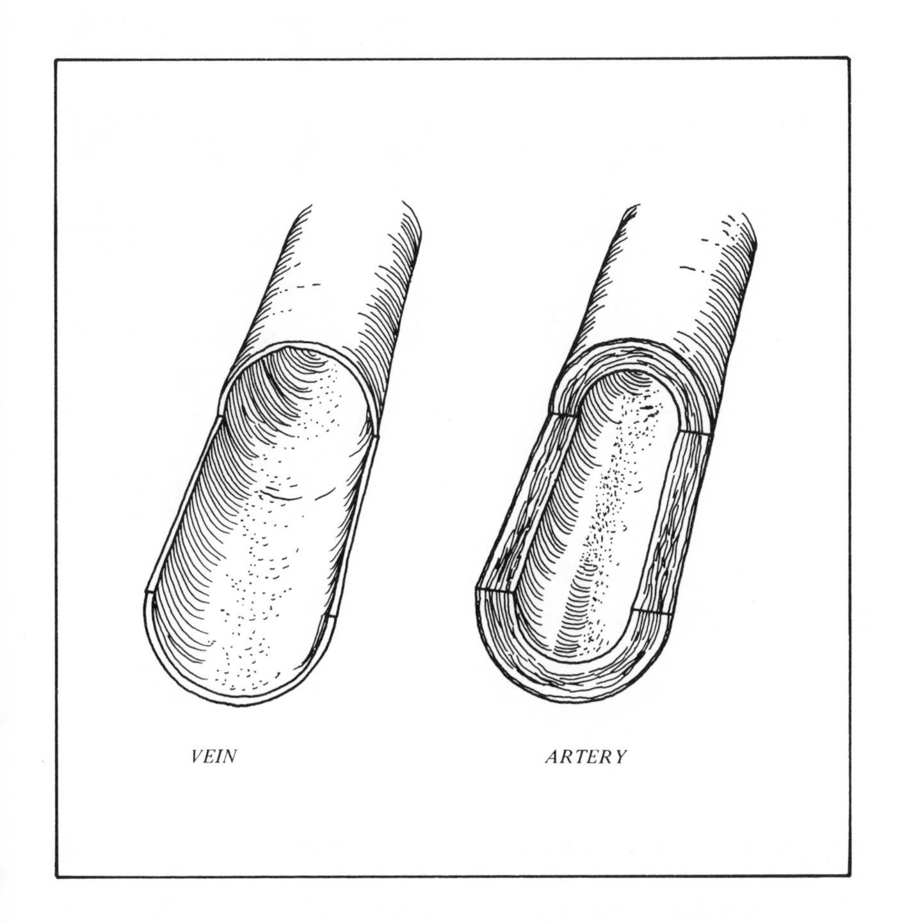

Vascular integrity is of prime importance. The moment vascular integrity is lost, the entire hemostatic mechanism must be initiated in order to minimize blood loss. In an attempt to limit this loss of vascular integrity, the human body has strengthened those vessels which experience either high pressure or frequent trauma.

---

1. *Vascular integrity is ______________.*	***crucial***
2. *Vessel stress is matched by vessel ______________.*	***strength***
3. *A large hole in a vessel may lead to ______________ bleeding, despite a normal coagulation system.*	***uncontrolled***

1. VASCULAR INTEGRITY
2. PLATELETS
3. COAGULATION CASCADE
4. CLOT LYSIS

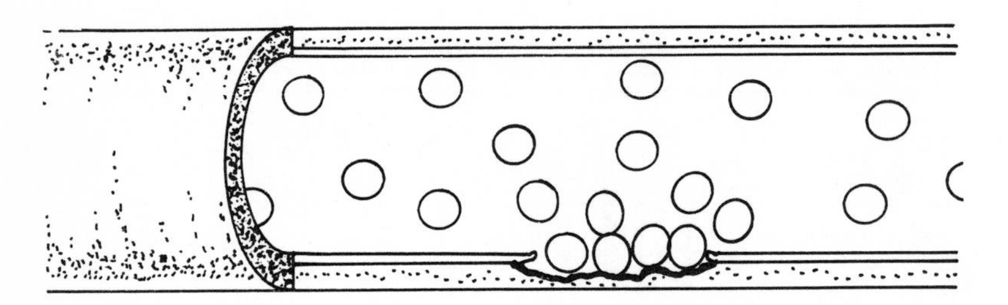

Platelets adhere to injured endothelial surface.

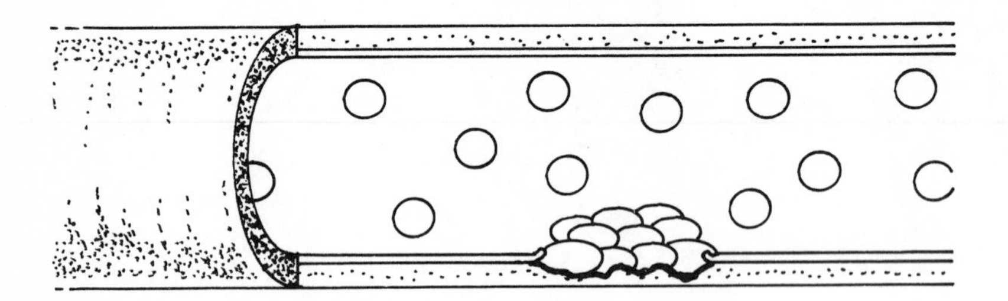

Platelets aggregate to form platelet plug.

Platelets play a crucial role in initiating and localizing clot formation. The platelet represents a complete hemostatic unit. The platelet's structure is directed to the function of localizing clot formation. Platelets circulate, making them available at any moment to form a cohesive mass of tightly aggregated platelets, to plug initially the break in the vascular tree.

(The mechanics of platelet interaction with the damaged vessel is further broken down by research scientists into: platelet contact; adhesion and spreading; release of ADP; and aggregation.)

---

1. *The first event usually triggering platelet action is a loss of vascular ____________ integrity.* — ***endothelial***
2. *Platelets then ____________.* — ***adhere***
3. *Additional platelets are then recruited to ____________.* — ***aggregate***

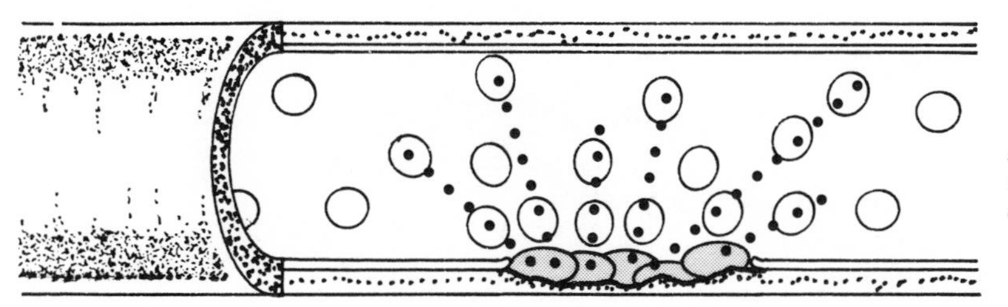

Aggregated platelets release ADP to recruit additional platelets.

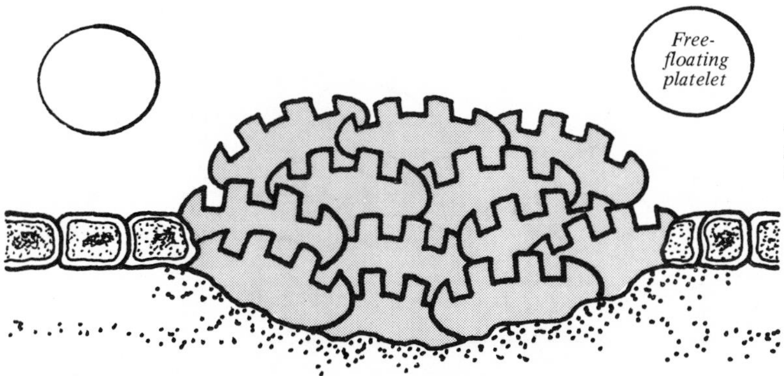

Aggregated platelets provide phospholipid surfaces for localizing coagulation cascade.

The major function of platelets is to circulate until they locate a break in vascular integrity. When platelets encounter a break in the endothelium (with the resultant exposure of subendothelial connective tissue, basement membrane, or collagen) they begin to adhere, and release ADP (adenosine diphosphate). The ADP recruits additional platelets to form the platelet plug.

In addition to providing the initial hemostatic plug, platelets also localize the formation of fibrin by the coagulation cascade. The rate-limiting step in the coagulation cascade is the availability of an appropriate phospholipid surface upon which to interact. Aggregated platelets display this appropriate phospholipid on their surface membrane.

1. *A primary action in platelet aggregation is the release of ______________.* **ADP**
2. *Platelets serve to localize thrombosis by localizing ______________ formation.* **fibrin**
3. *Aggregated platelets make available a platelet ______________.* **phospholipid**

1. VASCULAR INTEGRITY
2. PLATELETS
3. COAGULATION CASCADE

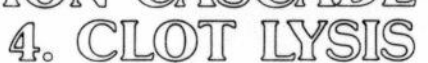

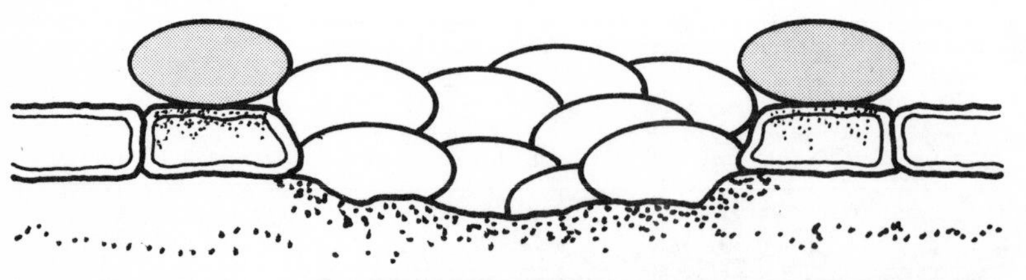

Aggregated platelets extend past site of denuded endothelium.

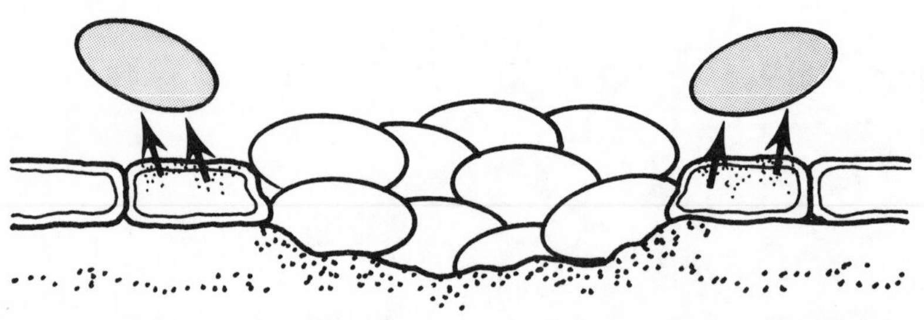

Prostacyclin produced by intact vessel wall inhibits further aggregation.

Prostacyclin may be produced in a blood vessel wall, upon contact with an activated platelet. Once the platelet plug extends past the site of denuded endothelium, the platelet interaction with normal vessel wall produces prostacyclin. This inhibits further platelet aggregation, localizing the platelet plug to the site of injury.

Foreign surfaces, such as artificial grafts used as vascular replacements, or cardiopulmonary bypass equipment, cannot, of course, produce prostacyclin. Thus the localization and inhibition capabilities of prostacyclin will not be available on the surface of artificial materials. Therefore, the platelet aggregation phenomenon can "snowball," and initiate graft thrombosis.

---

1. *Prostacyclin is produced when ____________ and platelets interact.* — ***endothelium***
2. *The action of prostacyclin inhibits platelet ____________.* — ***aggregation***
3. *Prostacyclin is not produced by ____________ surfaces.* — ***artificial***

1. VASCULAR INTEGRITY
2. PLATELETS
3. COAGULATION CASCADE
4. CLOT LYSIS

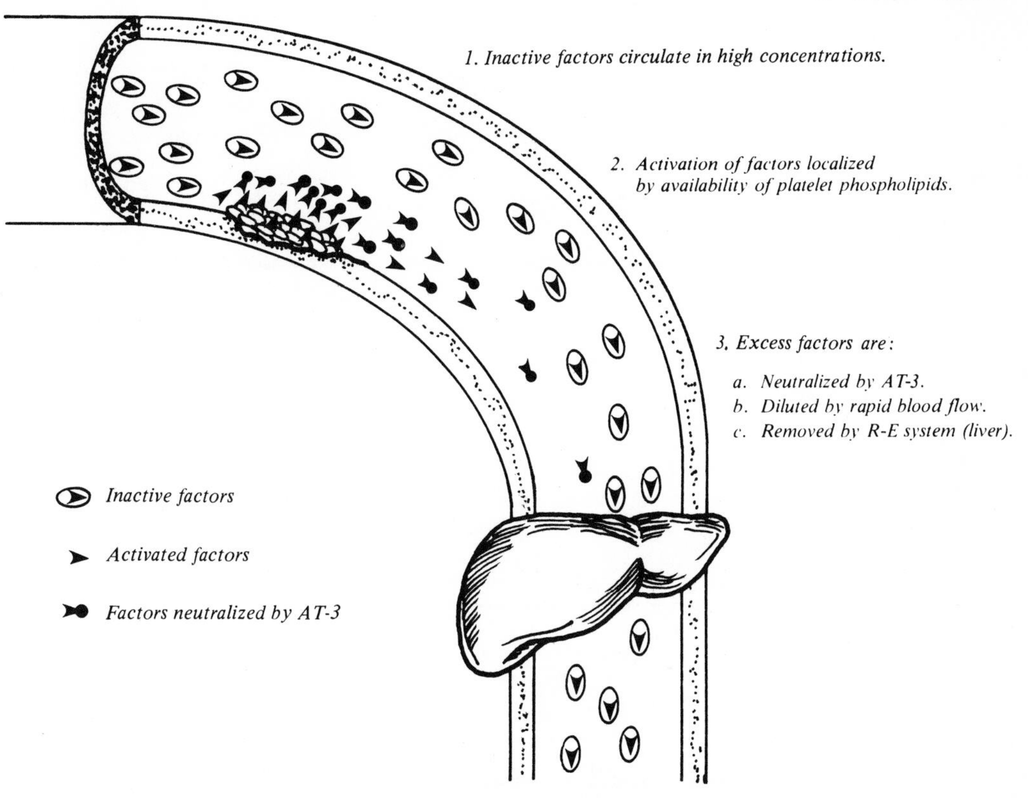

The coagulation factors circulate in inactive (precursor) forms in high concentrations. The rate-limiting step in the coagulation cascade is the availability of an appropriate phospholipid surface upon which to interact. Aggregated platelets and injured tissue cells may both provide such phospholipids.

Once the factors are in active form and producing fibrin, their action is localized to the site of injury by three major mechanisms. The activated factors are: diluted by rapid blood flow; removed by the reticulo-endothelial (R-E) system; and neutralized by a circulating protein called anti-thrombin 3 (AT-3).

In the next few pages we will discuss the neutralization of active proteases by anti-thrombin 3.

---

1. *Activated factors are ____________ by rapid blood flow.* **diluted**
2. *Activated factors are ____________ by the reticulo-endothelial system, especially the liver.* **removed**
3. *Activated factors are ____________ by a circulating protein called anti-thrombin 3.* **neutralized**

Anti-Thrombin 3 (AT-3)

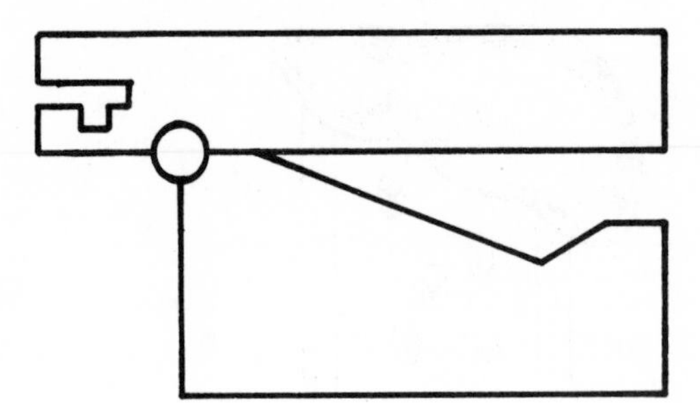

Anti-thrombin 3 (AT-3) is a normal physiological inhibitor of the coagulation cascade. This inhibitor consists of a single polypeptide chain with a molecular weight of 65,000, and is produced in the liver.

---

1. Activated factors have a natural ______________.	**inhibitor**
2. This inhibitor protein is called ______________.	**anti-thrombin**
3. Anti-thrombin is one of several mechanisms used to ______________ fibrin deposition.	**localize**

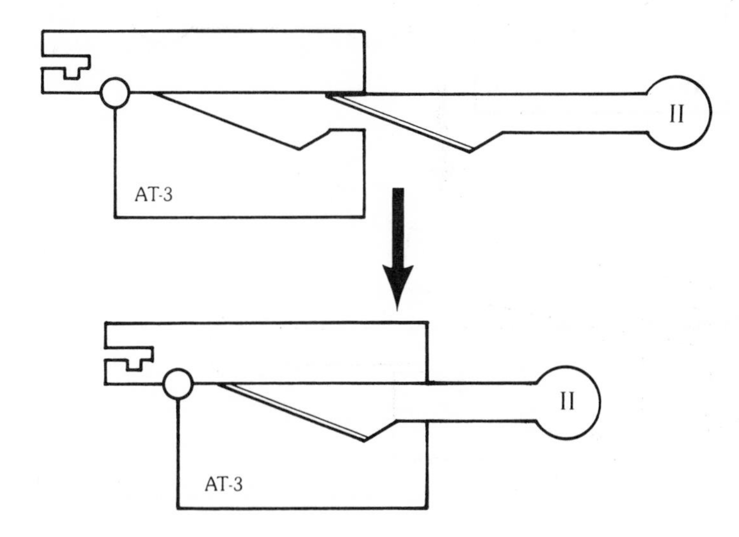

Anti-thrombin 3 (AT-3) is the principle plasma antagonist of the active proteases. Thus, it can bind thrombin (which is the activated form of prothrombin), and other activated proteases.

(Note: Inactive serine proteases are not neutralized by anti-thrombin 3 because inactive proteins cannot bind to anti-thrombin.)

This binding of anti-thrombin 3 and thrombin normally occurs at a slow rate. Is there a way to speed up this process?

---

1. *Anti-thrombin 3 is a protein found normally in __________.* — **plasma**
2. *Anti-thrombin 3 binds activated __________ to neutralize their activity.* — **proteases**
3. *Anti-thrombin 3 binds to __________ at its active center.* — **thrombin**

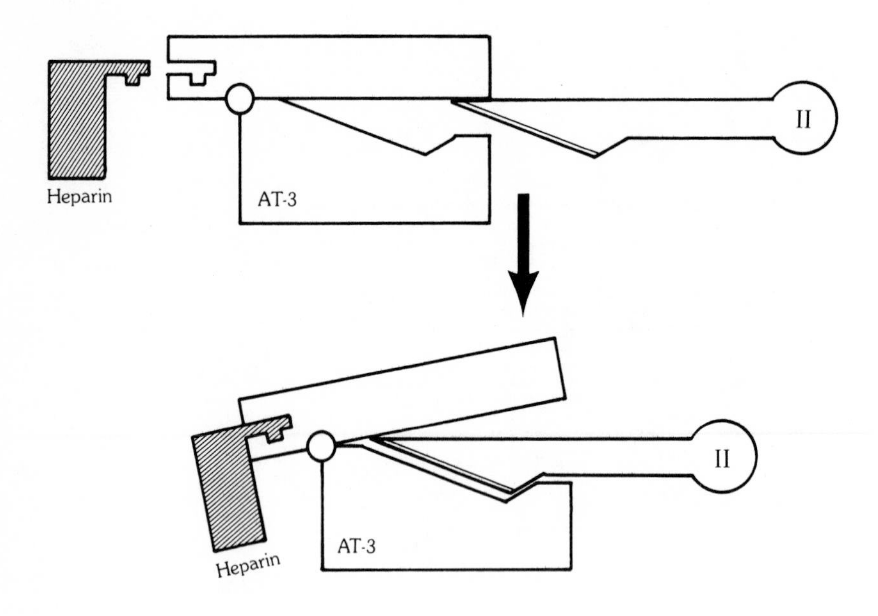

Yes.

Heparin may bind to anti-thrombin 3 (AT-3), causing a conformational change in anti-thrombin 3, which results in a more accessible binding site for activated serine proteases, of which thrombin is an example. Thus, the presence of heparin "opens up" anti-thrombin 3 so that it can rapidly bind to any activated serine protease, such as thrombin.

Is anti-thrombin 3's binding specific?

---

1. *Heparin produces a change in the ______________ of anti-thrombin 3.* — ***structure***
2. *The ability of anti-thrombin 3 to bind to thrombin is accelerated by ______________.* — ***heparin***
3. *Anti-thrombin 3 may bind any active ______________.* — ***serine protease***

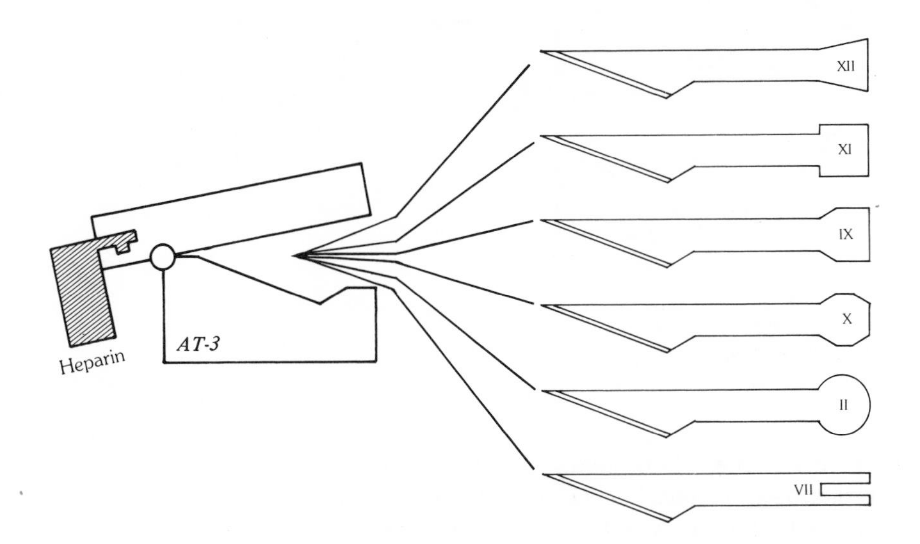

No. Above is a diagrammatic example of the capability of (heparin-activated) anti-thrombin 3 to bind with multiple coagulation factors (all the activated serine proteases).

NOTE: Heparin-activated anti-thrombin 3 binds to any available activated serine protease, of which thrombin (IIa) is the most obvious example.

[Factors V, VIII and fibrinogen (I) are not serine proteases, and are not directly affected by heparin.]

---

1. *Anti-thrombin 3 is made more active by the action of __________.* — ***heparin***
2. *Anti-thrombin 3 binds any active __________.* — ***serine protease***
3. *Several of the factors are not bound by anti-thrombin. These are factors __________.* — ***VIII, V, and I***

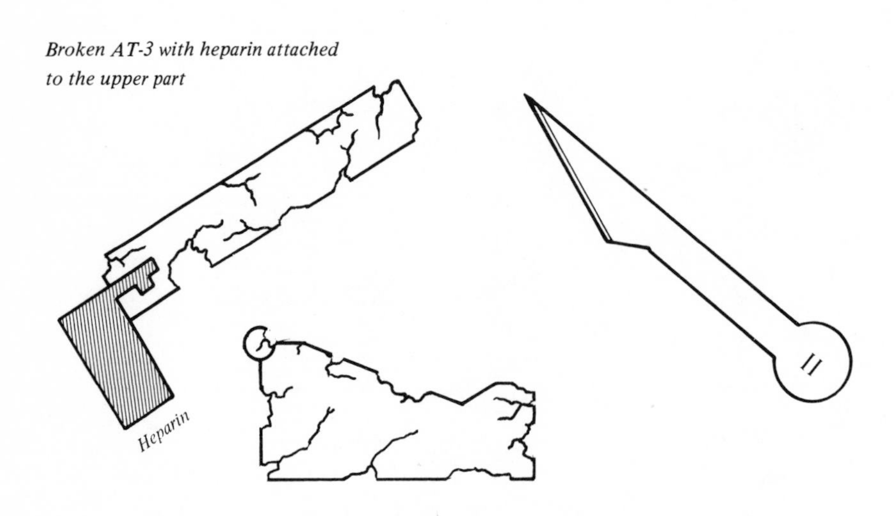

Heparin has no inherent anticoagulant properties. It is ineffective without functional AT-3.

Congenital reduction in anti-thrombin 3 (AT-3) levels, if severe, results in fatal thrombosis. Acquired deficiencies of AT-3 also result in relatively unopposed thrombin activity, and thus increased fibrin deposition. Acquired deficiencies of AT-3 can be seen in DIC (where AT-3 is destroyed by circulating proteins) and occasionally in women receiving oral contraceptive drugs (where production is decreased). Here again, fibrin deposition in uninjured vessels may result in morbidity and, occasionally, mortality.

Since heparin activity depends on adequate AT-3 levels (it enhances AT-3 activity), heparin will be ineffective in these circumstances. Heparin has no inherent anticoagulant properties.

(These conditions will be discussed in more detail later.)

---

1. *Deficiencies of AT-3 results in relatively ________ thrombin activity.*	***unopposed***
2. *If AT-3 levels are decreased, ________ activity will be ________.*	***heparin*** ***reduced***
3. *If AT-3 levels are reduced, as in DIC or in certain patients receiving oral contraceptives, ________ will be relatively more active and ________ deposition may result.*	***thrombin*** ***fibrin***

1. VASCULAR INTEGRITY
2. PLATELETS
3. COAGULATION CASCADE
4. CLOT LYSIS

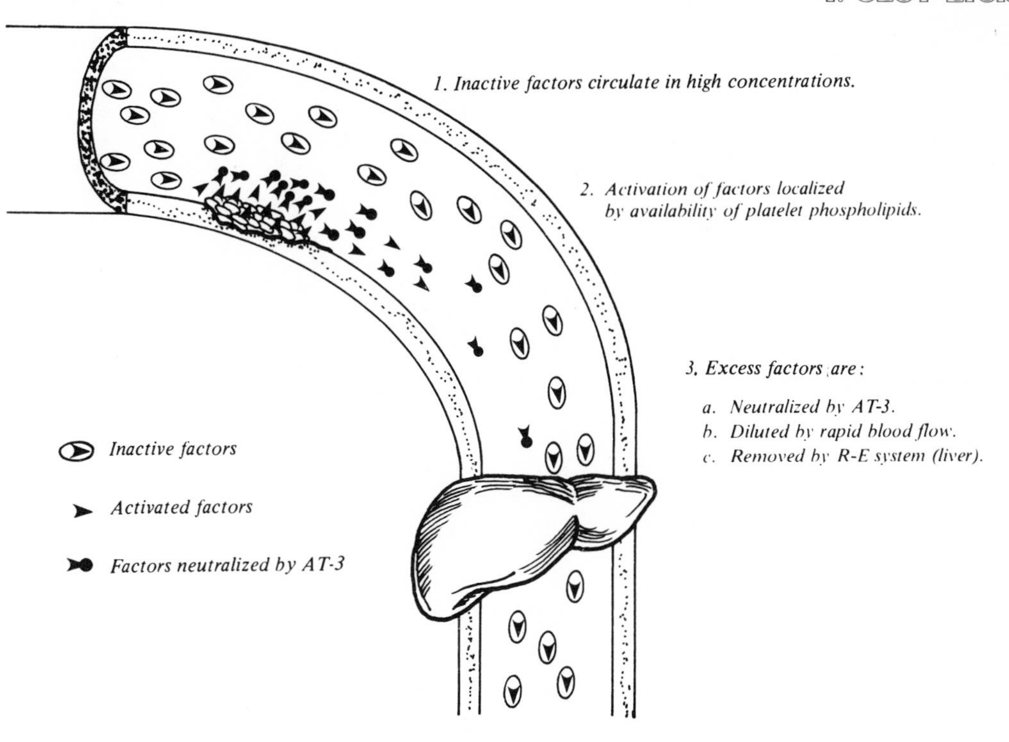

Review of localization of fibrin deposition:

The coagulation cascade is prevented from continuously exploding and forming a fibrin clot by several ingenious means:

- The coagulation proteins circulate in high concentrations, but in an inactive form.
- The inactive factors require a platelet phospholipid or tissue phospholipid upon which to intract, and be sequentially activated.
- Active factors are:
  - — diluted by rapid blood flow
  - — removed by the R-E system (liver)
  - — neutralized by a circulating protein, called anti-thrombin 3, which binds activated factors.

---

1. *Inactive factors circulate in ______________ concentration.* — ***high***
2. *Inactive factors interact on aggregated ______________.* — ***platelets***
3. *Active factors are localized to the site of injury by ______________, ______________, and ______________.* — ***dilution removal neutralization***

1. VASCULAR INTEGRITY
2. PLATELETS
3. COAGULATION CASCADE
4. CLOT LYSIS

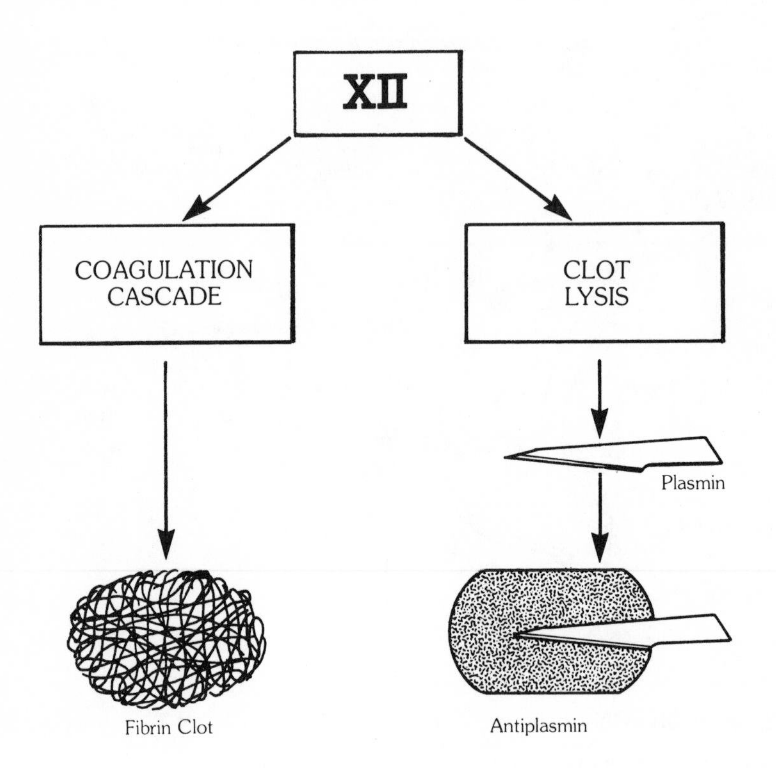

Clot lysis is localized by two mechanisms:

- Factor XII initiates both the coagulation cascade and clot lysis. Since the first steps are the same in both systems, clot lysis is initiated at the same time and place as clot formation.

- Plasmin is rapidly inactivated by a circulating protein (antiplasmin), which binds plasmin.

Obviously, the factors which have been discussed previously regarding localization of the entire clotting process will indirectly also help to localize the lytic process under normal circumstances.

---

1. Clot lysis normally can be _______________ because factor XII activation is localized. — ***localized***

2. The presence of _______________ is therefore normally localized. — ***plasmin***

3. _______________ rapidly inactivates circulating plasmin. — ***Anti-plasmin***

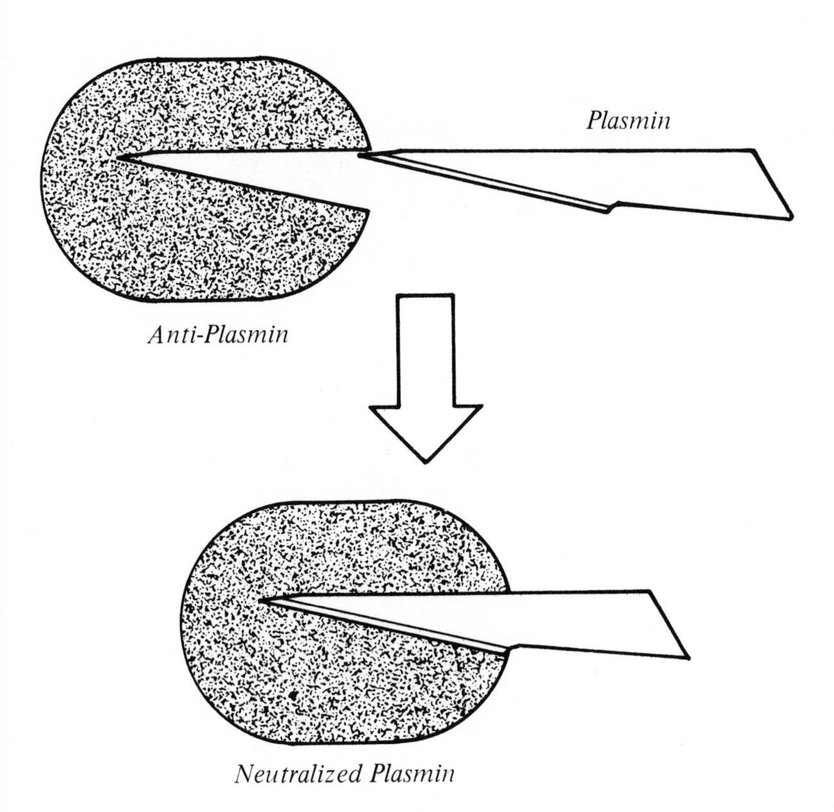

Anti-plasmin, an inhibitor of plasmin, binds active plasmin in a manner identical to anti-thrombin 3 binding of thrombin. Unlike anti-thrombin 3, anti-plasmin is not made more avid by heparin.

---

1. Anti-plasmin can only bind ____________ plasmin.	***activated***
2. Anti-plasmin is ____________ made more active by heparin.	***not***
3. The addition of ____________ does not alter anti-plasmin's activity.	***heparin***

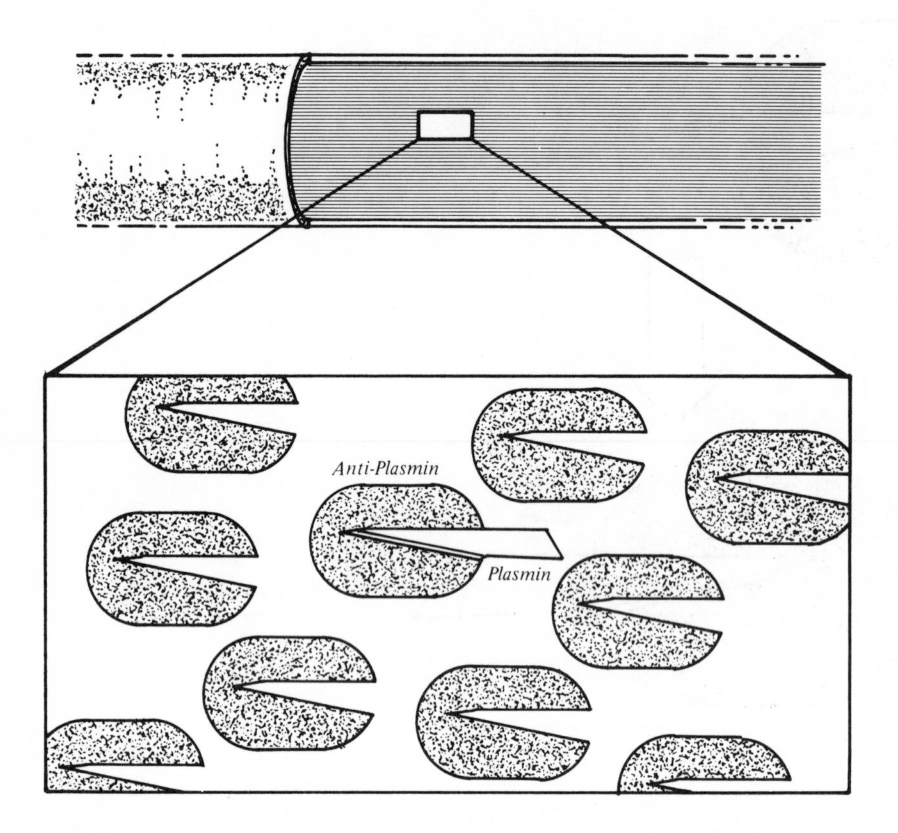

The blood concentration of the inhibitor protein, anti-plasmin, normally is 10 times that of plasmin. Activated plasminogen (plasmin) is thus neutralized very quickly.

---

1. Plasmin is quickly __________ by anti-plasmin.	***neutralized***
2. This complex is similar in its basic concept to the complex formed by thrombin and __________.	***anti-thrombin 3***
3. Anti-plasmin circulates in __________ concentrations, relative to plasmin.	***high***

1. VASCULAR INTEGRITY
2. PLATELETS
3. COAGULATION CASCADE
4. CLOT LYSIS

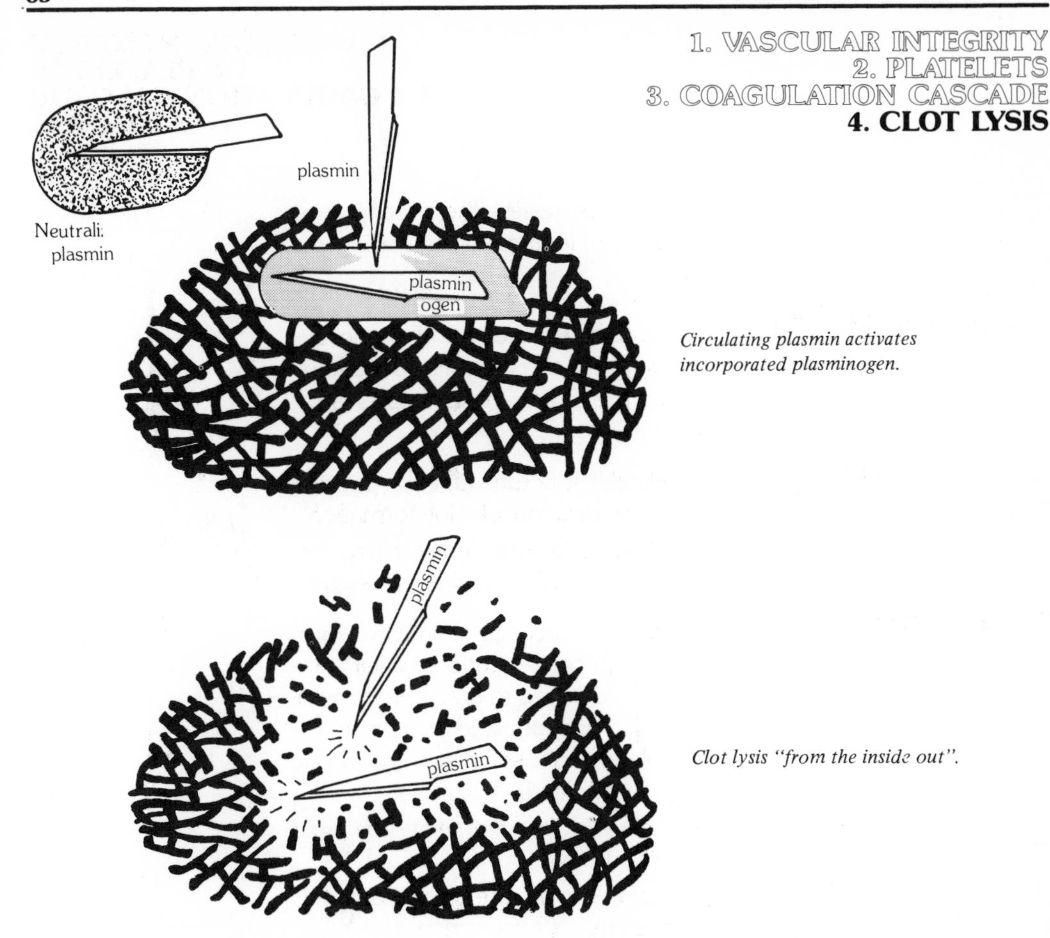

Circulating plasmin activates incorporated plasminogen.

Clot lysis "from the inside out".

Since activation of the plasminogen-plasmin system is immediately blocked by anti-plasmin, physiologic fibrinolysis is not based on the action of circulating plasmin. Instead, plasmin is activated locally within the fibrin clot, where it is protected from anti-plasmin.

Plasminogen is initially incorporated within the fibrin clot during its formation. The surrounding fibrin effectively protects the plasmin from inactivation by anti-plasmin. The consequence is clot lysis "from the inside out".

(Occasionally plasminogen activation to plasmin is massive, overpowering anti-plasmin neutralization. The result is circulating plasmin. The consequences of this situation are discussed under disorders of clotting and lysis.)

---

1. _______ is incorporated within a normal clot.	***Plasminogen***
2. Within the clot, plasminogen may be activated to _______.	***plasmin***
3. The presence of plasminogen inside a clot protects plasmin from _______.	***anti-plasmin***

1. VASCULAR INTEGRITY
2. PLATELETS
3. COAGULATION CASCADE
4. CLOT LYSIS

Let us review the mechanisms involved in localization of clotting and lysis.

VASCULAR INTEGRITY

Variation in structural and connective tissue strength of vessels, depending upon the stress these vessels must tolerate.

PLATELETS

1. Platelet structure, function directed to localization of clot formation.
2. Platelets provide rate-limiting factor (PF3) of coagulation cascade.

COAGULATION CASCADE

1. Factors circulate in inactive form in high concentrations. Their activity is localized to areas where available phospholipid is present—(platelet phospholipid and tissue phospholipid).
2. Active factors are diluted by rapid blood flow.
3. Active factors are removed by R-E system.
4. Active factors are neutralized by a circulating protein called antithrombin (AT-3) which becomes more avid in neutralizing active factors when exposed to heparin.

CLOT LYSIS

1. Initiation by Factor XII simultaneously with initiation of coagulation cascade.
2. Rapid neutralization of plasmin by anti-plasmin.
3. Plasminogen is incorporated into clot at the time of clot formation. Thus, when plasminogen is activated to plasmin, inside a fibrin clot, the plasmin is protected from anti-plasmin by the fibrin meshwork.

Let us now turn our attention to evaluation and testing of clotting and lysis.

Chapter 4
COAGULATION TESTING

This chapter is designed to acquaint the reader with the methods currently used in testing hemostasis. It is our intention to have these tests understandable and derivable from the information presented in Basics (Chapter 2). In addition, an understanding of testing will enable the reader to comprehend clearly the details presented in the next chapter on **disorders** of coagulation and lysis.

Two concerns need special emphasis. **First**, the bleeding time is one of the most misunderstood tests. It evaluates platelet function, and is unaffected by deficiencies of the coagulation cascade with one exception, which we will cover in detail in the next chapter. **Second**, for most readers, testing the coagulation cascade is especially confusing. We hope to clarify this area by encouraging you to visualize and use the diagram of the coagulation cascade presented in the Basics Chapter.

1. VASCULAR INTEGRITY
2. PLATELETS
3. COAGULATION CASCADE
4. CLOT LYSIS

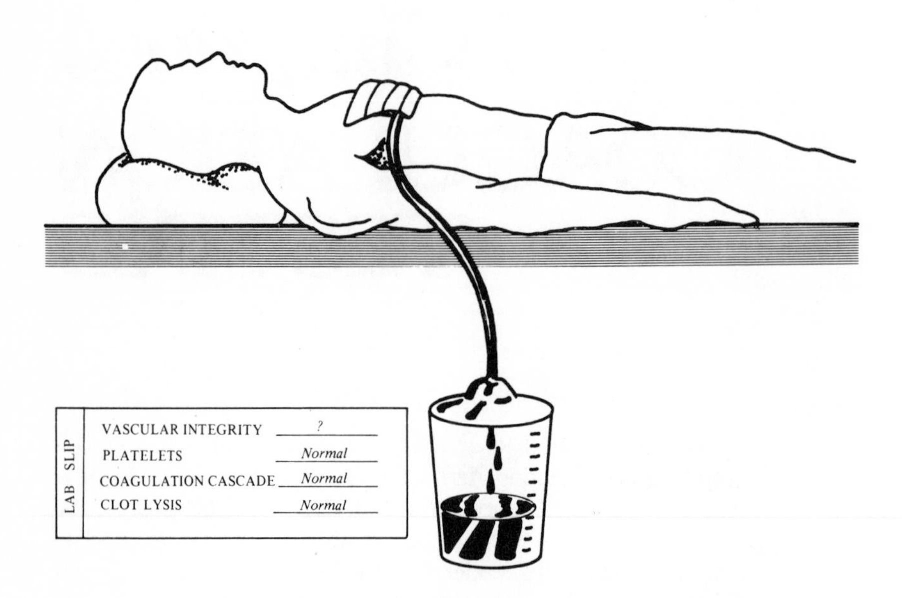

Vascular integrity is tested by visual inspection of a surgical operative field or area of trauma. Other diagnostic procedures may lead to a diagnosis of loss of vascular integrity. Examples of these might be endoscopic examinations, angiography, and computerized axial tomography (CAT scan). At present, vascular defects are not reliably assessed in the laboratory.

By testing the other three components of the hemostatic system (platelets, coagulation cascade, and clot lysis) and finding them to be within the normal range, the diagnosis of loss of vascular integrity becomes the diagnosis by exclusion.

Warning: Professionals often minimize the importance of testing vascular integrity. To diagnose a defect in vascular integrity requires acumen, a high index of suspicion, and proper inspection.

---

1. *Vascular integrity is tested by ____________.* **inspection**
2. *In the postoperative patient, bleeding of large volumes from a surgical site ____________ a loss of vascular integrity.* **suggests**
3. *Testing the other components of the hemostatic mechanism (platelets, coagulation cascade, clot lysis), and finding them normal, suggests a defect in ____________.* **vascular integrity**

1. VASCULAR INTEGRITY
2. PLATELETS
3. COAGULATION CASCADE
4. CLOT LYSIS

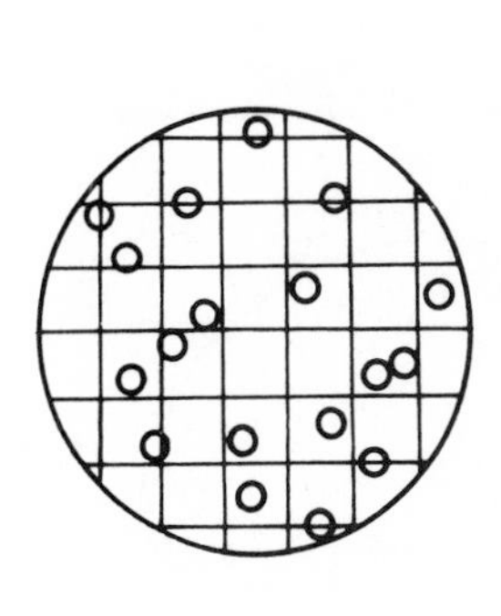

Platelet count 150-350,000

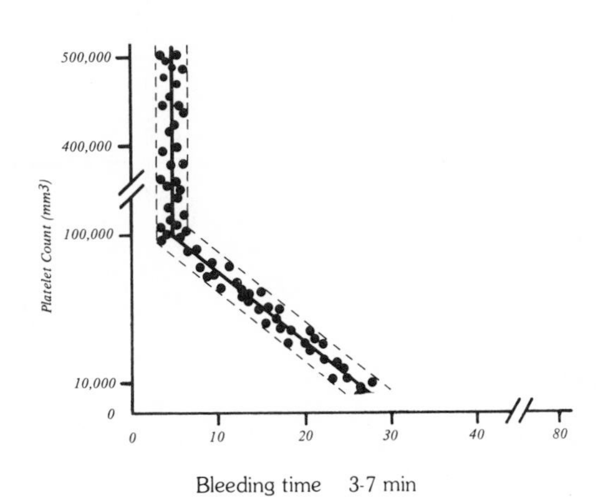

Bleeding time 3-7 min

PLATELET TESTING

The **platelet count** and the **bleeding time** are the mainstays of platelet testing. The platelet count tests only the **quantity** of platelets. The bleeding time tests both quantity and quality of platelets. We will discuss both of these tests in the following pages.

(There are specialized tests of platelet function performed in medical center research laboratories. They are designed primarily to diagnose hereditary defects of platelet function, namely abnormalities of contact, adhesion, spreading, release, and aggregation. These tests require consultation with a hematologist.)

---

1. *The platelet count tests only platelet __________.* ***quantity***
2. *The bleeding time tests the number and the __________ of platelets.* ***quality***
3. *Specialized tests of platelet function require consultation with a __________.* ***hematologist***

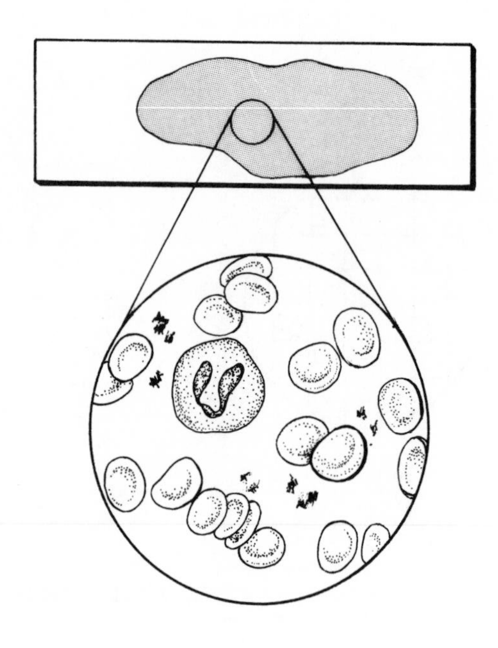

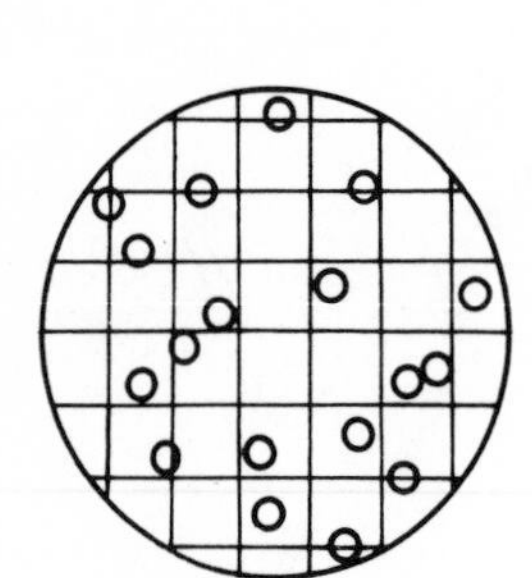

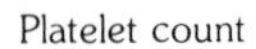

Platelet count

Blood smear

The platelet count is often the screening test used in platelet assessment, though it reveals only platelet quantity and not quality. An estimate of the platelet count can be determined from the blood smear. 10-15 platelets per high power field indicates a platelet count of approximately 150,000-350,000/mm^3, assuming the blood specimen is a representative sample. Precise determination of platelet number is accomplished by phase contrast microscopy hemocytometer counts.

---

1. *A normal value for platelet count is ____________ platelets/mm^3.* — ***150,000-350,000***
2. *A platelet count does **not** test platelet ____________.* — ***quality***
3. *An estimate of the platelet count is available on a ____________.* — ***blood smear***

1. VASCULAR INTEGRITY
2. PLATELETS
3. COAGULATION CASCADE
4. CLOT LYSIS

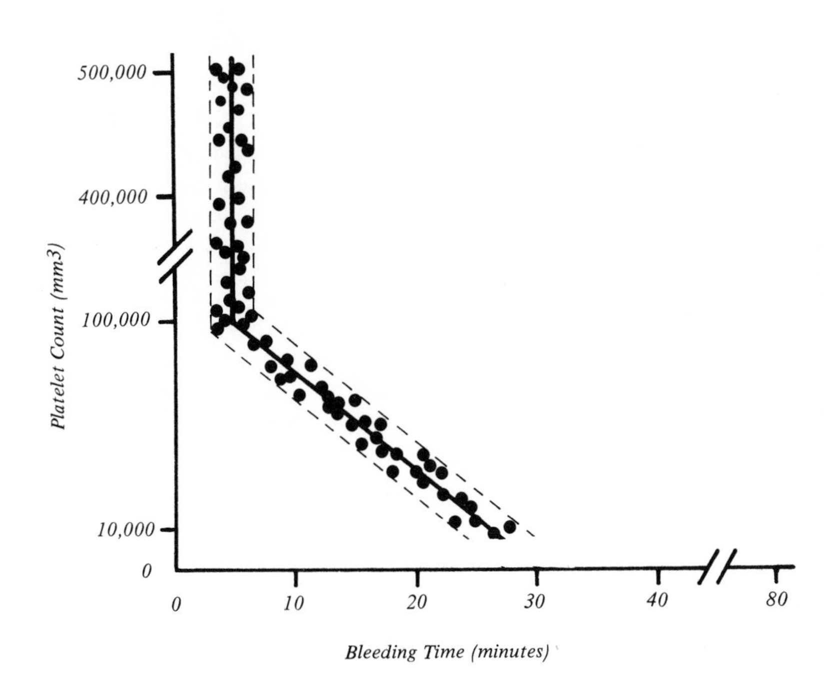

The bleeding time measures both platelet quality and quantity. The bleeding time is normal when platelets are present in a concentration of at least 100,000 platelets/mm^3 and are of normal quality. Between 10,000 platelets/mm^3 and 100,000/mm^3, the bleeding time is linearly related by the equation:

$$\text{Bleeding time (minutes)} = 30.5 - \frac{\text{Platelet Count}}{3{,}850}$$

---

1. *A bleeding time of 4.5 minutes would indicate at least __________ platelets/mm^3.* ***100,000***
2. *A bleeding time of 30.5 minutes would indicate that there are no more than __________ platelets/mm^3 if platelets are qualitatively normal.* ***10,000***
3. *The bleeding time tests both platelet __________ and __________.* ***quality quantity***

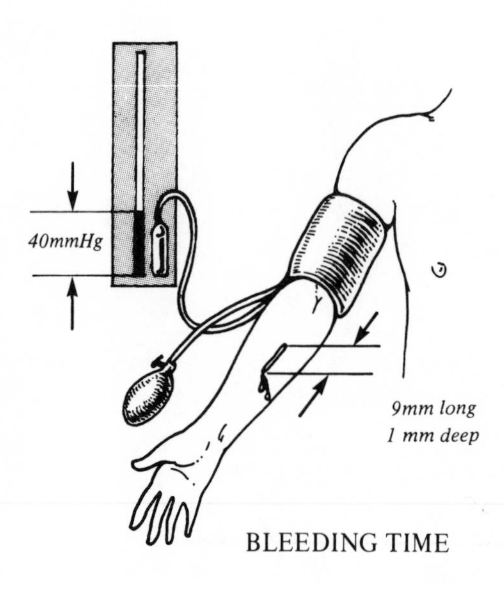

BLEEDING TIME

How is the bleeding time performed? Note that this is **not** an **in vitro** laboratory test; it is performed directly on the patient, **in vivo**, as follows:

A. Blood pressure cuff inflated to 40 mmHg (torr).
B. Standardized incision 1 mm deep, 9 mm long on the flexor aspect of the forearm.
C. Blot every 30 seconds until no serum is blotted.
D. Bleeding time is from incision to absence of serum.
E. Normal value is approximately 4.5 minutes.

1. VASCULAR INTEGRITY
2. PLATELETS
3. COAGULATION CASCADE
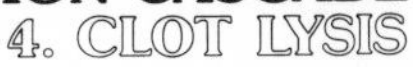
4. CLOT LYSIS

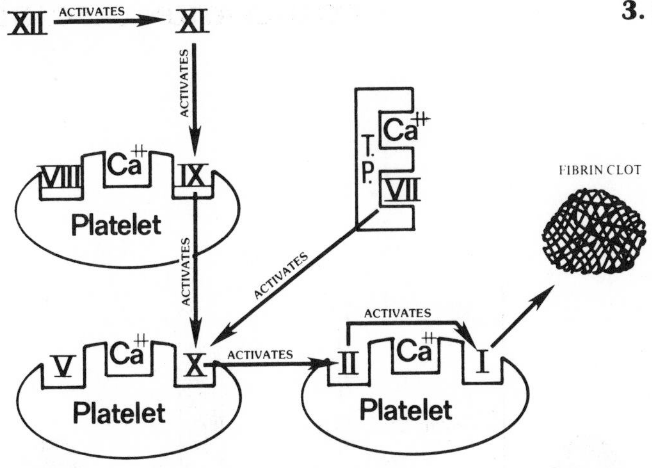

Testing the coagulation cascade is often confusing. We hope to clarify this area by urging you to visualize and use the basic diagram of the coagulation cascade. Three basic points about testing the coagulation cascade must be appreciated:

A. At present, all tests of the coagulation cascade depend on the conversion of fibrinogen (I) to fibrin (Ia), to provide an end-point for the test. The fibrin clot may be examined visually, or detected with the use of photoelectric cells, light beams, magnets, etc. What is important is that the end-product, fibrin, is the end-point of all tests of the coagulation cascade. Thus, a sufficient amount of normal fibrinogen is required to perform any test of the coagulation cascade.

B. All the tests performed in the laboratory have a calcium chelating agent in the collection tube, and are therefore devoid of available calcium (this is done to prevent the specimen from clotting while enroute to the lab). Calcium must be re-added to the plasma to perform many of the tests.

C. Artifacts are easily introduced into the testing system. For example, tissue fluids (phospholipid) may contaminate a specimen during difficult venipuncture. Heparin may contaminate a specimen drawn from an intravascular cannula, if heparin flush systems are employed. Delay in placing the specimen in the appropriate collection tube, inappropriate shaking of the specimen, and personnel technical differences also may influence the testing results.

---

1. *The end-product for all tests evaluating the coagulation cascade is ______________.* — ***fibrin***
2. *Fibrin is produced from ______________.* — ***fibrinogen***
3. *There are ______________ methods for evaluating the formation of the fibrin clot.* — ***many***

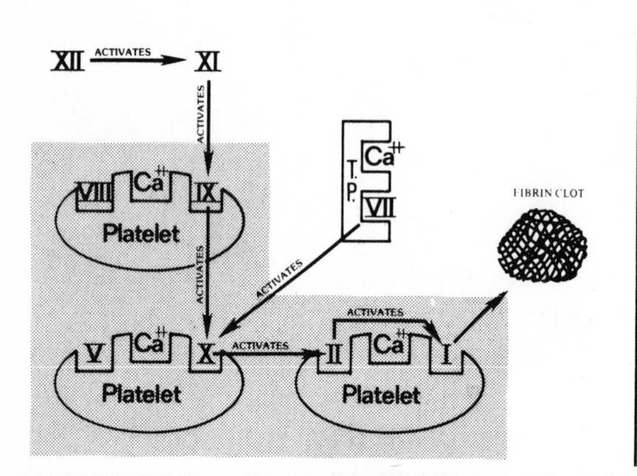

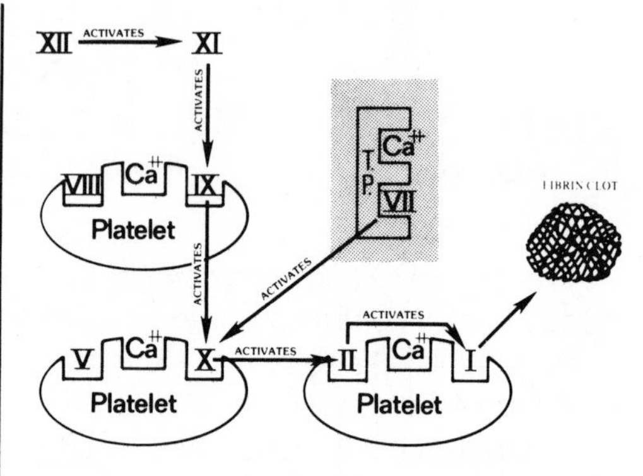

The basic difference between the intrinsic and extrinsic pathways is the phospholipid—the platelet phospholipid vs. the tissue phospholipid. By adding a different phospholipid to different test tubes, we can initiate and test separately the two pathways.

By adding **platelet phospholipid** and Ca^{++}, the long, intrinsic pathway is tested. The most common test for this pathway has a long name—**partial thromboplastin time (PTT)**. If factors XII and XI are surface activated prior to the addition of platelet phospholipid and calcium, the test is called the activated PTT (aPTT).

By adding **tissue phospholipid** and Ca^{++}, the short, extrinsic pathway is tested. The common test for this pathway has a shorter name—**prothrombin time (PT)**.

---

1. The intrinsic pathway is tested by adding _____________ phospholipid. — ***platelet***

2. A common intrinsic pathway test is the _____________. — ***aPTT***

3. The extrinsic pathway is tested by adding _____________ phospholipid. — ***tissue***

4. A common extrinsic pathway test is the _____________. — ***PT***

1. VASCULAR INTEGRITY
2. PLATELETS
3. COAGULATION CASCADE
4. CLOT LYSIS

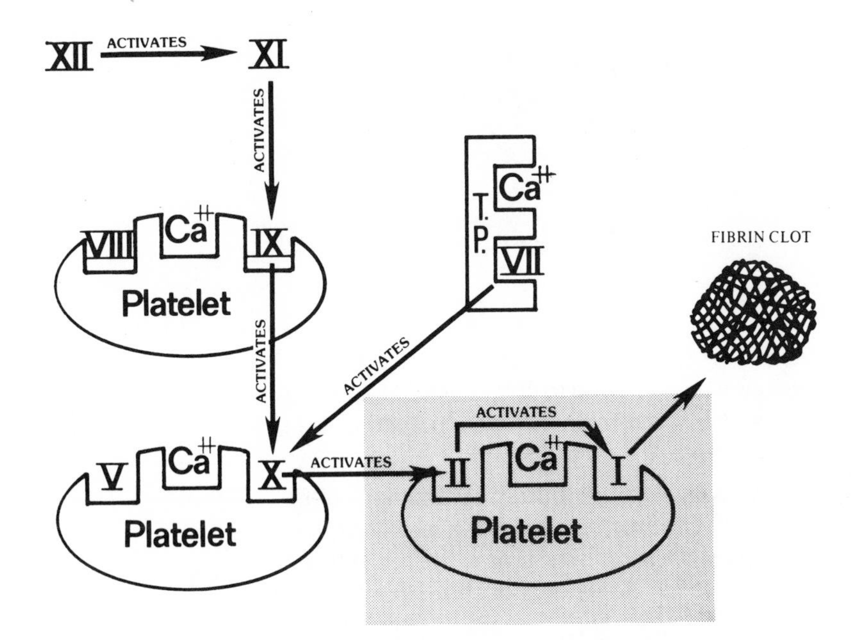

The thrombin time (TT) and fibrinogen determination are performed by adding **activated** factor. **This process bypasses all of the previous steps in the coagulation cascade.** Any of the abnormalities "further back" in the cascade become inconsequential, since the formation of fibrin is "artificially" triggered at the end stage. Thus, an isolated defect of either the intrinsic or extrinsic pathway (such as factor VIII or VII deficiencies respectively) would **not** by tested.

---

1. *The TT and fibrinogen level are different from the aPTT and PT in that ____________ factor is added.* ***activated***
2. *The TT and fibrinogen level ____________ the previous steps in the cascade.* ***bypass***
3. *Steps in the coagulation cascade prior to factor II are ____________ by the TT and fibrinogen level.* ***not tested***

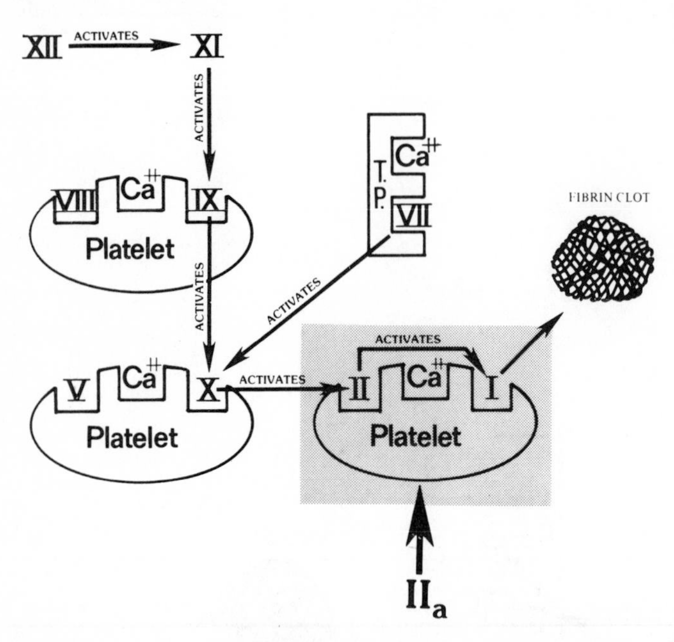

The thrombin time (TT) is performed by adding thrombin (IIa) to the specimen. Fibrinogen will be converted to fibrin unless insufficient or abnormal fibrinogen exists, or thrombin inhibitors (heparin, fibrin split products, etc.) are present.

The fibrinogen determinataion is performed by adding a huge **excess** of thrombin (IIa) to "overpower" any thrombin inhibitors. The more fibrinogen in the sample, the shorter the time to the appearance of a fibrin clot. A standard curve for the amount of fibrinogen present vs. time to appearance of a fibrin clot is performed for comparison. This time will be reduced if the fibrinogen concentration is low or the fibrinogen is an abnormal type.

[There is a modification of the thrombin time, called the Reptilase time (R.T.), which is used to distinguish thrombin inhibitors from abnormalities of fibrinogen. Details are found in the appendix on testing.]

Let us look now at several **representative deficiencies** which could cause abnormalities of each of the tested pathways.

---

1. *The TT measures the conversion of fibrinogen to ______________.* — ***fibrin***
2. *The TT will be abnormal if there are ______________, or a ______________ or ______________ fibrinogen.* — ***thrombin inhibitors***, ***low***, ***abnormal***
3. *The fibrinogen level measures the ______________ of fibrinogen, or presence of abnormal ______________.* — ***quantity***, ***fibrinogen***

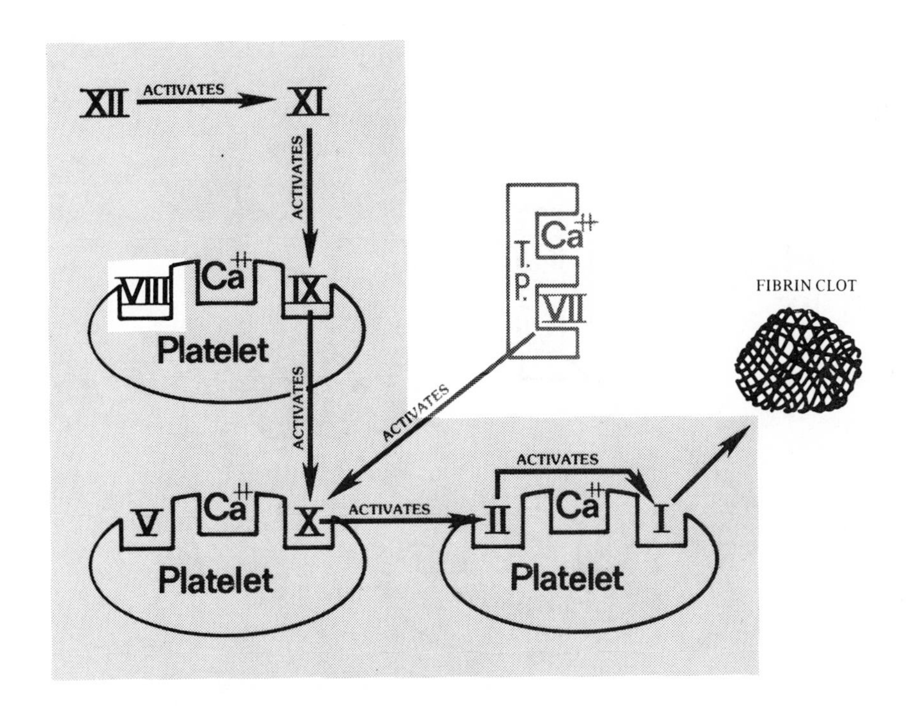

An **isolated deficiency of factor VIII** would result in an:

Abnormal aPTT

Normal PT
TT
Fibrinogen

The **long** intrinsic pathway is tested by the **long** name test, **activated partial thromboplatin time (aPTT).** Factor VIII is in the long, intrinsic pathway, and thus tests of the intrinsic system would show abnormalities. The extrinsic and end stage tests do not contain factor VIII, so their tests (PT, TT, Fibrinogen) would be **normal.**

---

1. An intrinsic test is the ____________. — ***aPTT***

2. A factor VIII deficit would demonstrate an abnormal ____________. — ***aPTT***

3. A factor VIII deficit would show a ____________ PT, TT, and fibrinogen. — ***normal***

1. VASCULAR INTEGRITY
2. PLATELETS
3. COAGULATION CASCADE
4. CLOT LYSIS

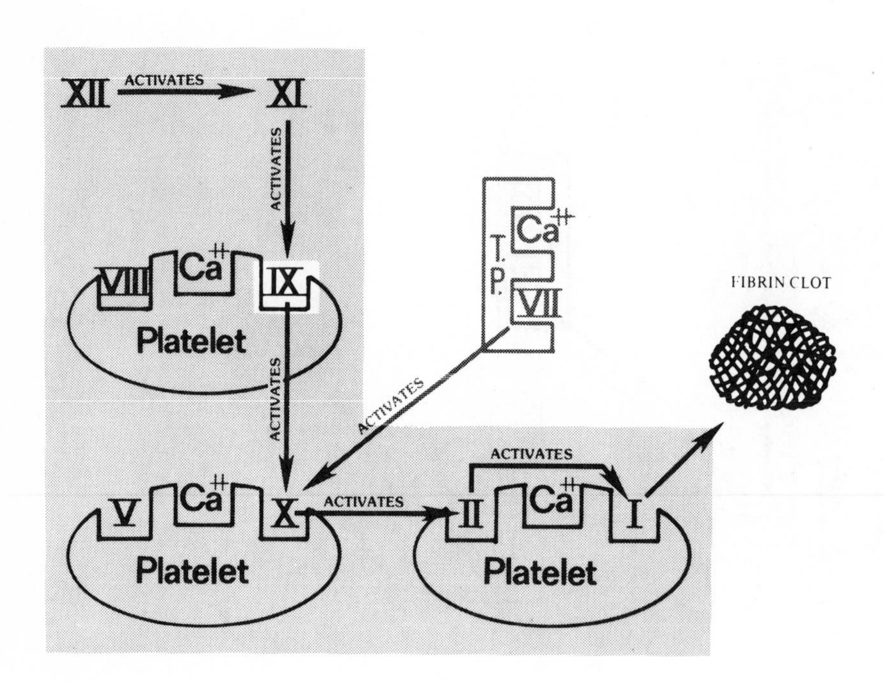

An **isolated deficiency of factor IX** would result in an:

Abnormal aPTT

Normal PT
TT
Fibrinogen

The **long** name test (aPTT) tests the long intrinsic pathway. Factor IX is in the long intrinsic pathway, so the **long**-named test (aPTT) would be abnormal when factor IX is deficient. The extrinsic and endstage tests do not require factor IX to be present, so their tests (PT, TT, fibrinogen) would be **normal**.

---

1. *A factor IX deficit would demonstrate an abnormal ____________.* — ***aPTT***
2. *A factor IX deficit would demonstrate a normal ____________.* — ***PT***
3. *The TT and fibrinogen would be ____________ in a factor IX deficit.* — ***normal***

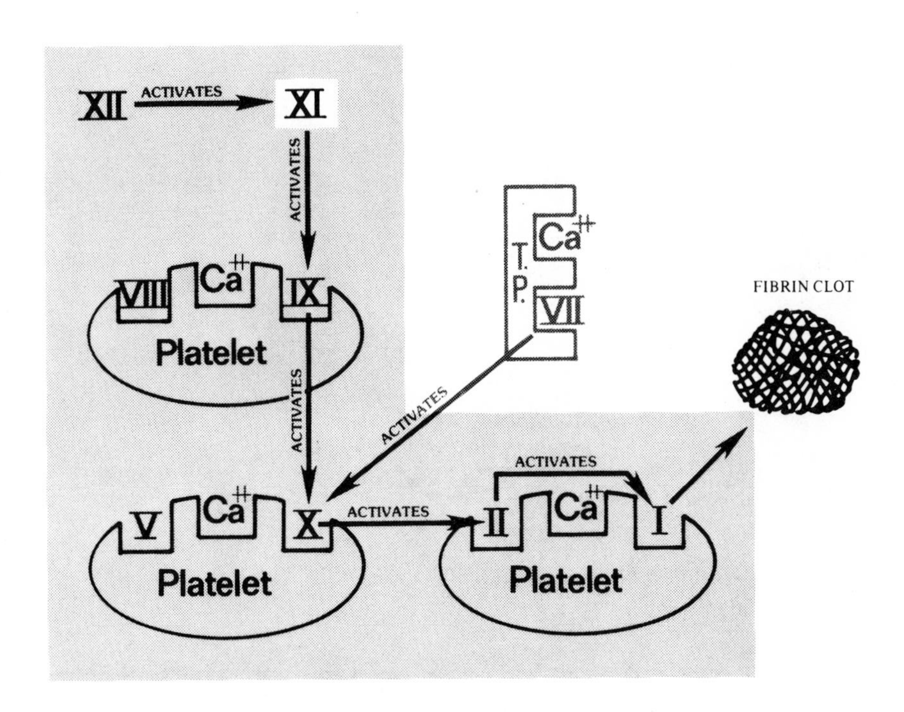

An **isolated deficiency of factor XI** would result in an:

Abnormal aPTT

Normal PT
TT
Fibrinogen

The **long** name test (aPTT) tests the long intrinsic pathway. Factor XI is in the long intrinsic pathway, so the **long**-named test (aPTT) would be abnormal when factor XI is deficient. The extrinsic and endstage tests do not require factor XI to be present, so their tests (PT, TT, fibrinogen) would be **normal**.

---

1. *A factor XI deficit would demonstrate an abnormal ______________.* — ***aPTT***
2. *A factor XI deficit would demonstrate a normal ______________.* — ***PT***
3. *The TT and fibrinogen would be ______________ in a factor XI deficit.* — ***normal***

1. VASCULAR INTEGRITY
2. PLATELETS
3. COAGULATION CASCADE
4. CLOT LYSIS

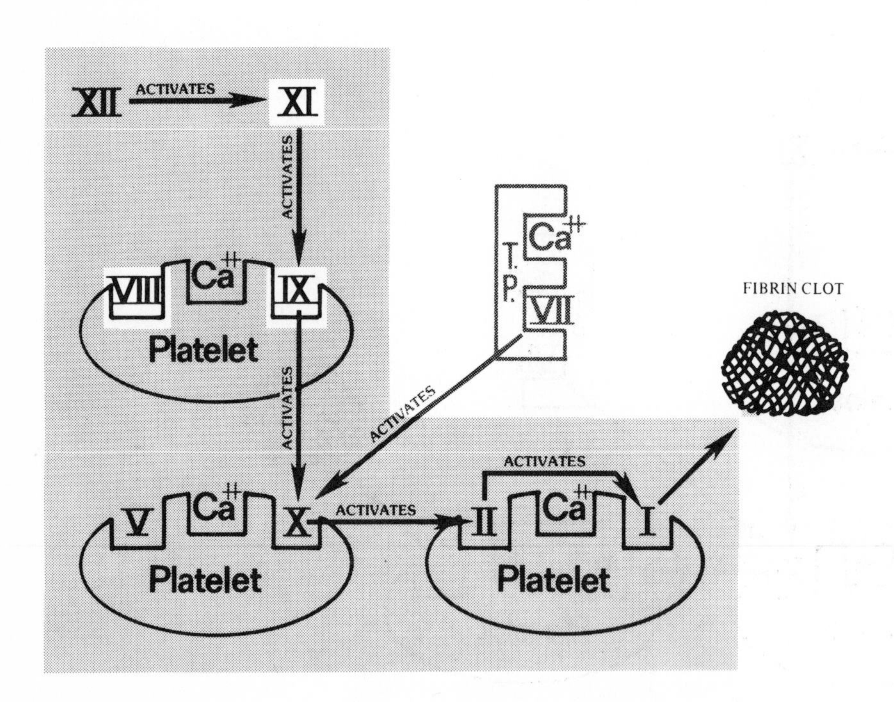

If **isolated** deficiencies of factors VIII, IX, and XI all show the same pattern of testing abnormality, namely an abnormal aPTT with a normal PT, TT, and fibrinogen, how are they differentiated? The aPTT, or other routine tests of the coagulation cascade, will not differentiate them from each other.

They are differentiated by mixing studies. In the laboratory, plasma which is known to be deficient in **each** of these abnormalities can be mixed with the patient's plasma. The plasma which does **not** correct the PTT performed on a mixed specimen, must also be deficient in that factor, and thus identifies the deficient factor. Serially diluted mixing studies are called factor assays, and are used to quantify a factor deficit.

---

1. ______________ separate intrinsic abnormalities from each other.	***Mixing studies***
2. Isolated deficiencies of factors in the intrinsic pathway are ______________ separated by the aPTT.	***not***
3. Isolated deficiencies of factors in the intrinsic pathway will demonstrate a ______________ PT, TT, and fibrinogen.	***normal***

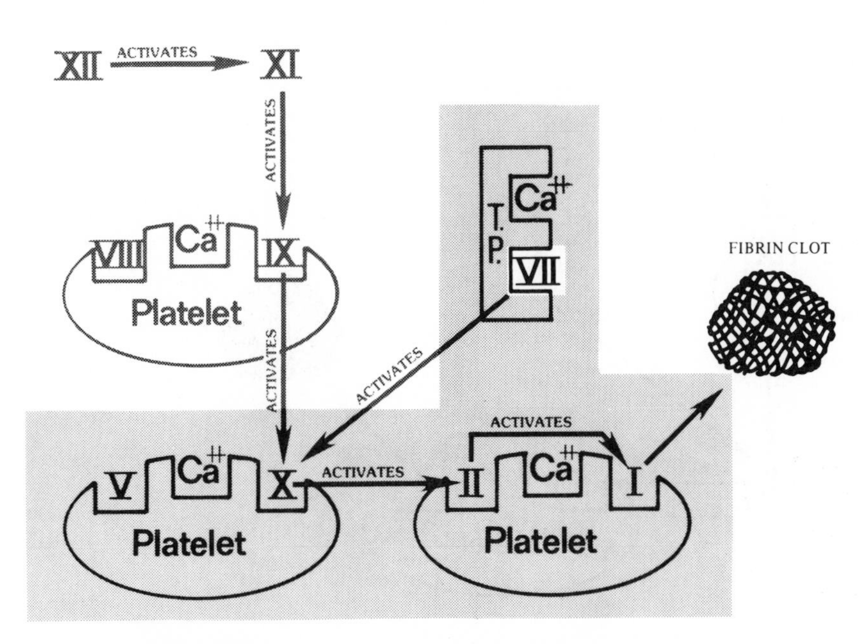

An **isolated deficiency of factor VII** would result in an:

Abnormal PT

Normal aPTT
TT
Fibrinogen

The **short** pathway is tested by the **short** named test—the **prothrombin time (PT)**. Factor VII is contained in the short, extrinsic pathway, thus extrinsic testing with the PT would be abnormal. The intrinsic system tests such as PTT would be normal, since factor VII is not in the intrinsic pathway. In like manner, since factor VII is not in the final common pathway, those tests such as the TT and fibrinogen level also would be **normal**.

(Note: There are modifications of the PT which can assist in discriminating factor VII deficiencies from the action of inhibitors. Please see testing details for the P&P test in the Appendix on testing.)

---

1. *Factor VII deficiency demonstrates an abnormal ____________.* ***PT***

2. *Factor VII deficiency demonstrates a normal ____________.* ***aPTT***

3. *The TT and fribrinogen level are ____________ in a factor VII deficiency.* ***normal***

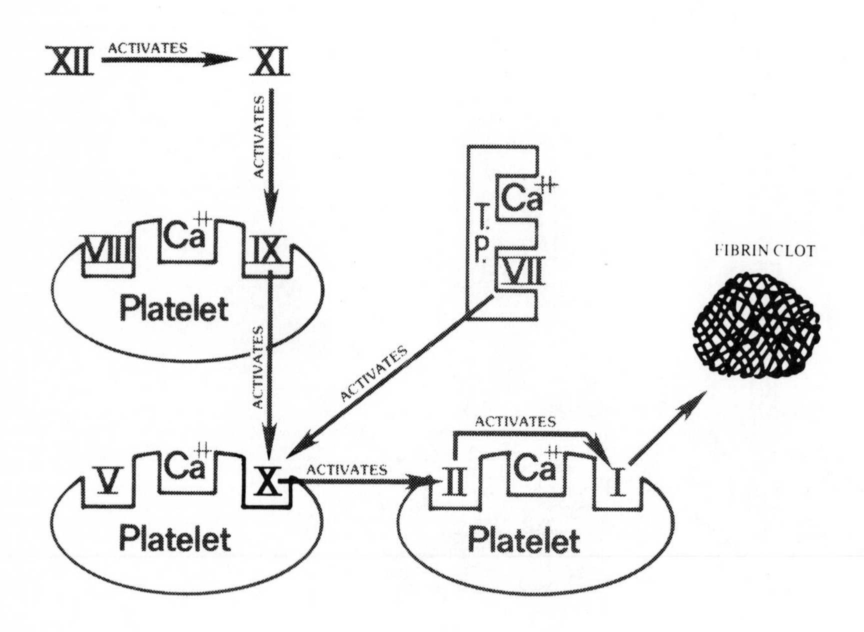

An **isolated deficiency of factor X** would result in an:

Abnormal: aPTT
PT

Normal: TT
Fibrinogen

Factor X is in **both** the **long** (intrinsic) and the **short** (extrinsic) pathways. Both tests thus become abnormal when factor X is deficient.

Since **activated** factor (IIa-thrombin) is added in performing the thrombin time and the fibrinogen determination, the cascade is triggered at a stage past factor X's involvement. So, the TT and fibrinogen would remain **normal** even with **no** factor X present. (An isolated factor X deficiency is rare.)

---

1. *Factor X deficiency demonstrates an abnormal ______ and ______.* — ***aPTT PT***
2. *Factor X deficiency demonstrates a normal ______ and ______.* — ***TT fibrinogen***
3. *The TT and fibrinogen level utilize the ______ factor ______ in performing these tests.* — ***activated thrombin***

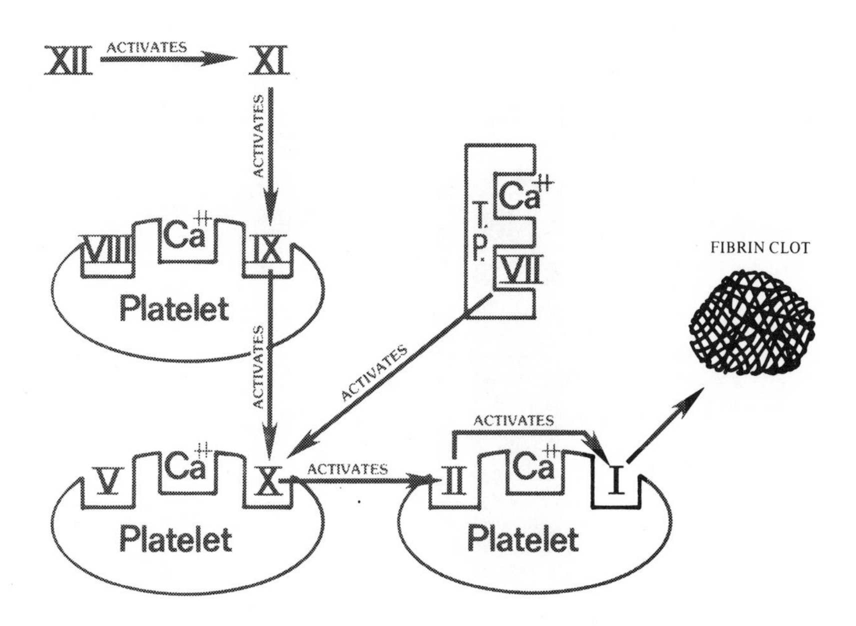

An **isolated deficiency of factor I (fibrinogen)** would result in:

Abnormal: aPTT
PT
TT
Fibrinogen

A decrease in the concentration of factor I (fibrinogen) to less than 100 mg%, results in an abnormal aPTT, PT, TT, and fibrinogen. Conversion of fibrinogen to fibrin is the end-point of all clinical tests of the coagulation cascade. A deficiency of fibrinogen thus results in abnormalities of **all** these coagulation tests.

---

1. *Fibrinogen conversion to fibrin is the ______________ of all tests of the coagulation cascade.* — ***end-point***
2. *A fibrinogen level less than ______________ prolongs all tests of the coagulation cascade.* — ***100 mg%***
3. *The aPTT, PT, TT, and fibrinogen level are all ______________ if factor I is deficient.* — ***abnormal***

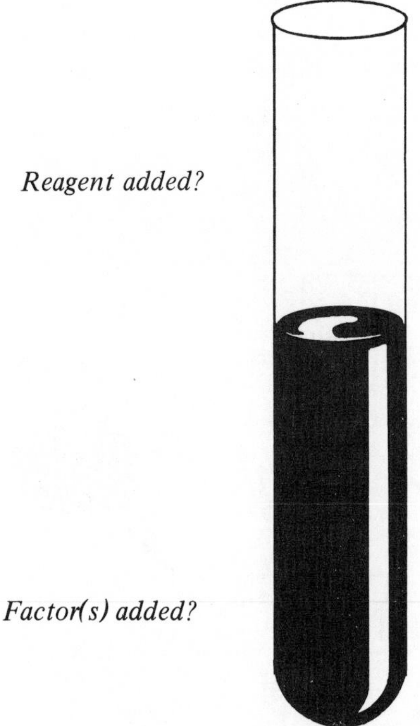

If you use our diagram of the coagulation cascade you should be able to **understand** any coagulation test, and be able to **evaluate** its use in the work-up of a bleeding patient.

The test results should be dissectable and understandable if you keep in mind:

reagents added to the collection tube to prevent clotting enroute to the laboratory (heparin, calcium chelating agents such as EDTA or citrate, etc.),

phospholipids added in the laboratory (platelet, tissue, or none), and

factors added in the laboratory (active or inactive).

The items or agents added during coagulation testing which may determine the test run, or results obtained, include:

1. ______ — ***reagents***

2. ______ — ***phospholipids***

3. ______ — ***factors***

1. VASCULAR INTEGRITY
2. PLATELETS
3. COAGULATION CASCADE
4. CLOT LYSIS

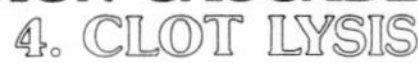

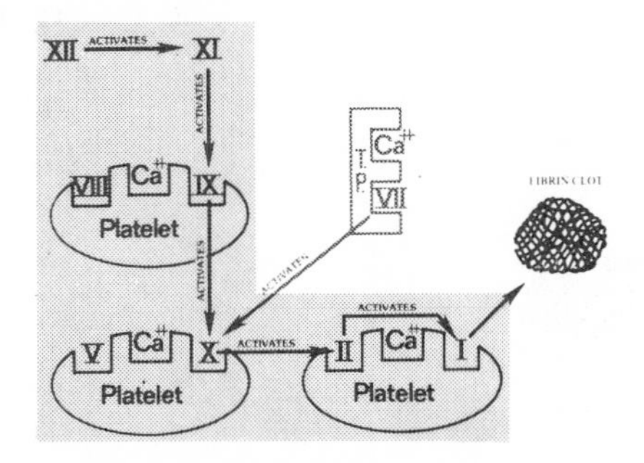

You should be aware that there are many tests of the intrinsic pathway. The variations in the tests which evaluate the long, intrinsic pathway basically involve differences in surface activation. The tests are termed aPTT, WBCT, and ACT.

aPTT (activated partial thromboplastin time)—The plasma is surface activated for 10-15 minutes to maximally activate factors XII and XI, and then the platelet-like phospholipid (PF-3) and Ca^{++} are added. By previously surface activating factors XII and XI, the test becomes more standardized and reproducible.

WBCT (whole blood clotting time, or Lee-White method) uses the glass surface of the test tube to surface-activate platelets and factor XII. Because of the variation in surfaces on different glass test tubes, and the variations in personnel test performance, this test has greatly variable results. The lack of reproducibility makes this test difficult to interpret.

ACT (activated coagulation time) standardizes surface-activation by adding celite (inert diatomaceous earth). The test is reproducible, and measures the same information as the PTT or aPTT. Since the information is readily determined at the bedside, it has become the test of choice in the operating room and many intensive care units.

One caveat in using the WBCT and ACT rather than the aPTT. The patient must have a sufficient number of platelets to supply the phospholipid (PF-3), on which coagulation proteins interact, since PF-3-like material is **not** added to the test tube, as it is in the aPTT.

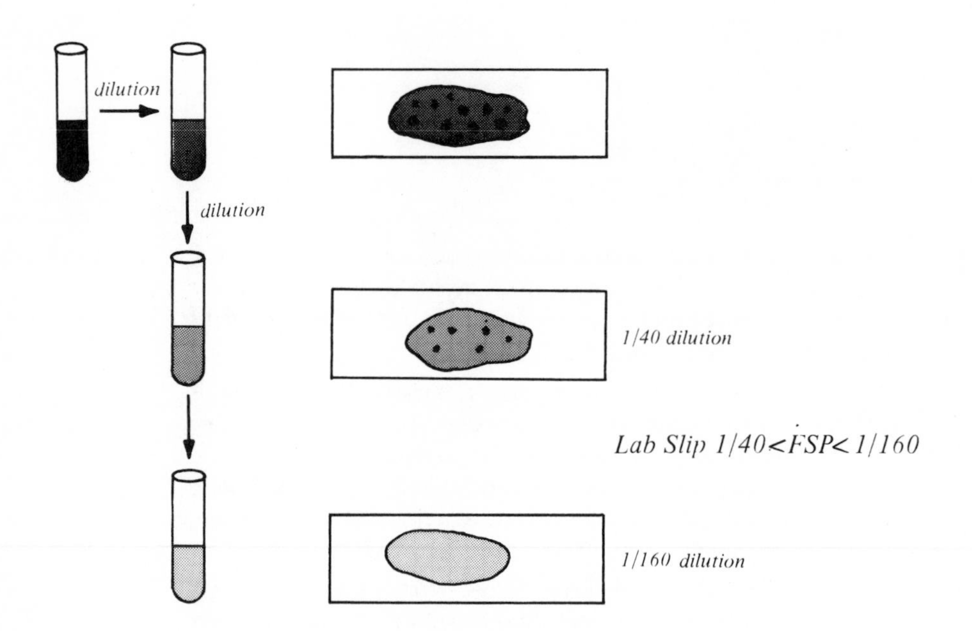

Clot lysis is detected by the presence of fibrin degradation products (fibrin split products, or FSP). The level of degradation products in plasma is quantitatively determined by mixing plasma with antibodies against the degradation products. Serial dilutions of plasma are mixed with the antibodies until **no visible clumping** is seen.

Normally there should be no (or very few) fibrin split products in the plasma. Their presence indicates the clot lysis is proceeding at faster than normal rates. The presence of fibrin split products **alone** does not establish a diagnosis of any particular clinical state. FSP determinations need to be utilized along with other coagulation tests, and analyzed in conjunction with an assessment of the patient's overall clinical state.

(See also the testing Appendix and the chapter on DIC.)

---

1. *Clot lysis is measured by the presence of ________ ________ (FSP).* — ***fibrin split products***

2. *The level of FSP is a balance between ________ and ________ of FSP.* — ***production removal***

3. *The presence of FSP does ________ establish a clinical diagnosis.* — ***not***

1. VASCULAR INTEGRITY
2. PLATELETS
3. COAGULATION CASCADE
4. CLOT LYSIS

Normal Values for Tests

Test	Normal Value
Platelet Count	150,000-350,000/mm^3
Bleeding Time	3-9 minutes
Activated Partial Thromboplastin Time (aPTT)	25-37 seconds
Activated Coagulation Time (ACT)	90-120 seconds (automated)
Prothrombin Time (PT)	Control ± 2 seconds (or >60%)*
Thrombin Time (TT)	Control ± 5 seconds
Fibrinogen Level	150-350 mg%
Fibrin Split Products (FSP)	Negative at greater than 1:4 dilution

These values are published normals (the New England Journal of Medicine 302:44-46, 1980). The reader should contact the local laboratory for normal values. In addition, please see the testing appendix for more details.

*When the PT is reported as a percentage of normal, it is derived by comparing the patient's PT with a standardized curve, produced by performing the PT on a series of dilutions of pooled plasma from normal donors.

1. VASCULAR INTEGRITY
2. PLATELETS
3. COAGULATION CASCADE
4. CLOT LYSIS

SUMMARY OF HEMOSTASIS TESTING

Hemostatic Area		Test	Item(s) Tested
Vascular Integrity		Inspection	Vascular Integrity
Platelets		Platelet count	Platelet number
		Bleeding time	Platelet number and quality
Coagulation Cascade			
	Intrinsic	aPTT ACT WBCT	Deficiencies of, or inhibitors of: XII, XI IX, VIII X, V II, I
	Extrinsic	PT	Deficiencies of, or inhibitors of: VII, X, V, II, I
	End-stage	TT	Deficiencies of, or inhibitors of: IIa, I
		Fibrinogen level	Deficiencies of, or abnormalities of: I
Clot Lysis		fibrin split products	Degradation Products of fibrin and fibrinogen

The fine points of using these coagulation tests will be developed further in the chapters to follow.

Chapter 5
DISORDERS OF COAGULATION

Disorders of hemostasis can result in either bleeding or thrombosis. In this chapter we will discuss those disorders which cause bleeding. Disorders causing thrombosis will be covered in chapter 9. However the major side-effect of drugs used to treat or prevent thrombosis is bleeding, we will discuss these drugs in this chapter.

1. VASCULAR INTEGRITY
2. PLATELETS
3. COAGULATION CASCADE
4. CLOT LYSIS

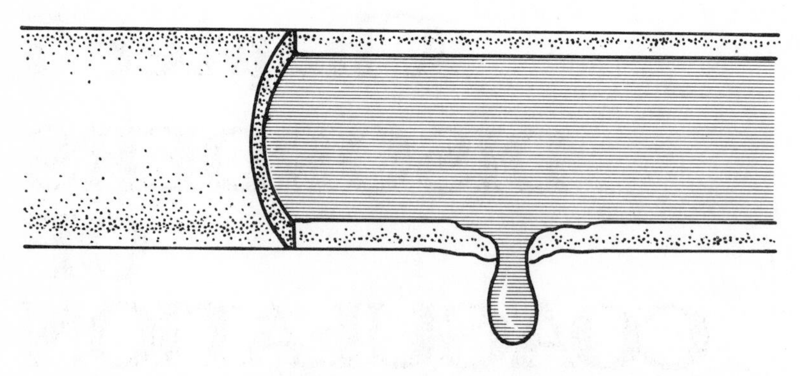

Normal vessel

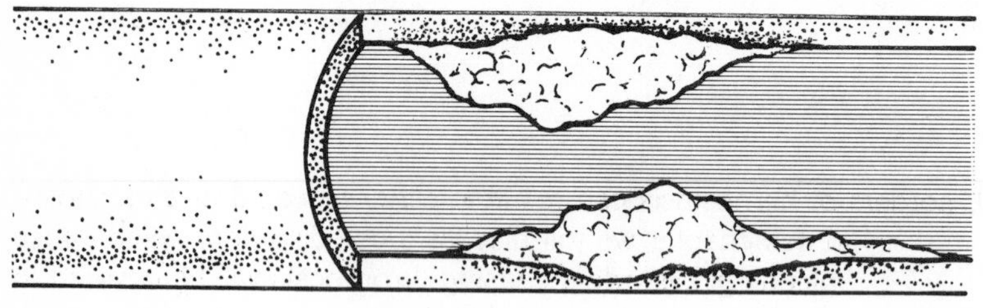

Abnormal vessel

Disorders of vascular integrity, can be divided conceptually into two categories:

- Normal vessels subjected to trauma—surgical or otherwise.
- Abnormal vessels—e.g., atherosclerosis
  cystic medial necrosis
  systemic steroid therapy
  vitamin C deficiency
  Marfan's syndrome
  Ealos-Danlos syndrome
  Osler-Weber-Rendue syndrome
  Inflammatory and immune-mediated vascular injury

---

1. *Normal vessels subjected to surgical trauma can ______________ despite normal platelets and coagulation cascade.* — ***bleed***
2. *Abnormal vessels can ______________ despite normal platelets and coagulation cascade.* — ***bleed***

1. VASCULAR INTEGRITY
2. PLATELETS
3. COAGULATION CASCADE
4. CLOT LYSIS

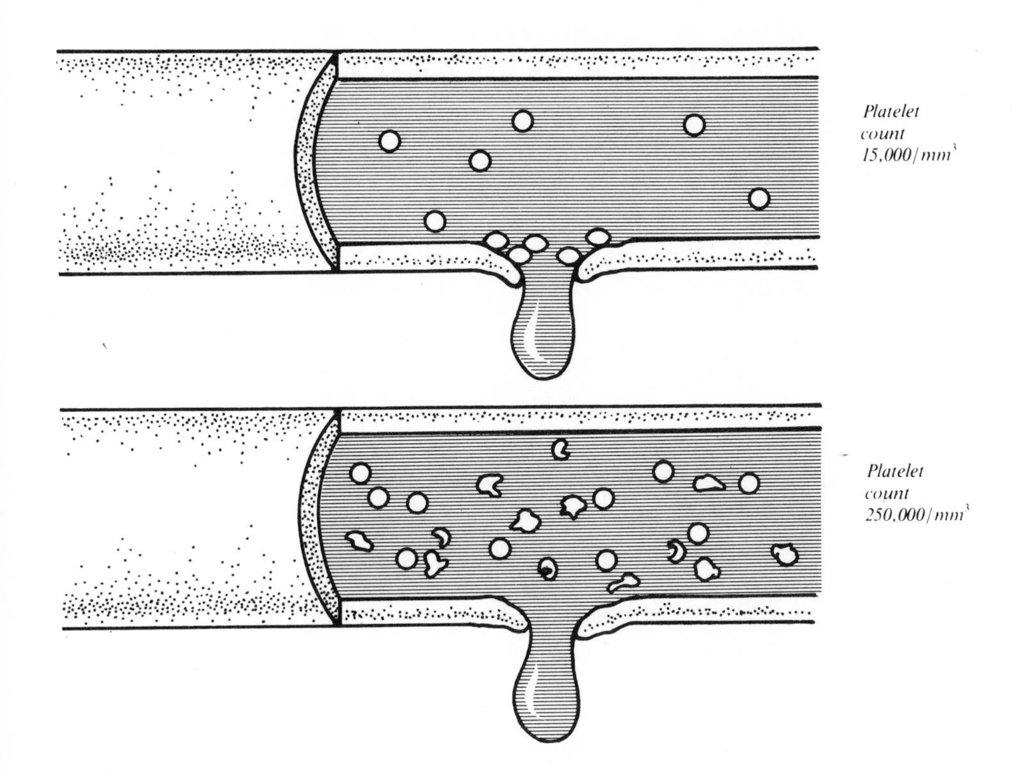

Platelets are the second component of hemostasis. Quantitative or qualitative platelet deficiencies, or both, can cause bleeding.

---

1. *Quantitative platelet disorders imply an inadequate ______________ of platelets.* — ***number***
2. *Qualitative platelet disorders imply an inadequate ______________ of platelets.* — ***function***
3. *Quantitative and qualitative disorders may occur ______________.* — ***simultaneously***

1. VASCULAR INTEGRITY
2. PLATELETS
3. COAGULATION CASCADE
4. CLOT LYSIS

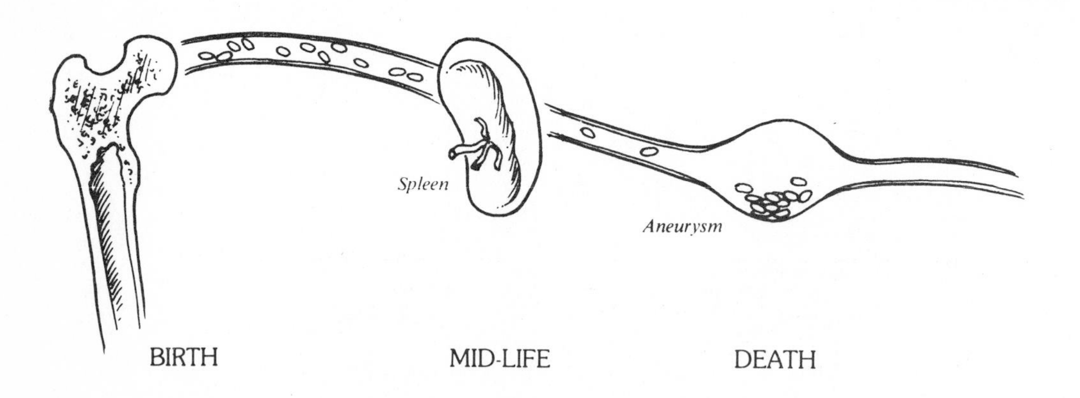

Categorizing the various quantitative platelet disorders (inadequate number of platelets) is easy, by imagining the dangers a platelet faces during its normal life cycle.

Birth: Production deficiency
Mid-life: Abnormal sequestration
Death: Destruction or removal

Platelet production is decreased if the bone marrow is infiltrated with tumor or has been destroyed by radiation or drugs. Congenital platelet production deficiency is seen rarely.

Excessive platelet sequestration is seen in hypersplenism, secondary to various etiologies. The number of circulating platelets usually increases after removal of the enlarged spleen.

Platelet destruction and removal is seen both on an immunologic and a non-immunologic basis. Immune destruction of platelets by antibodies directed against platelets is seen after multiple platelet transfusions. Immune destruction can be idiopathic, and is then termed idiopathic thrombocytopenia purpura (ITP). Non-immunologic removal of platelets occurs because of massive platelet consumption in DIC, or because of platelet washout during massive tıansfusions with platelet-poor banked blood or crystalloid. (After 24 hours bank blood is devoid of functioning platelets. A 15 unit blood transfusion will effectivetly reduce the platelet number to critical levels.)

---

1. Platelet production defects cause an inadequate ______________ of platelets to be produced. **number**

2. Sequestration of platelets by large spleens causes an inadequate ______________ of circulating platelets. **number**

3. Platelet removal by the immune system or during massive transfusions cause an inadequate ______________ of circulating platelets. **number**

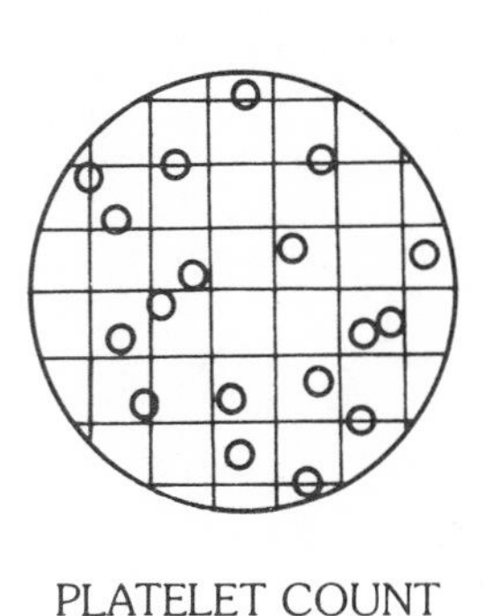

PLATELET COUNT

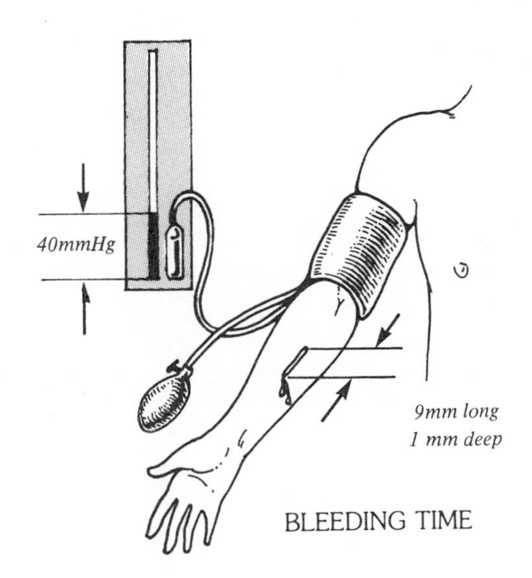

BLEEDING TIME

Qualitative platelet disorders (poor function despite adequate number) are diagnosed by comparing a bleeding time with a simultaneously drawn platelet count. A comparison of the bleeding time and platelet count will readily demonstrate whether the platelets "fit" the expected relationship. If not, they are not functioning normally.

If platelet malfunction is suspected and the platelet count is greater than 100,000, a bleeding time should be ordered. Platelet malfunction is produced by:

- Congenital lesions of platelet mechanics
- Drugs:
  - ASA
  - Dextran
  - Aminoglycosides
  - Protamine
  - Nitroprusside
- Storage of platelets
- Uremic plasma
- Fibrin split products
- Cirrhotic liver disease

---

1. Platelet dysfunction is termed a ______ platelet disorder.	***qualitative***
*2. The **sine quo non** of diagnosing a qualitative platelet defect is the ______.*	***bleeding time***
3. Many ______ produce platelet dysfunction.	***drugs***

1. VASCULAR INTEGRITY
2. PLATELETS
3. COAGULATION CASCADE
4. CLOT LYSIS

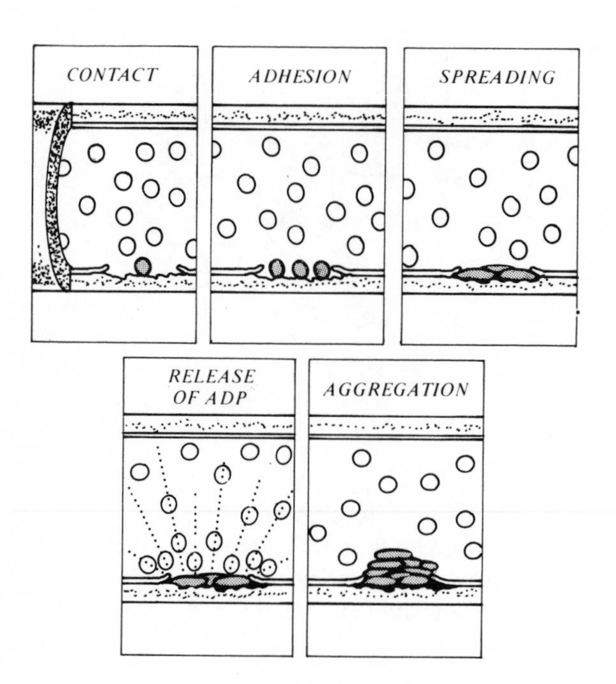

The mechanism of platelet disorders due to congenital lesions follows the five steps in platelet mechanics. Therefore, there are congenital lesions defined for:

platelet contact
platelet adhesion
platelet spreading
platelet release
platelet aggregation

Only highly specialized studies can define the exact location of the platelet defect. However an abnormal bleeding time without thrombocytopenia is still the **sine quo non** for establishing the initial diagnosis of platelet dysfunction.

---

1. *Congenital platelet disorders occur in each of the sequential __________ of platelet mechanics.* — ***five steps***
2. *Establishing that a congenital bleeding disorder is due to platelet dysfunction requires an abnormal __________, and a normal platelet count.* — ***bleeding time***

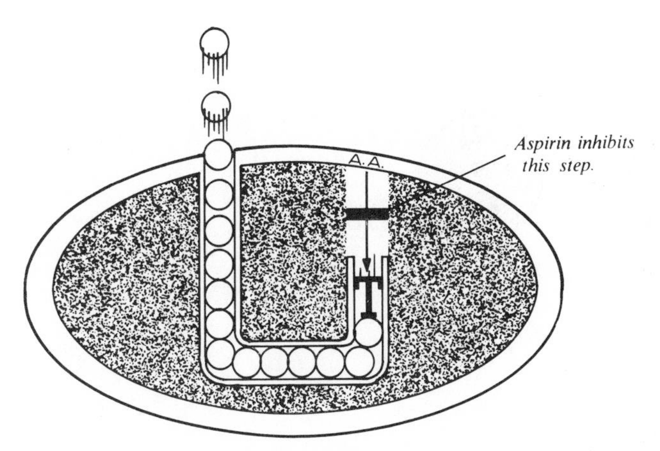

Thromboxane is synthesized by arachidonic acid(AA) in activated platelet cell membrane.

The mechanism of platelet dysfunction after ingestion of aspirin (ASA) is the inhibition of prostaglandin synthesis. The major prostaglandin produced in the platelet is thromboxane A_2, which evokes ADP release and platelet aggregation.

Platelets "poisoned" by ASA do not aggregate properly because of an inability to synthesize thromboxane A_2. As with other qualitative defects of platelets, the defect is demonstrated clinically by a prolonged bleeding time in the presence of an adequate number of circulating platelets. ASA "poisoned" platelets, while unable to release ADP themselves, are able to help form a platelet plug, if non-ASA "poisoned" platelets are present to release ADP to signal platelet aggregation. Transfusion of two units of normal platelets is sufficient to initiate platelet plug formation and result in enough ADP release to signal ASA "poisoned" platelets to help continue plug formation.

Since the normal daily production of platelets is approximately 10% of the total body pool of platelets, and the plasma half-life of ASA is only 30 minutes, platelet function will usually normalize within several days after discontinuing ASA.

(Note: If a patient is actively bleeding with ASA "poisoned" platelets, more than two units of platelets may be necessary, because the transfused units may be **consumed** rapidly in the bleeding patient.)

---

1. *Aspirin inhibits ______________ synthesis.* — ***prostaglandin***
2. *Aspirin treated platelets cannot synthesize ______________.* — ***thromboxane*** A_2
3. *Aspirin treated platelets thus cannot release ______________.* — ***ADP***

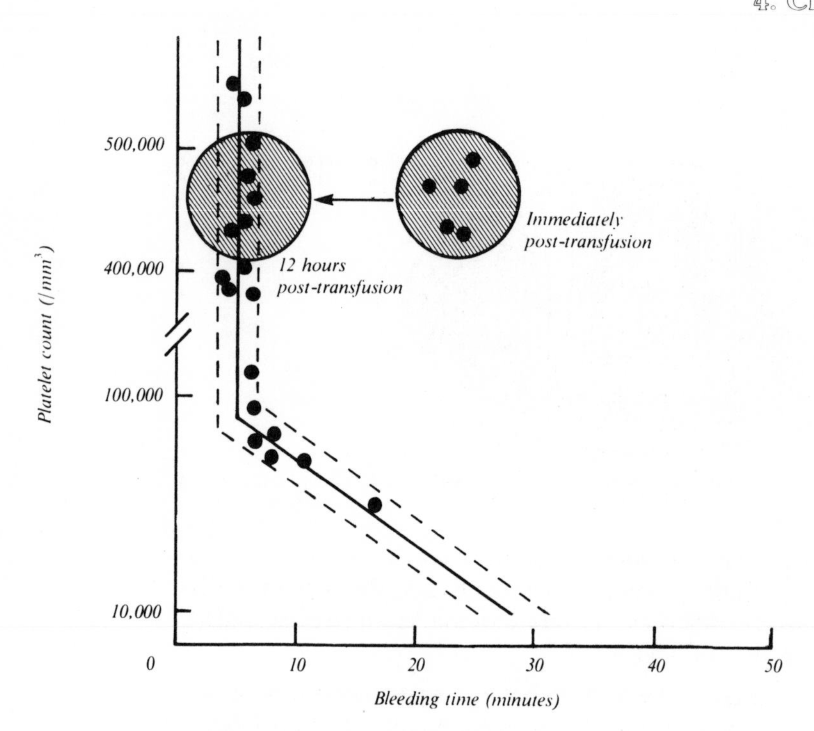

The mechanism of platelet dysfunction after storage of platelets is due to a depletion of energy stores, specifically ATP. This reduces the rate of production of ADP for platelet aggregation until the platelets circulate long enough to replete their energy stores.

Therefore, transfused platelets have a storage defect which develops during storage greater than four hours. This defect is characterized by the bleeding time not being fully corrected immediately after an apparently adequate transfusion of platelets. The storage defect affects the platelets for 8-20 hours post-transfusion. A comparison of the bleeding time and platelet count will demonstrate readily whether the platelets "fit" the expected relationship. When the platelet count and the bleeding time correlate, the storage defect has been corrected.

---

1. *Platelets used in transfusions have a ______________ defect.*	***storage***
2. *It takes ______________ hours for transfused platelets to function normally.*	***8-20***
3. *The storage defect is detected by comparing the ______________ and the ______________.*	***bleeding time*** ***platelet count***

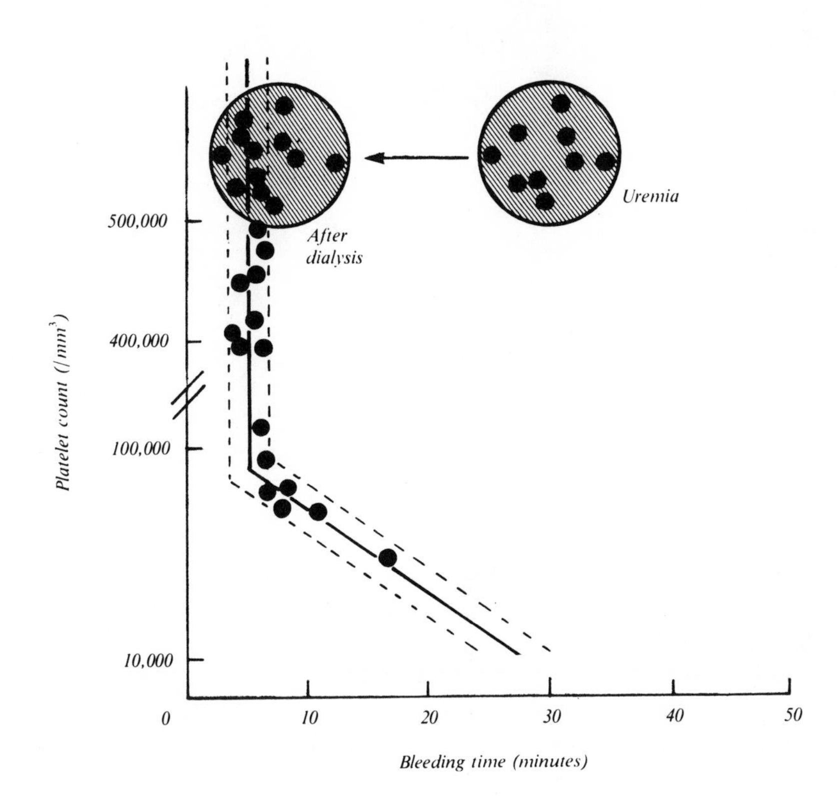

The mechanism of platelet dysfunction when platelets are exposed to uremic plasma is not fully understood, but it is known that the chemical(s) causing the dysfunction is (are) dialyzable. Oxalo-succinic acid may be the chemical responsible.

Hemodialysis returns platelet function, and thus the bleeding time, towards normal.

---

1. *The chemical causing platelet dysfunction in a uremic patient may be ______________.* **oxalo-succinic acid**
2. *Platelet dysfunction caused by uremia is corrected by ______________.* **dialysis**
3. *The bleeding time in a uremic patient normalizes after ______________.* **dialysis**

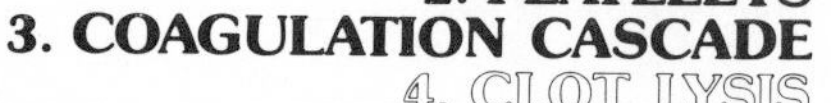

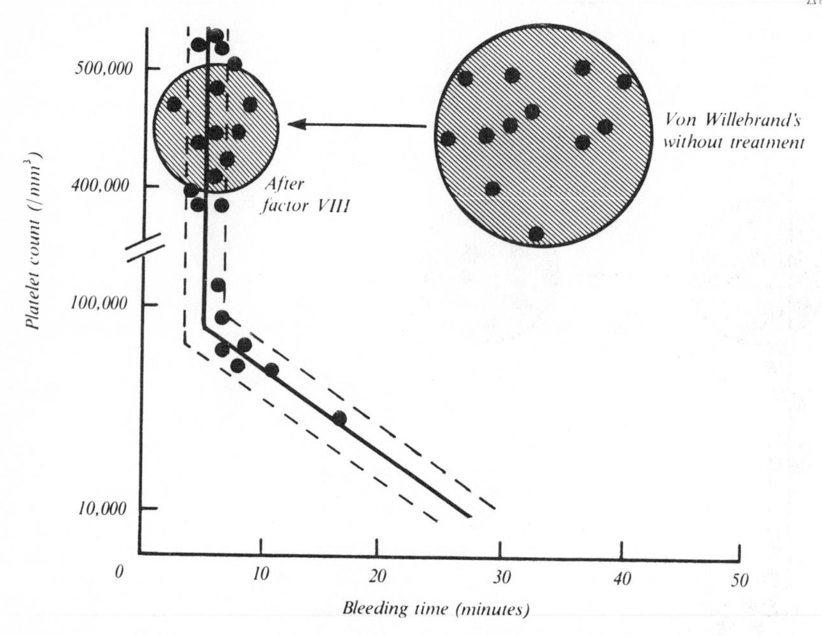

The mechanism of platelet dysfunction in Von Willebrand's disease is a deficiency of factor VIII. Von Willebrand's disease is unique in that platelet dysfunction is due to a coagulation factor deficiency. Therefore it is placed appropriately in this text at the junction between disorders of platelets and disorders of the coagulation cascade.

Von Willebrand's disease is probably the most common congenital disorder of the hemostatic system, with an incidence greater than classic hemophilia. It is characterized by:

- prolonged bleeding time despite an adequate number of platelets;
- correction of bleeding time and clinical bleeding by administration of factor VIII (Cryoprecipitate or FFP);
- factor VIII **activity is low,** but factor VIII related **antigen** is markedly diminished or absent.

The relationship between **factor VIII activity** and **factor VIII antigen** is not fully understood.

---

1. *Von Willebrand's disease is characterized by a prolonged ______________.* — ***bleeding time***
2. *The platelet defect in Von Willebrand's disease is corrected by transfusion of ______________.* — ***factor VIII***
3. *Factor VIII has two biological components, factor VIII activity and factor VIII related ______________.* — ***antigen***

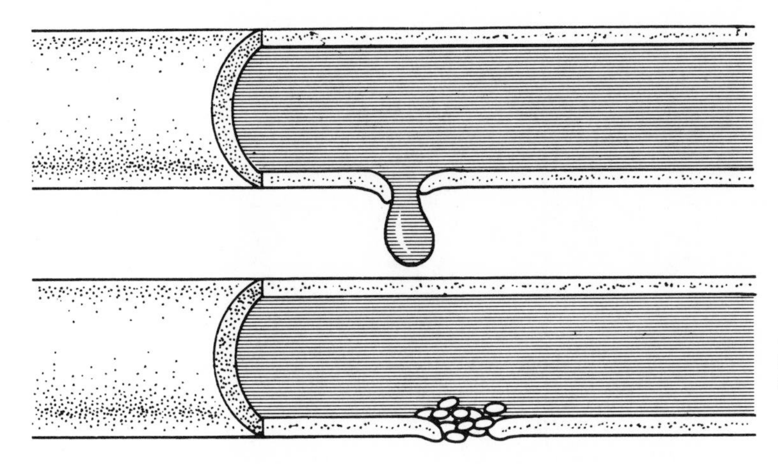

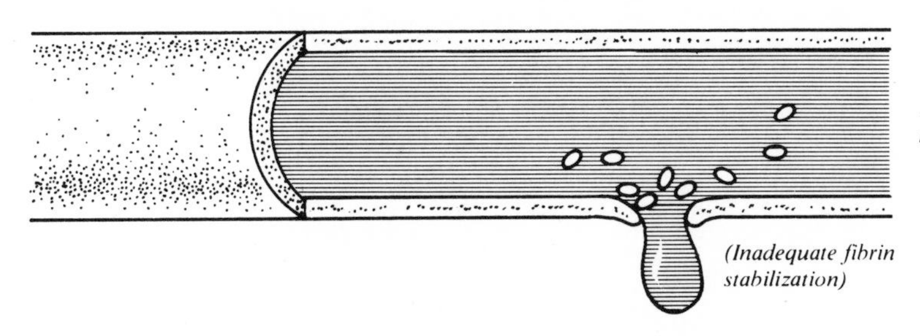

Disorders of the coagulation cascade present with a unique clinical picture. Vascular injury always precedes bleeding. The bleeding from the injury stops initially (assuming platelet function is normal). However, within several hours, bleeding starts again, because of inadequate fibrin stabilization of the platelet plug. Disorders of the coagulation cascade display abnormalities in the screening tests of the intrinsic and extrinsic pathways, namely the aPTT and PT, as previously presented.

The bleeding time, however, is usually normal, since it tests platelet plug formation and not fibrin stabilization of the platelet plug.

---

1. *Disorders of the coagulation cascade result in inadequate ______________ stabilization of the platelet plug.* — ***fibrin***
2. *The screening tests of the coagulation cascade are the ______________ and ______________.* — ***aPTT, PT***
3. *Disorders of the coagulation cascade do not usually prolong the ______________.* — ***bleeding time***

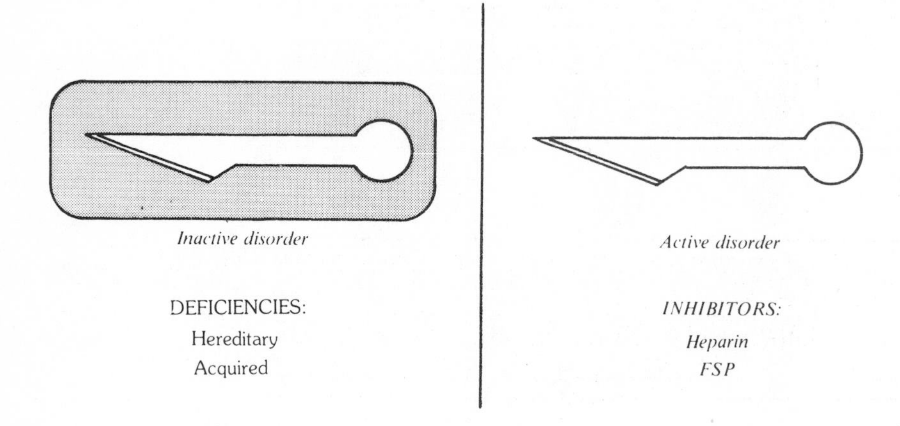

DEFICIENCIES:
Hereditary
Acquired

INHIBITORS:
Heparin
FSP

Disorders of the coagulation cascade can be divided into two categories for therapeutic decision:

Disorders of inactive factors
Disorders of active factors

We have categorized these disorders for ease of understanding and continuity, and will approach them in the following order:

- Inactive factor disorders:
  - Hereditary disorders
  - Acquired disorders
    - Antibodies
    - Production decreased—hepatic disease
      —vitamin K deficiency
    - Consumption/Dilution
- Active factor disorders:
  - Inhibition by heparin
  - Inhibition by fibrin split products

Let us begin with inactive factor deficiencies.

---

1. *Disorders of the coagulation cascade can be divided into disorders of ________ factors, and disorders of ________ factors.* — ***inactive***, ***active***
2. *Inactive factor deficiencies are further divided into hereditary disorders and ________ disorders.* — ***acquired***
3. *Active factor disorders are due to inhibition of active factors by ________ or ________.* — ***heparin, FSP***

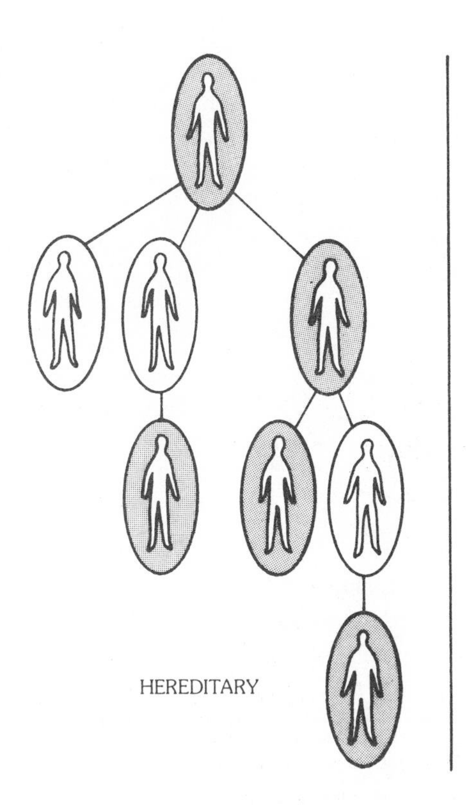

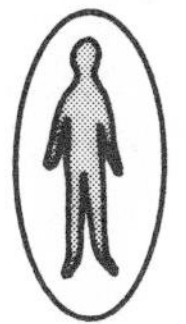

ACQUIRED

We have divided inactive factor deficiencies into two categories: hereditary disorders and acquired disorders.

The two categories are contrasted below.

Hereditary	**Acquired**
Single factors involved	Multiple factors involved
Rare	Common
Life long history	Sudden onset of bleeding

---

1. *Inactive factor deficiencies are either ______________ or ______________.* — ***hereditary*** ***acquired***
2. *Hereditary inactive factor deficiencies usually involve a ______________ factor.* — ***single***
3. *Acquired inactive factor deficiencies usually involve ______________ factors.* — ***multiple***

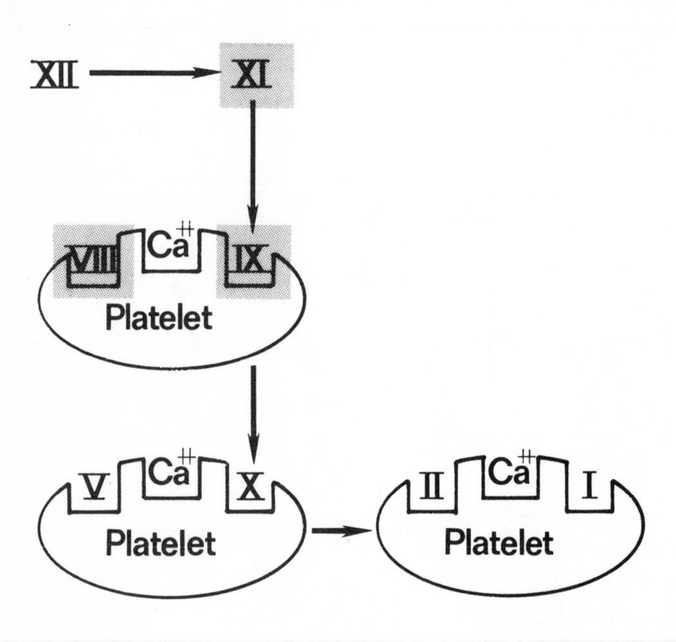

Disease	Factor Deficiency	Incidence
Hemophilia A	Factor VIII	1/25,000
Hemophilia B	Factor IX	1/100,000
Hemophilia C	Factor XI	1/1,000,000

A hereditary deficiency of each factor has been described. The three most common are termed Hemophilia A, B, and C represented by low concentrations of Factor VIII, IX, and XI, respectively. We will cover Hemophilia A (Factor VIII deficiency) in some detail in the next few pages. The other factor deficiencies resemble Factor VIII deficiency by having practically identical manifestations. In addition, they cannot be differentiated by the standard laboratory tests. However, differentiation of the three most common factor deficiencies (VIII, IX, and XI) can be accomplished by specific factor assays that are available in special laboratories at medical centers. The differentiation is therapeutically crucial and justifies the expense and expertise of special factor studies, when standard coagulation studies demonstrate a severe abnormality. These studies require consultation with a hematologist.

---

1. *Hemophilia A, B, and C all demonstrate __________ clinical manifestations.* — ***similar***
2. *Standard coagulation tests __________ the three hemophilias from each other.* — ***cannot differentiate***
3. *The hemophilias are diagnosed specifically by __________ __________.* — ***factor assays***

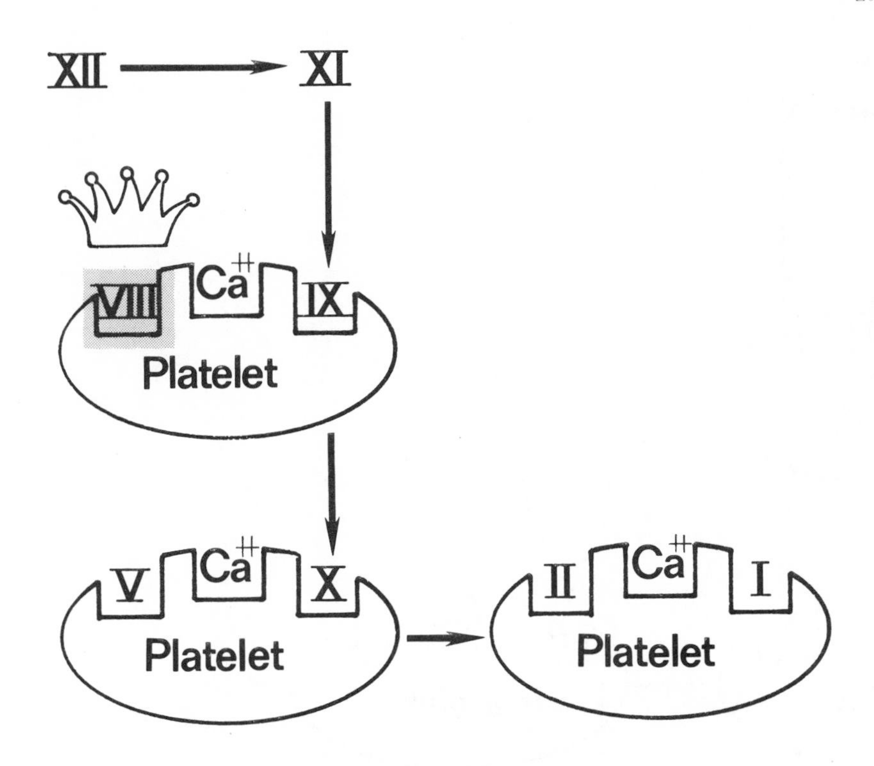

The most common and important hereditary factor deficiency is in Factor VIII activity (Hemophilia A), a sex linked abnormality. This deficiency was made famous by its not uncommon appearance in several European royal families, after much inbreeding. The severity of the bleeding disorder is related to the plasma concentration of Factor VIII activity.

Factor VIII Activity % Normal	Type of Bleeding
50-100	None
25-50	Tendency to bleed after major trauma
5-25	Severe bleeding after surgical operations and some bleeding after minor trauma
1-5	Severe bleeding after minor injury Occasional spontaneous hemorrhages
1	Severe crippling hemophilia with spontaneous bleeding into joints or muscles

(Specific treatment of Factor VIII deficiency is found in the chapter on treatment.)

(Biggs, pg 238, table 21.)

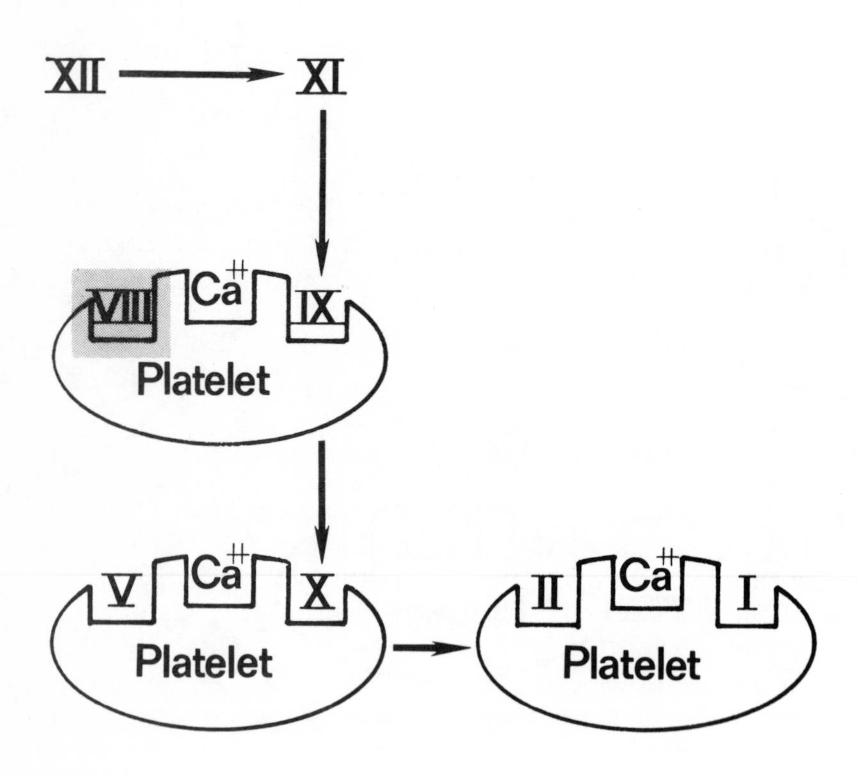

The transition in this text from hereditary to acquired inactive factor deficiencies is facilitated by the disorder induced by antibodies against inactive factors. While the disorder caused by antibodies against inactive factors is an acquired disorder it is similar clinically to the hereditary factor deficiency of the same factor, except in its age of onset.

For example, the clinical disorder induced by antibodies against Factor VIII is identical to that of hereditary deficiency of Factor VIII, the only difference being that of the age of onset. With the hereditary deficiency of Factor VIII, the bleeding disorder is life-long. In contrast, antibodies against Factor VIII result in a rather sudden onset of bleeding.

---

1. *Antibodies against factor VIII occur frequently if ______________ is given to treat hemophilia A.* — ***factor VIII***
2. *Antibodies against coagulation factors produce a clinical picture which is identical to the ______________ deficiency of that factor.* — ***hereditary***

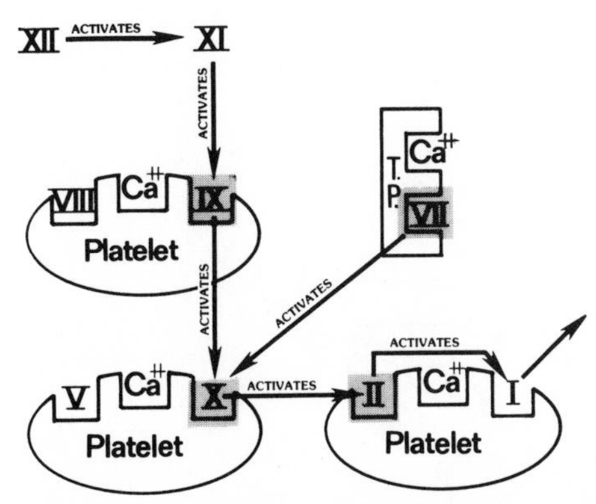

Most acquired deficiencies of inactive coagulation factors (in contrast to the hereditary deficiencies) are common, involve multiple factors rather than a single factor, and have a sudden onset rather than lifelong bleeding tendency. The acquired deficiencies of cogulation factors have, as a common mechanism, production deficits. Production deficiency can occur at the site of synthesis or at the site of factor modification. Since the liver is the production site of all the coagulation cascade proteins except Factor VIII, liver disease from various etiologies may result in a deficiency of inactive factors. Consumption or dilution also may result in factor deficiencies.

Since vitamin K enzymatically modifies four coagulation factors (enabling them to bind to phospholipids) a deficiency of vitamin K from any etiology will result in an insufficient plasma concentration of the modified form of factors II, VII, IX, and X.

- Liver disease
  - Acute hepatitis
  - Alcoholic liver disease
  - Chronic liver congestion (cardiac, cirrhotic, etc.)
- Vitamin K deficiency
  - Malabsorption
  - Antibiotic destruction of intestinal flora which produce vitamin K
  - Coumadin poisoning or treatment (more on this in the next few pages)

---

1. *Inactive factor disorders are __________.* — ***common***
2. *Inactive factor disorders often involve __________.* — ***multiple factors***
3. *Inactive factor disorders are common with __________ and __________ deficiency.* — ***hepatic disease***, ***vitamin K***

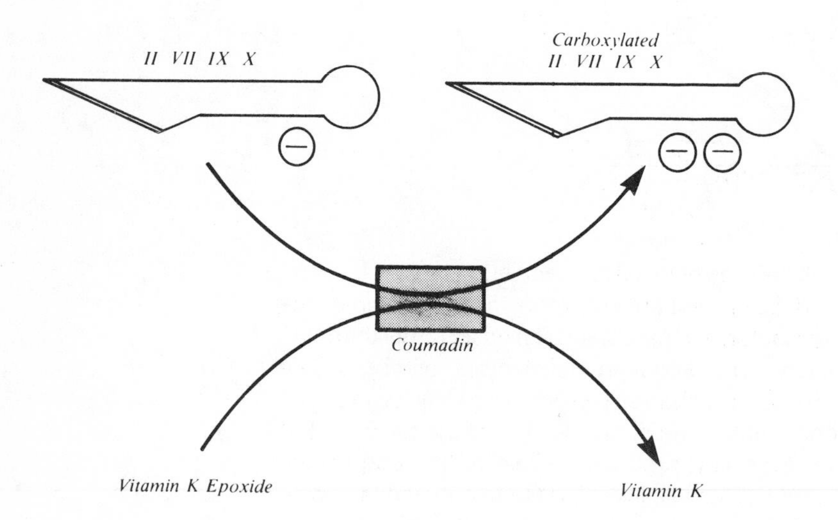

One area of the acquired inactive factor deficiencies which we would like to emphasize is the effect of coumadin. Coumadin basically produces a deficiency of vitamin K. Since a vitamin K deficiency results in an insufficient plasma concentration of the **modified** form of factors II, VII, IX, and X, coumadin, in effect, produces the same deficiency.

Note: Coumadin stops the vitamin K dependent addition of gamma carboxyl to factors II, VII, IX, and X, which enable these factors to bind via Ca++ to the phospholipids. These four factors are still being produced, they just aren't **functional**. That is, without the additional carboxyl group, they cannot bind to the platelet or tissue phospholipids and therefore do not become involved in the coagulation cascade.

(Details of treatment for coumadin-induced disorders are discussed in the treatment chapter.)

---

1. Coumadin produces a deficiency of ______________.	***vitamin K***
2. Coumadin overdose can be removed by the administration of ______________.	***vitamin K***
3. Coumadin blocks the vitamin K addition of a carboxyl group to factors ______________.	***II, VII, IX, X***

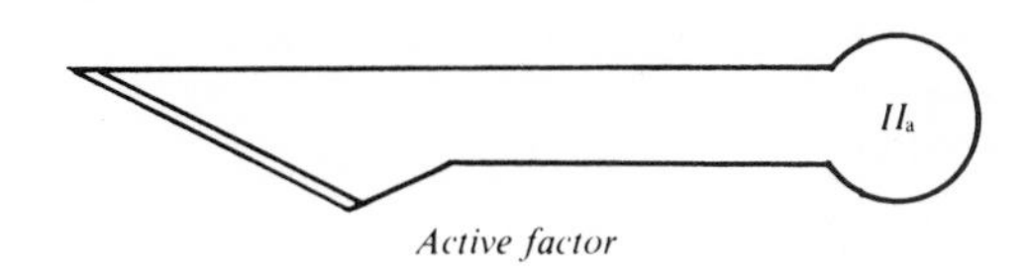

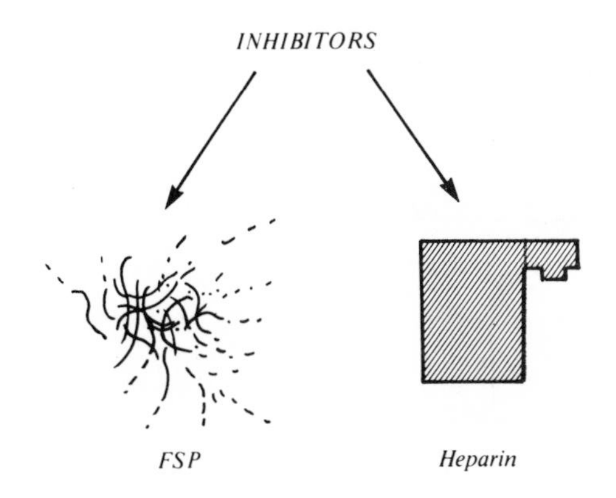

Now let us turn our attention to disorders of the coagulation cascade caused by inhibiting **active** factors. Disorders of active factors are caused by either heparin or fibrin split products.

---

1. *Disorders of the coagulation cascade can be divided into ________ and ________ disorders.*	***inactive factor active factor***
2. *________ and ________ are two chemicals which can cause active factor disorders.*	***Heparin, fibrin split products***

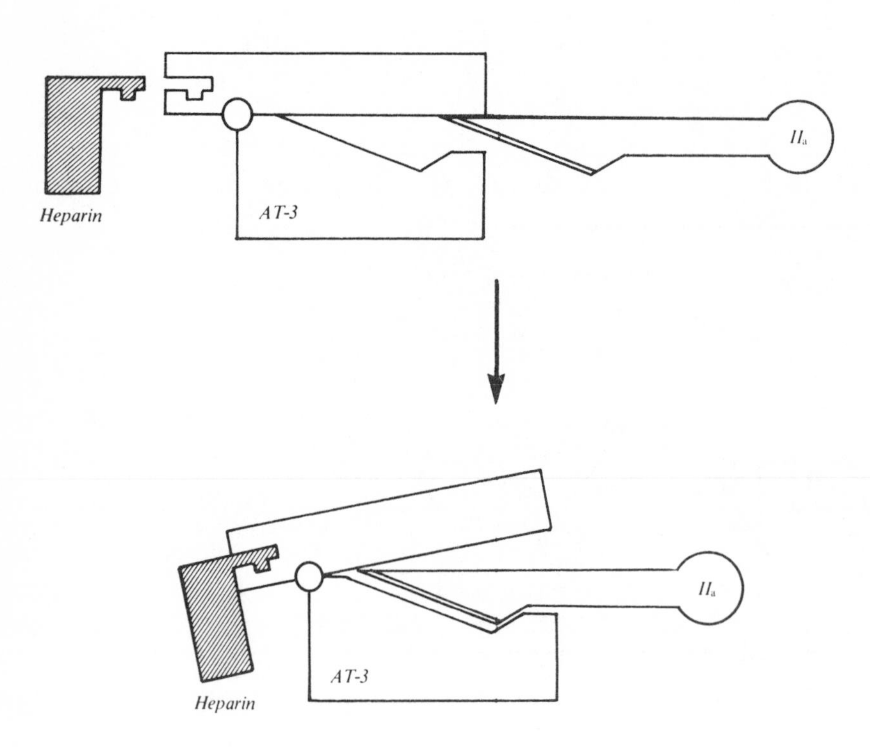

Heparin as a cause of bleeding is always due to exogenous administration of the drug. To review, heparin "anticoagulates" by making an endogenous protein, anti-thrombin 3 (AT-3), more avid in its binding of **activated** serine proteases. The greater the concentration of the heparin/AT-3 complex, the greater the level of "anticoagulation". Obviously the level of anticoagulation depends upon the concentration of heparin, the concentration of AT-3, and the concentration of the resulting complex.

---

1. *Heparin requires ____________ to be effective in "anticoagulating".* — ***AT-3***
2. *Heparin, a normal chemical found in the body, only causes bleeding if the drug is given ____________.* — ***exogenously***

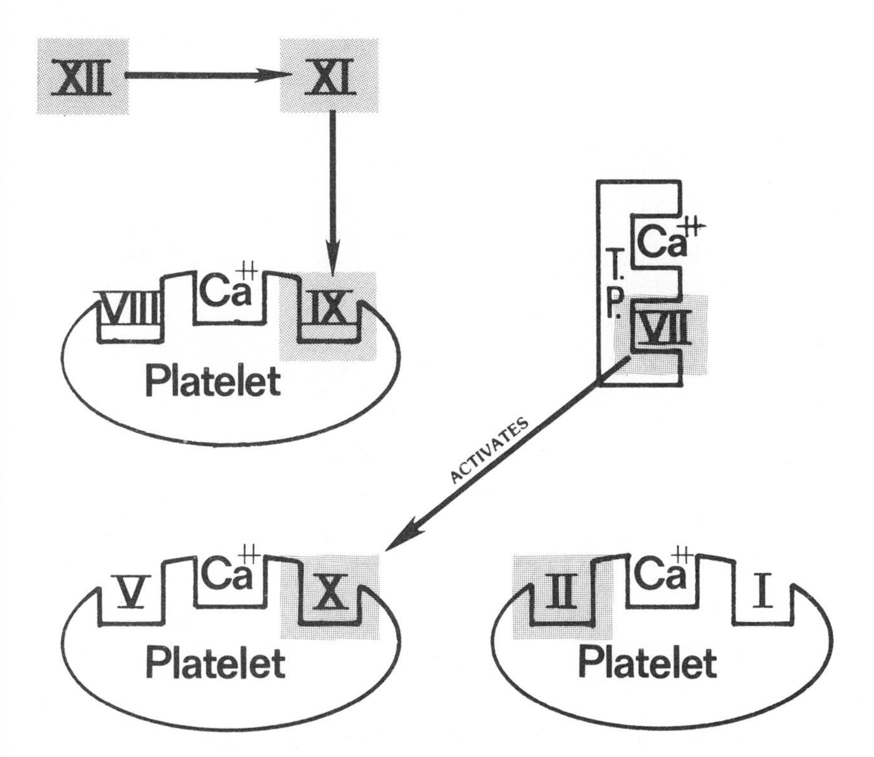

Heparin, via its effect on AT-3, can prolong any test of the coagulation cascade since it affects every factor except factors V, VIII, I. As previously mentioned, the TT is the most sensitive assay of the presence of heparin, the aPTT and ACT being intermediate assays, and the PT the least sensitive assay. As a rule, the TT is prolonged at minidose heparin (5000 units sc q12h). The aPTT is prolonged at therapeutic doses of heparin, usually a loading dose of 2,000-10,000 units then 500 units every hour via IV. The PT is prolonged only after the massive doses of heparin such as those used for cardiopulmonary bypass.

---

1. *The most sensitive assay of heparin is the ______________.* — ***thrombin time***
2. *The ______________ is an intermediate assay of heparin and becomes prolonged with therapeutic doses of heparin.* — ***aPTT***
3. *The ______________ becomes prolonged only after massive doses of heparin, such as those used for cardiopulmonary bypass.* — ***PT***

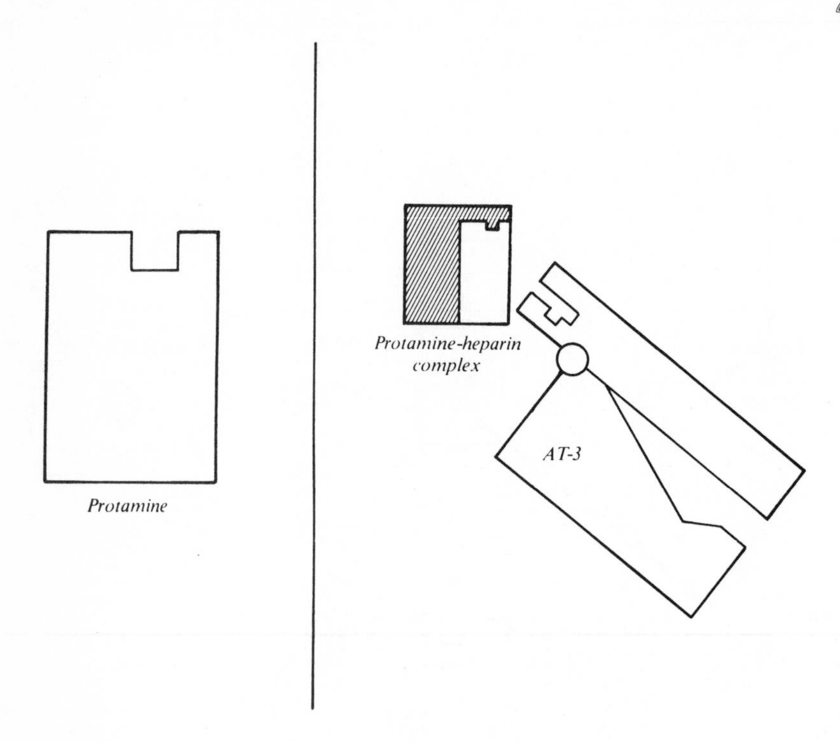

If heparin is the cause of bleeding, its effect is usually reversed "naturally" by simply discontinuing the drug, thus allowing the concentration to decrease by metabolism. If large doses of heparin have been administered, such as in surgery involving cardiopulmonary bypass, the reversal can be accomplished by using protamine. Details of protamine reversal of heparin therapy is found in the chapter on treatment, and Appendix F.

Protamine is used to antagonize the effects of heparin by forming a complex with heparin. Protamine competes with anti-thrombin for available heparin. As heparin is bound by protamine, less heparin is available to make AT-3 more avid in its binding of activated serine proteases, and the coagulation cascade returns to a more normal state.

---

1. *Protamine __________ the anticoagulation induced by heparin.* — **antagonizes**
2. *A __________ forms when heparin and __________ interact.* — **complex**, **protamine**
3. *Protamine "ties up" heparin, leaving anti-thrombin less avid, and thus __________ and other proteases will be available to continue the cascade system to completion.* — **thrombin**

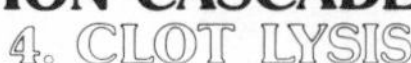

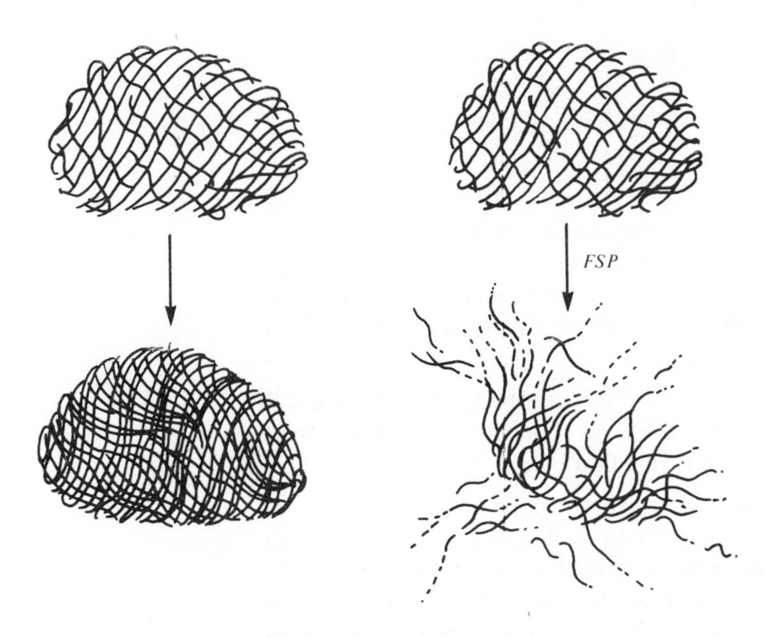

Fibrin split products (FSP), the natural breakdown products of a fibrin clot, in high concentrations inhibit the cross-linking of fibrin monomers. Fibrin split products contain the same amino acids as fibrin and therefore can compete with the sites of fibrin cross-linking.

---

1. *FSP are the natural breakdown products of a ______________.* — ***fibrin clot***
2. *FSP compete with the ______________ sites on fibrin monomer.* — ***cross-linking***

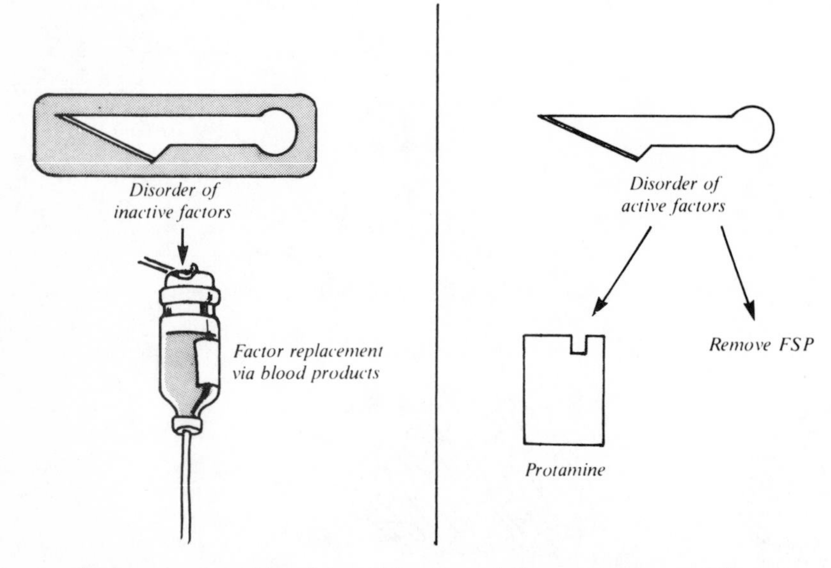

Before leaving disorders of the coagulation cascade, we will emphasize why we have divided the disorders of the coagulation cascade into inactive factor disorders and active factor disorders. Basically, all disorders of **inactive factors** can be treated with fresh frozen plasma or other blood products containing factors.

Disorders of active factors, on the other hand, are not treated with factor replacement but rather either with heparin reversal via protamine, or with removal of fibrin split products.

Differentiating inactive factor deficiency from an active factor disorder is best done with a thrombin time. If both the PT and aPTT are prolonged and a thrombin time is abnormal, then heparin effect is the likely cause of the disorder, and can be treated appropriately with protamine. If, on the other hand, the thrombin time is normal, despite an abnormal aPTT and PT, then heparin effect is ruled out (the TT is the most sensitive assay of heparin), and the inactive factor deficiency can be treated with the appropriate blood products.

---

1. *Inactive factor disorders are treated with ______.* — ***factor replacement***
2. *Active factor disorders are treated with ______ or ______.* — ***protamine***, ***removal of FSP***
3. *The ______ is the best test to differentiate active from inactive factor disorders.* — ***thrombin time***

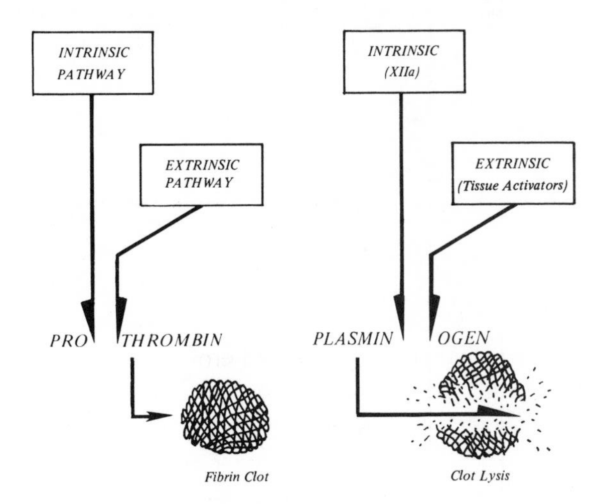

Fibrin Clot

Clot Lysis

Disorders of clot lysis, the fourth component of our conceptual framework of hemostasis, include:

- Abnormal fibrinolysis
- Normal but increased fibrinolysis secondary to diffuse intravascular coagulation (DIC)

We will discuss abnormal fibrinolysis in this chapter, and then discuss DIC in the following chapter.

---

1. *Disorders of clot lysis comprise the ________ component of hemostasis.*	***fourth***
2. *Increased fibrinolysis can be normal or ________.*	***abnormal***
3. *Increased fibrinolysis is a normal sequelae of increased ________.*	***fibrin formation***

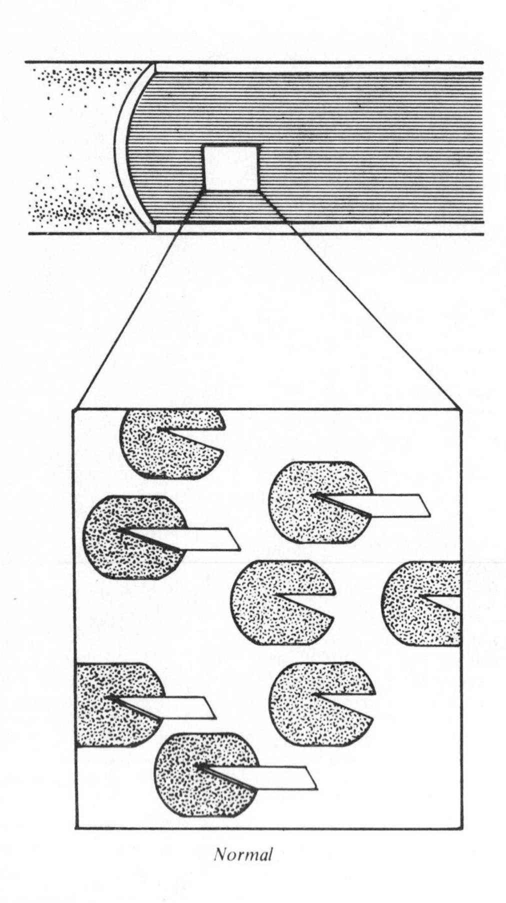

Normal

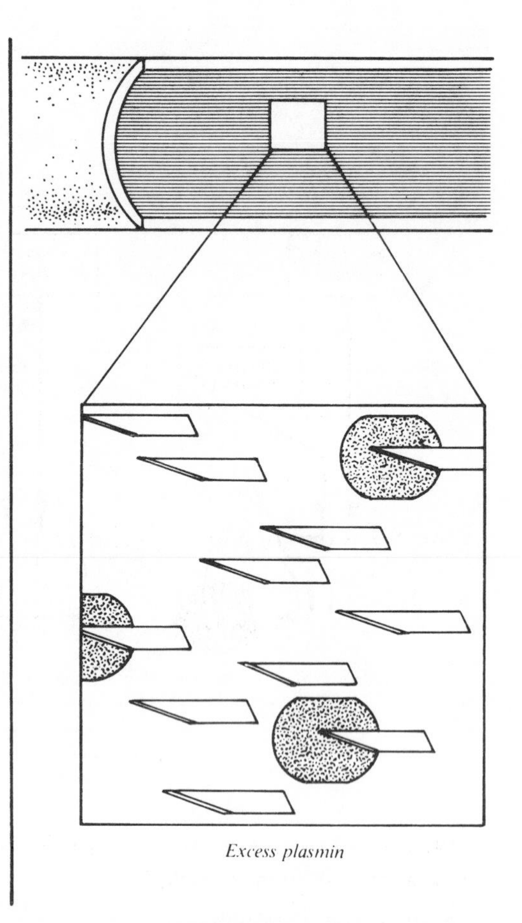

Excess plasmin

Abnormal fibrinolysis means **circulating** plasmin. Normally there is no circulating plasmin because it is neutralized immediately by antiplasmin. There are circumstances, however, when this localization of plasmin to the site of clot formation goes awry because of massive plasminogen activation.

---

1. *Abnormal fibrinolysis occurs when there is ____________ plasmin.* — ***circulating***
2. *Normally plasmin is localized to the site of clot formation by ____________.* — ***antiplasmin***
3. *Massive plasminogen activation may overpower antiplasmin's ability to neutralize ____________.* — ***plasmin***

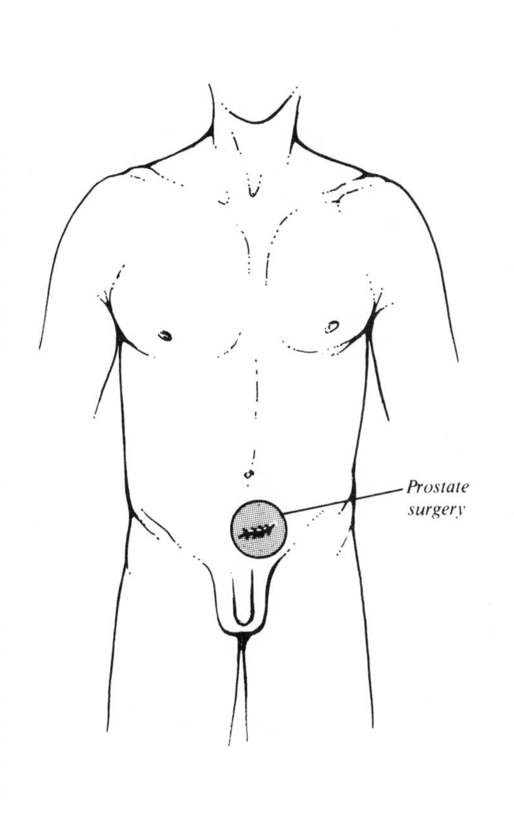

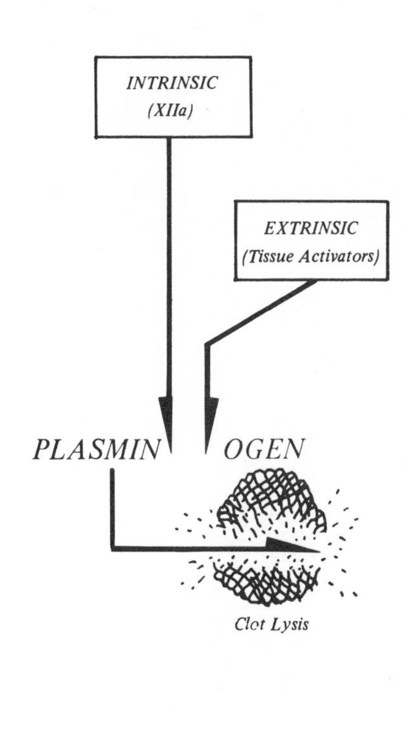

Urologic surgery, especially when it involves the prostate gland, may result in release of large amounts of tissue plasminogen activators into the blood stream. This can result in massive tissue activation of plasminogen to plasmin, and thereby overpower the neutralizing ability of antiplasmin. This results in abnormal fibrinolysis. Lysis of clots appropriately plugging areas of surgical vascular injury may result in uncontrollable bleeding.

---

1. *Prostatic surgery may release large amounts of ____________ ____________ of plasminogen into the blood stream.* — ***tissue, activators***
2. *Massive action of plasminogen to plasmin may result in ____________ plasmin.* — ***circulating***
3. *Circulating plasmin results in abnormal ____________.* — ***fibrinolysis***

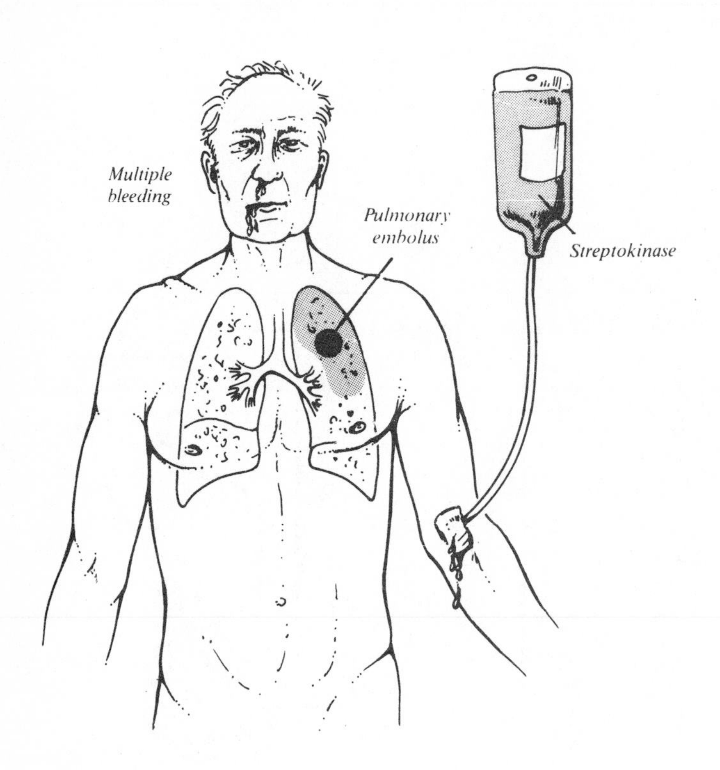

Abnormal fibrinolysis also occurs after intravenous administration of streptokinase and urokinase. These agents are administered to lyse the clots forming pulmonary emboli (PE) and deep vein thrombi (DVT). Streptokinase and urokinase both are tissue activators of plasminogen to plasmin. The massive doses used in treating PE and DVT result in circulating plasmin. However, the circulating plasmin not only lyses the unwanted clots in the lungs and/or veins, it also lyses clots formed appropriately at sites of vascular injury. Bleeding is a frequent event during threatment with these agents. Monitoring therapy with streptokinase and urokinase is not routinely performed. Instead, a standard dose regimen often is used.

---

1. *Abnormal fibrinolysis occurs from intravenous administration of ______________ and ______________.* — ***streptokinase, urokinase***
2. *Streptokinase and urokinase activate plasminogen to ______________.* — ***plasmin***
3. *______________ is a frequent complication after treatment with tissue activators.* — ***Bleeding***

SUMMARY

Disorders of hemostasis which produce bleeding can be summarized according to the four components of hemostasis:

Vascular Integrity	Normal vessels subjected to trauma Abnormal vessels caused by disease processes of many etiologies
Platelets	Quantitative Disorders (number) Nonproduction, Dilution, Sequestration, Destruction Qualitative Disorders (dysfunction) Drugs (ASA), Uremia, Storage Defect, Fibrin Split Products, Mechanics Combinations of the above Von Willebrand's Disease (VIII)
Coagulation Cascade	Inactive Factors Disorders Hereditary Disorders (VIII, IX, XI)
Acquired Disorders	Antibodies Production problems (esp. II, VII, IX, X) hepatic disease, vitamin K deficiency (coumadin) Consumption/Dilution Active Factors Disorders Heparin Fibrin Split Products
Clot Lysis	Abnormal Fibrinolysis Plasminogen activators (urokinase, streptokinase) Increased Fibrinolysis Secondary to increased Fibrin Formation

Now let us turn our attention to one disorder which we discuss separately and in greater detail—DIC.

Chapter 6
DISSEMINATED INTRAVASCULAR COAGULATION

It is important that you understand that all of the **localized** hemostatic processes can become uncontrolled. When clotting becomes widespread, various coagulation constituents become utilized more rapidly than they can be replaced. Such a clinical condition used to be called "consumption coagulopathy"—a term actually quite descriptive and accurate. Now the term disseminated intravascular coagulation (DIC) is used more commonly. (In other texts, you may find this process termed "defibrination syndrome". Do not be confused by the terminology, nor minor differences in various authors' descriptions or definitions. Be concerned only with an understanding of the process.)

The loss of localization of the clotting process is, in general, the basis for a **disseminated** clotting process, **disseminated intravascular coagulation**. The lytic process is diffusely initiated as well, but this is **NOT** a primary lytic disease. The "defect" is not in the lytic system, as the accelerated lytic system is only a consequence of diffuse clotting.

1. VASCULAR INTEGRITY
2. PLATELETS
3. COAGULATION CASCADE
4. CLOT LYSIS

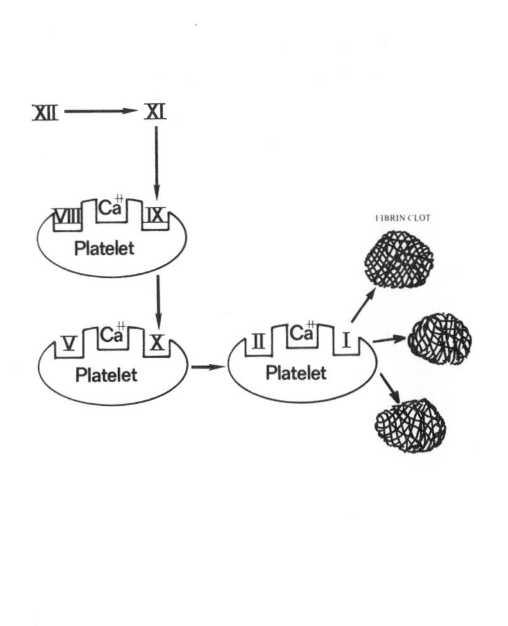

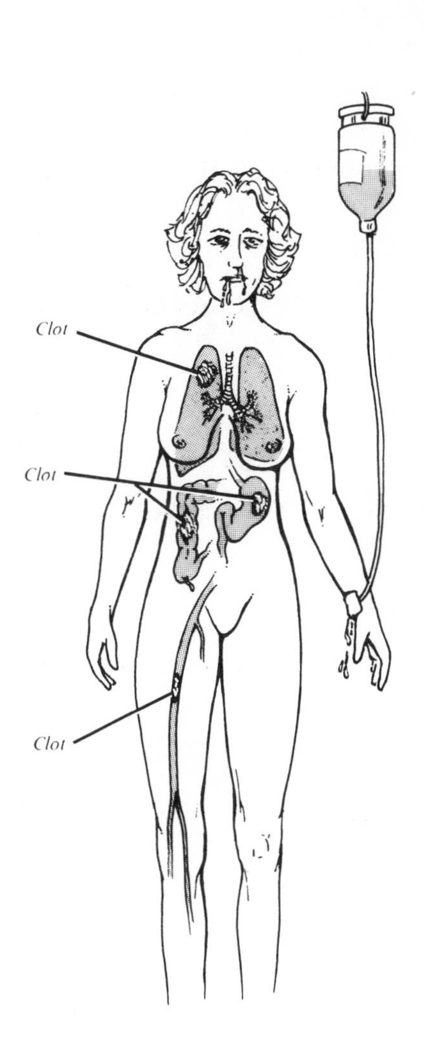

Disseminated intravascular coagulation (DIC) is a term we use when the body is forming, and then lysing, fibrin clot in a **diffuse** manner, rather than in the normal physiological localized manner.

---

1. The process of diffuse clotting is a ______________ process.	***disseminated***
2. A general term for this process is ______________.	***DIC***
3. DIC inkvolves a ______________ lytic process, not a primary lytic process.	***secondary***

1. VASCULAR INTEGRITY
2. PLATELETS
3. COAGULATION CASCADE
4. CLOT LYSIS

Let us review briefly the mechanisms involved in **localization** of clotting and lysis.

VASCULAR INTEGRITY

Variation in structural and connective tissue strength of vessels, depending upon the stress these vessels must tolerate.

PLATELETS

1. Platelet structure and function are directed to localization of clot formation.
2. Platelets provide a rate-limiting phospholipid (PF-3) for the coagulation cascade.

COAGULATION CASCADE

1. Factors circulate in **inactive** form in high concentration. Their activity is localized to areas where available phospholipid is present—(platelet phospholipid and tissue phospholipid).
2. Active factors are **diluted** by rapid blood flow.
3. Active factors are **removed** by the reticuloendothelial system.
4. Active factors are **neutralized** by a circulating protein called antithrombin (AT-3) which becomes more avid in neutralizing active factors, when exposed to heparin.

CLOT LYSIS

1. Lysis is initiated by Factor XII (Intrinsic), simultaneously with initiation of the coagulation cascade.
2. Plasmin normally is rapidly neutralized by antiplasmin.
3. Plasminogen is incorporated into a clot at the time of clot formation. Thus, plasminogen is protected from anti-plasmin.
4. Fibrin split products are removed from the circulation by the hepatic Kupffer cells, thus limiting their systemic effects.

1. VASCULAR INTEGRITY
2. PLATELETS
3. COAGULATION CASCADE
4. CLOT LYSIS

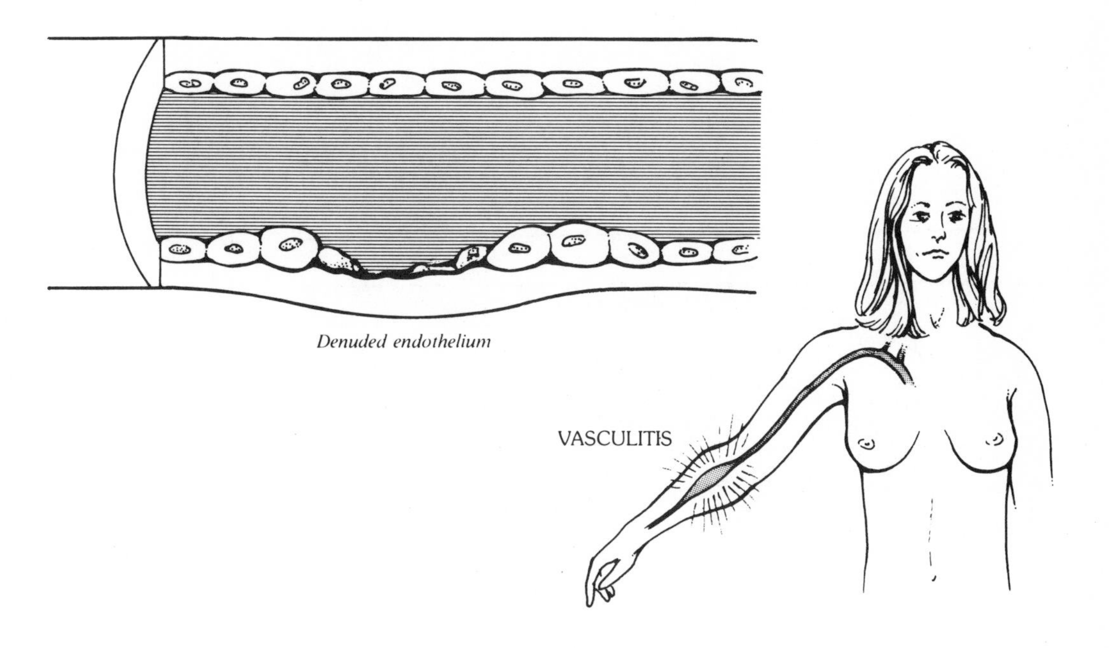

Localization ceases to exist in some disease states. Which abnormalities might be expected to initiate the process of DIC?

Remember that each time we approach a problem, we should analyze each of the four components of hemostasis. We won't always find perfect and exact separations for each disease entity, but having an available system for analyzing the etiology is important. Thus, the first area in which to search for a cause of DIC is:

VASCULAR INTEGRITY—the common element in the disorders below is the obvious presence of large surfaces of **denuded** vascular endothelium:

Vasculitis
Burns
Dissecting aortic aneurysm

Examples of disorders of vascular integrity which may involve DIC are:

1. ______________
2. ______________
3. ______________

vasculitis
burns
dissecting aortic aneurysm

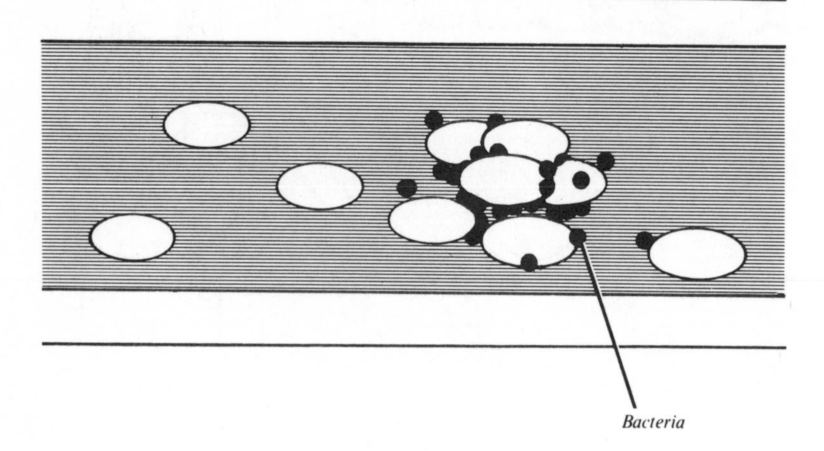

The second area is, of course:

PLATELETS—The diffuse presence of immune complexes or bacteria will cause platelets to aggregate in many areas of the body, in the absence of vascular injury. This may initiate a diffuse clotting process, and consumption of platelets. Several such disorders are:

Immunological complex disease processes
Toxemia of pregnancy—immune complexes
Sepsis
- Viremia
- Bacteremia

---

1. *Immune complexes cause ____________ clumping in DIC.* **platelet**
2. *____________ may cause platelets to aggregate, initiating DIC.* **sepsis**
3. *In DIC, platelets are ____________ rapidly.* **consumed**

1. VASCULAR INTEGRITY
2. PLATELETS
3. COAGULATION CASCADE
4. CLOT LYSIS

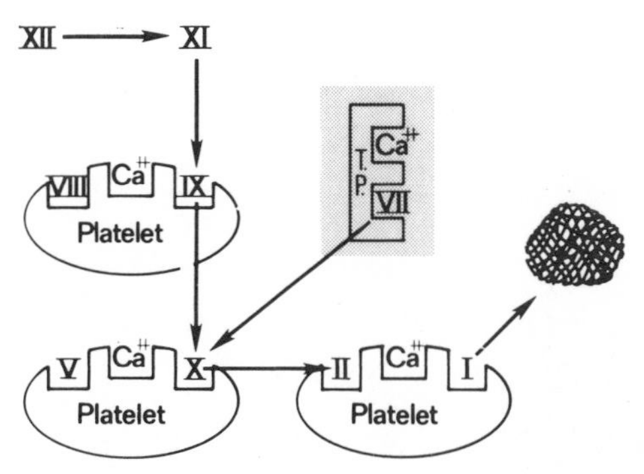

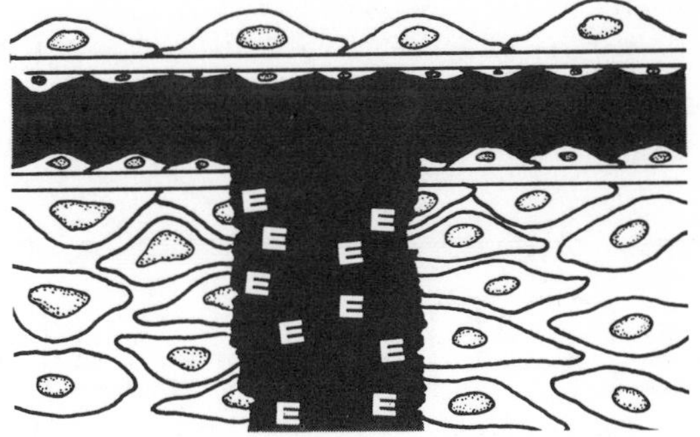

The third area of importance is:

COAGULATION CASCADE—In each of the instances below, you will notice the intravascular presence of large quantities of tissue phospholipids:

Tissue phospholipid from massive crush injuries
Tissue phospholipid from necrotic malignant tissue
Obstetrical Complications
 Amniotic fluid or tissue (especially if embolized)
 Retained (dead) fetal tissue
 Placental rupture or abruptio
Red cell hemolysis from any cause, which releases red cell membrane phospholipid

---

1. *DIC may be involved in processes which release ______________.* — **tissue phospho-lipids**

2. *Intravascular tissue phospholipid is present after massive ______________, necrosis of ______________ tissue, and after hemolytic transfusion reactions which release ______________ phospholipid.* — **crush injuries**, **malignant**, **red cell**

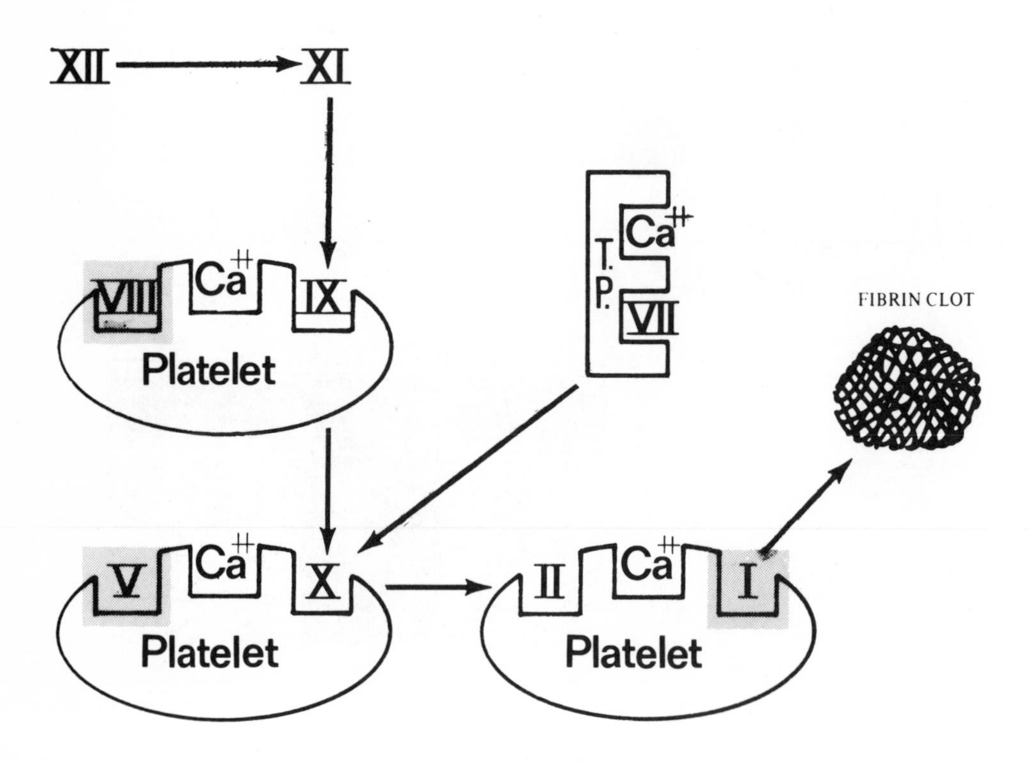

The initiation of the coagulation cascade by any of the disease processes presented on the previous page will lead to the formation of fibrin. If this process is a widely disseminated one, a consumption of coagulation cascade factors may occur. The labile factors (cofactors) V and VIII will be greatly decreased, as will the end product, fibrinogen. Cofactors V and VIII, and fibrinogen, are used once and destroyed, in contrast to the activated serine proteases such as IX and X which catalyze multiple reactions. Thus a "consumption coagulopathy" will result.

---

1. *The cofactors __________ and __________ may be consumed in DIC.* — ***V, VIII***
2. *The factor __________ may also be consumed.* — ***fibrinogen***
3. *During DIC, __________ will be consumed during the clotting process.* — ***platelets***

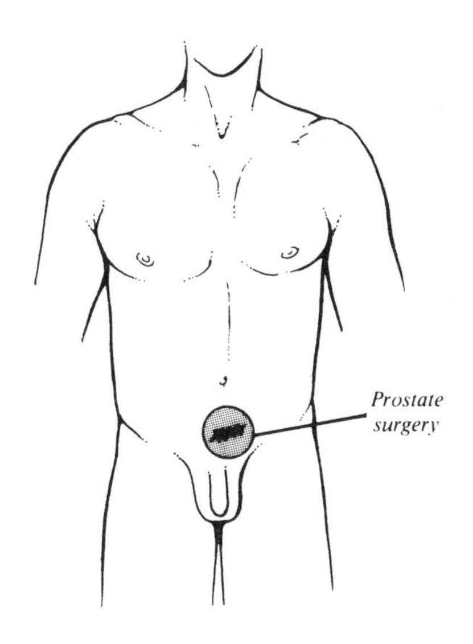

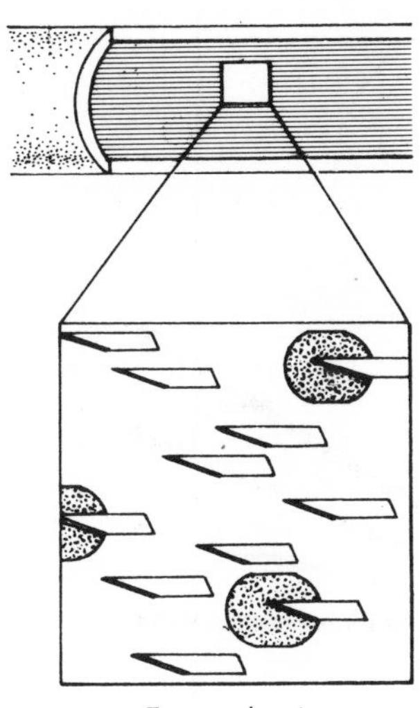

Excess plasmin

And finally, the fourth component:

CLOT LYSIS

When large amounts of clot have been formed, the lytic process will also have been initiated in the area of each clot. The degradation of large amounts of fibrin produces large quantities of **fibrin split products** (FSP). These protein fragments have physiological activity—the more serious of which are to inhibit fibrin cross-linking, and to produce platelet dysfunction. The balance between FSP formation and FSP removal by the hepatic Kupffer cells determines the concentration of FSP circulating. High production rates will lead to high circulating concentrations.

An increase in the presence of FSP also may occur in other processes. If fibrinolysis is initiated by agents such as urokinase or streptokinase, FSP will be increased. The clinical picture will be identical to that seen in DIC.

---

1. *Degradation of fibrin produces ______________.* — ***FSP***
2. *The concentration of circulating FSP is a balance between FSP ______________ and FSP ______________.* — ***production***, ***removal***
3. *The production of FSP secondary to urokinase or streptokinase may resemble ______________.* — ***DIC***

1. VASCULAR INTEGRITY
2. PLATELETS
3. COAGULATION CASCADE
4. CLOT LYSIS

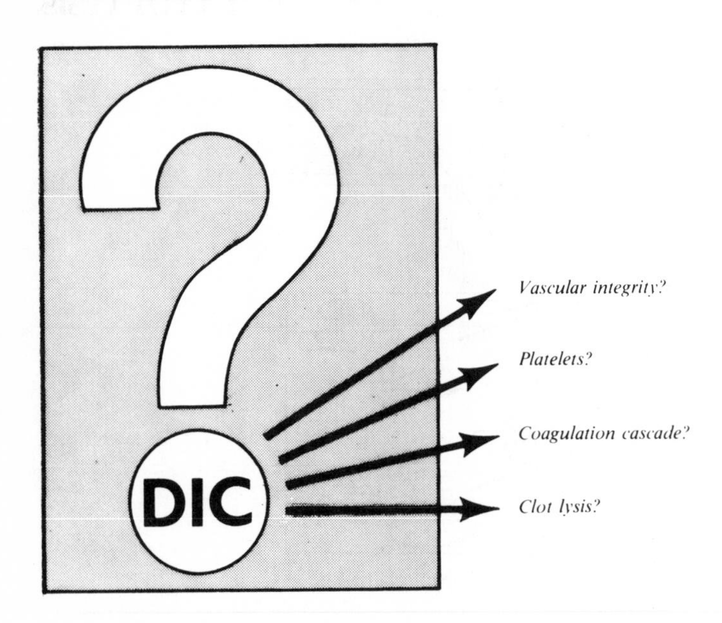

In general, how might we diagnose DIC?

First of all—be suspicious! Then ask the following questions in the four component areas:

Hemostasis Component	Question
Vascular Integrity	Is a vessel broken? Is the endothelium damaged?
Platelets	Are platelets being consumed? Is there platelet dysfunction?
Coagulation Cascade	Are factors V, VIII and fibrinogen being consumed?
Clot Lysis	Are FSP being produced at faster than normal rates? Are there signs of FSP inhibition of fibrin cross-linking?

---

1. *The diagnosis of DIC can be suspected by using the four ______ of hemostasis for a framework.*	***components***
2. *DIC consumes ______.*	***platelets***
3. *DIC consumes coagulation factors ______, ______, and ______.*	***VIII, V, I***
4. *DIC may involve the presence of high concentrations of ______.*	***fibrin split products***

1. VASCULAR INTEGRITY
2. PLATELETS
3. COAGULATION CASCADE
4. CLOT LYSIS

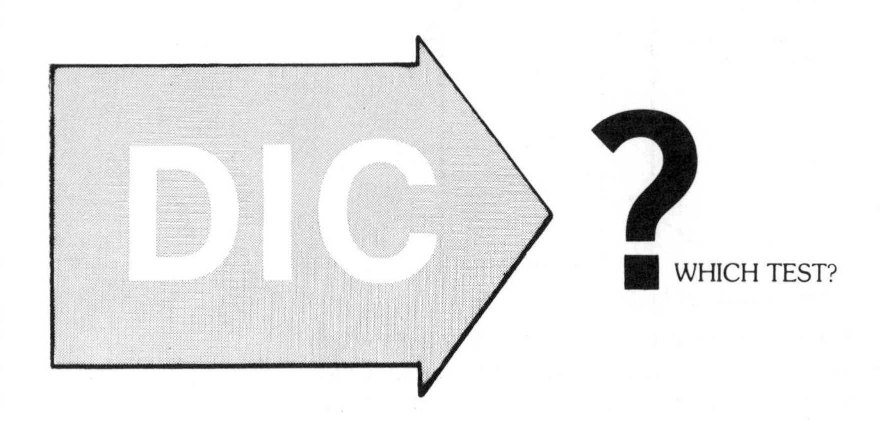

How, then MIGHT each of these be tested and diagnosis confirmed?

Hemostasis Component	Test
Vascular Integrity	
If a surgical patient—	Inspect surgical site
If a trauma patient—	Inspect trauma site
If inflammatory disease—	Inspect inflamed area
Platelets	
Quantity—	Perform serial platelet counts
Quality—	Perform serial bleeding times
Coagulation Cascade	
Consumption of V, VIII, I—	Perform an aPTT
Consumption of I—	Perform a fibrinogen level
Inhibition of fibrin cross-linking—	Perform a TT and RT
Clot Lysis	
Increased fibrinolysis—	Perform a FSP determination

---

1. *The diagnosis of a vascular integrity abnormality as a cause of DIC involves ______________.* — ***inspection***
2. *DIC diagnosis may be facilitated by serial tests of platelet ______________ and ______________.* — ***quantity, quality***
3. *The diagnosis of DIC is facilitated by testing the coagulation cascade for ______________ of factors, and ______________ of fibrin crosslinking.* — ***consumption***, ***inhibition***
4. *The diagnosis of DIC may be facilitated by the presence of high concentrations of ______________.* — ***FSP***

1. VASCULAR INTEGRITY
2. PLATELETS
3. COAGULATION CASCADE
4. CLOT LYSIS

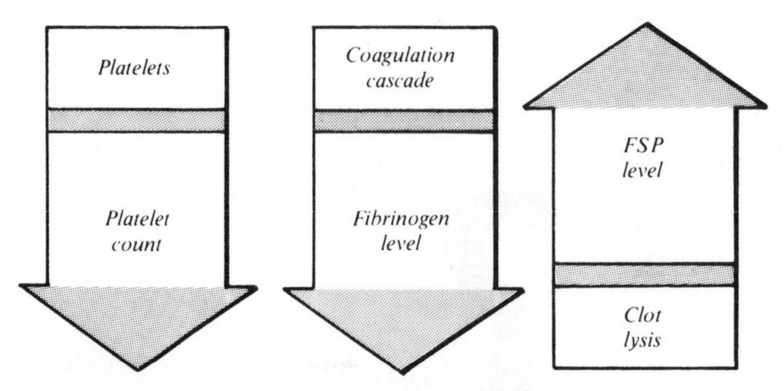

Which tests become abnormal first?

Platelets and fibrinogen decrease initially, and thus tests which evaluate platelet number and fibrinogen concentration are early indicators. It is very helpful to have baseline values for more accurate analysis. If the test results decrease by half, this may be significant (thus, a platelet count of 200,000/mm^3 might be significant if the count started at 400,000/mm^3, even though 200,000/mm^3 is within the normal range). Serial bleeding times performed concomitantly with serial platelet counts will demonstrate platelet dysfunction caused by the presence of FSP.

Hourly platelet counts and fibrinogen levels reflect activity of the process. The plasma half life of platelets and fibrinogen is normally 4-5 days. Since production is not "geared up" to replace sudden losses, the platelet and fibrinogen levels directly reflect activity of intravascular coagulation, through consumption of constituents. The prolonged activated partial thromboplastin time (aPTT) is due to Factors V, VIII, and fibrinogen (I) depletion. This test is less sensitive in evaluating minute-to-minute changes, but is a guideline to the effectiveness of clot formation. Comparison of the thrombin time and reptilase time will demonstrate the effect of FSP on fibrin cross-linking.

The concentration of fibrin (and fibrinogen) split products (FSP) reflects both the ability of the reticular-endothelial system to remove FSP, and the concomitant rate of production of FSP by the lytic process. FSP concentrations may be decreased during DIC if fibrinogen has been consumed.

---

1. *Early indicators of the DIC process are decreasing ____________ counts, and ____________ concentration.* — ***platelet fibrinogen***
2. *Hourly platelet counts and fibrinogen determinations reflect the ____________ of DIC.* — ***activity***
3. *The FSP concentration reflects both FSP ____________ and FSP ____________.* — ***production removal***

1. VASCULAR INTEGRITY
2. PLATELETS
3. COAGULATION CASCADE
4. CLOT LYSIS

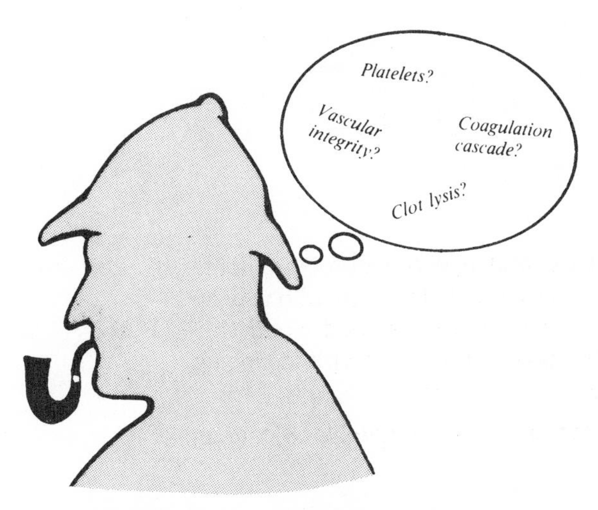

There are three basic steps in the successful treatment of DIC. The first is to locate and **treat the inciting cause**. This will be the mainstay of therapy, and if performed properly, will lead to a "winding down" of the entire process. This first step **CANNOT BE OVEREMPHASIZED**. Failure to perform it, or to find the cause, will make further treatment most difficult, and survival for the patient very unlikely.

Thus—remember the classification system for causes of DIC we have previously mentioned, and for:

Vascular Integrity	Maintain good circulation Stop or repair vascular injury
Platelets	Find cause of sepsis, immunologic abnormality, etc., and appropriately treat
Coagulation Cascade	Find damaged, necrotic, or circulating tissue phospholipids and remove
Clot Lysis	Find additional causes, if any, for increased fibrinolytic activity

Remember also to treat secondary problems arising from the initial cause (such as appropriate treatment of hypoxemia from pulmonary embolism of amniotic fluid, etc.)

What is step two?

---

1. Step number one in DIC treatment is to locate and treat the ______. — ***cause***

2. If the cause cannot be found, ______ is unlikely. — ***survival***

3. Treat ______ as they occur. — ***secondary problems***

1. VASCULAR INTEGRITY
2. PLATELETS
3. COAGULATION CASCADE
4. CLOT LYSIS

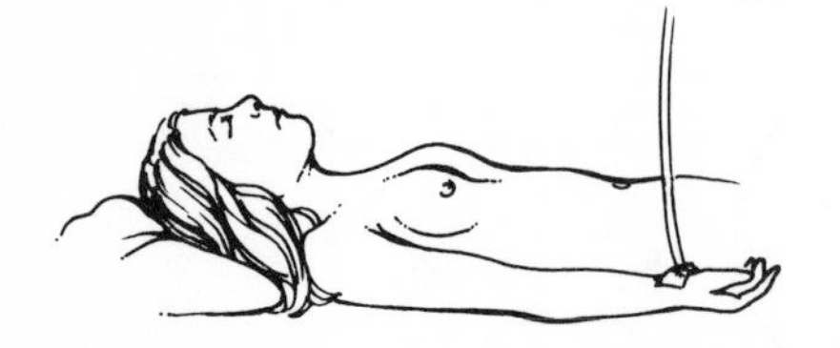

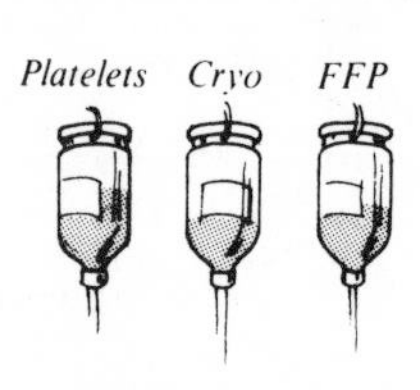

Once the cause of DIC is located and treated, the process should slow down and eventually stop. However, until that control has been achieved, one must temporarily replace the consumed blood constituents, so that fibrin may be laid down where needed, and clotting returned to a more normal state.

Thus, step two is the **replacement of consumed blood constituents:**

Consumed Constituents	Replacement Component	Goal
Platelets	Platelets	Platelet count above 100,000/mm^3 (preferably 125,000/mm^3)
Factors V, VIII	Fresh Frozen Plasma (or cryoprecipitate for VIII)	aPTT or ACT normal
Fibrinogen	Cryoprecipitate or fresh fresh frozen plasma	Fibrinogen level 200 mg %

Therapy is governed by evaluation of these laboratory tests, performed approximately 20 minutes after administration of the replacement components. To monitor effectiveness of therapy, the balance sheet should demonstrate that replacement is proceeding faster than consumption.

What is step three?

Replace consumed constituents:

______ *platelets*
______ *factors V, VIII*
______ *fibrinogen*

1. VASCULAR INTEGRITY
2. PLATELETS
3. COAGULATION CASCADE
4. CLOT LYSIS

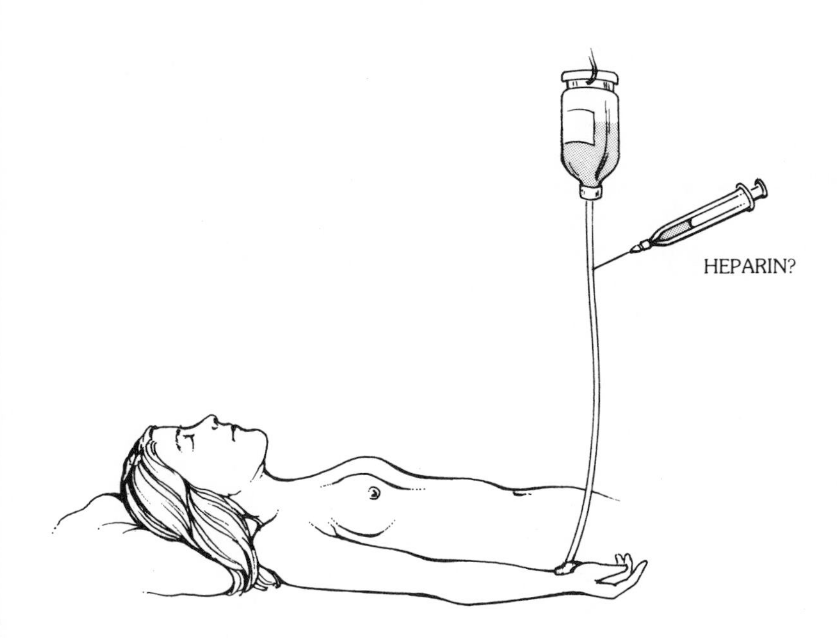

Step three is the controversial one, and involves the possible administration of drugs which modulate either the coagulation cascade, or fibrinolysis, or both. **If step one has been utilized effectively, and step two used as needed, step three is almost always unnecessary.**

If the etiology of DIC is the **intravascular** presence of tissue phospholipid, which triggers the extrinsic pathway, then treatment which inhibits the coagulation cascade is treatment of the primary cause. Heparin therapy represents such treatment, and may be indicated until such time as tissue phospholipid can be removed from the intravascular space. This is a double-edged sword, however. While heparin will limit fibrin deposition, such fibrin deposition may be required in the area of injury. Thus while "shutting down" the cascade system is a generalized way, the **local** area of injury may be deprived of the benefit of fibrin clot.

---

1. Step one of DIC treatment is to ____________. — ***treat the cause***

2. Step two of DIC treatment is to ____________. — ***replace consumed components***

3. Step three of DIC treatment may include the use of ____________. — ***heparin***

1. VASCULAR INTEGRITY
2. PLATELETS
3. COAGULATION CASCADE
4. CLOT LYSIS

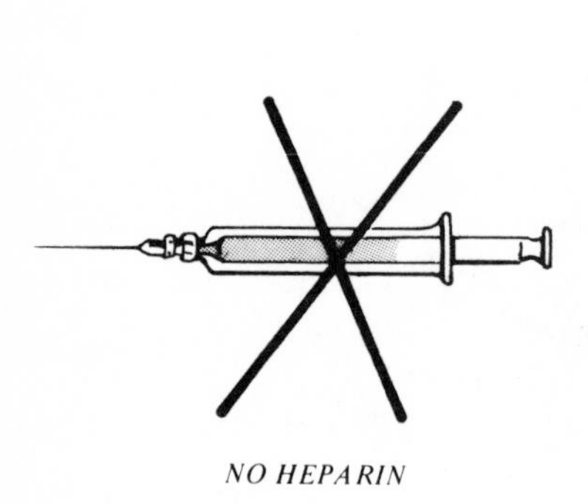

NO HEPARIN

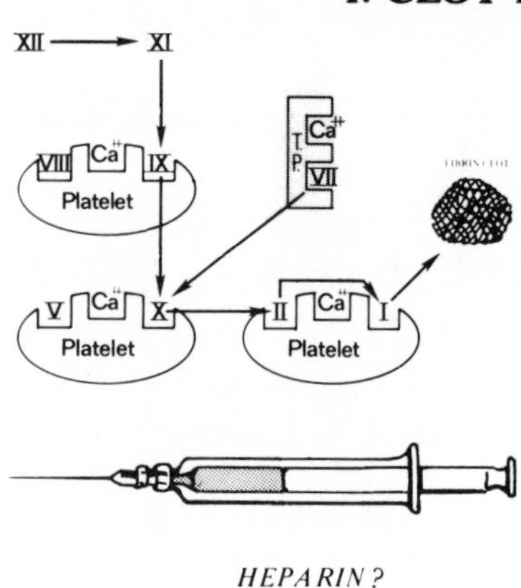

HEPARIN ?

If the primary cause of DIC is in the area of disorders of vascular integrity or platelets, heparin does not treat the primary cause, it only modifies a subsequent process. The vascular or platelet process would continue unchecked and DIC would continue despite heparin therapy.

In summary:

Vascular Disorders—burns, vasculitis, etc. NO HEPARIN

Platelet Disorders—sepsis, immune disease, toxemia, etc. NO HEPARIN

Coagulation Cascade Disorders— CONSIDER HEPARIN*

Clot Lysis Disorders— CONSIDER HEPARIN*

[Since heparin's activity with anti-thrombin allows anti-thrombin to bind **plasmin**, heparin may offer some controlled "anti-lytic" effects along with "anti-clotting" effects.]

Thus if the coagulation cascade has been triggered by intravascular tissue phospholipid, and steps one and two have failed, heparin might be tried.

***If this is considered, we would strongly recommend consultative advice from a qualified hematologist.**

---

1. *If DIC is initiated by vascular or platelet disorders, heparin is ______________ indicated.* ***not***
2. *If DIC involves primary initiation of the coagulation cascade, ______________ may be indicated.* ***heparin***
3. *The use of heparin in DIC should involve the advice of a ______________.* ***hematologist***

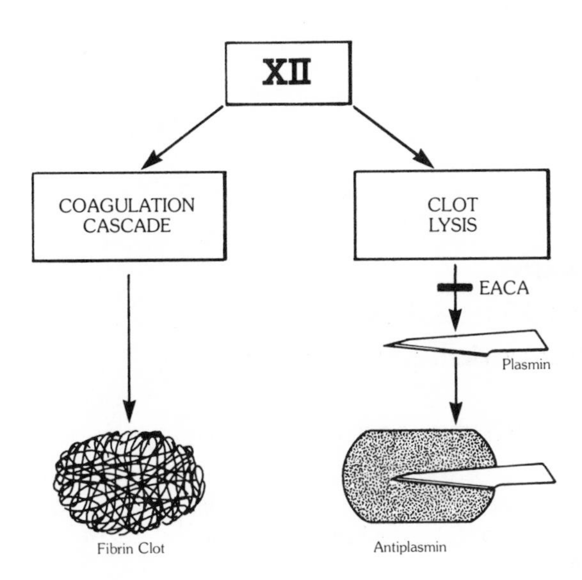

One other drug needs to be mentioned—epsilon aminocaproic acid (EACA). EACA blocks the formation of plasmin in the fibrinolytic system.

Use of EACA will produce an imbalance in the clotting vs. lysis general scheme. If clotting continues, and lysis is prevented, generalized severe thrombosis may result. Vital organs may be impaired because of thrombosis of supplying vessels. Clearly, in continued clotting, this is **not** desirable. (If EACA is given, heparin should be administered first, and its effects demonstrated prior to EACA administration.)

If the lytic process has been activated by such agents as urokinase and streptokinase, and clotting itself is **not** active, then EACA may be indicated.

[Again, if either heparin or EACA are considered, we strongly recommend consultation with a qualified hematologist.]

---

1. *Blocking the fibrinolytic system can be achieved with the use of ______________.* — ***EACA***
2. *EACA may be indicated if clotting is not active, and lysis has been initiated by either ______________ or ______________.* — ***urokinase***, ***streptokinase***
3. *EACA may be associated with the complication ______________.* — ***thrombosis***
4. *The use of EACA requires advice from a ______________.* — ***hematologist***

1. VASCULAR INTEGRITY
2. PLATELETS
3. COAGULATION CASCADE
4. CLOT LYSIS

SUMMARY

Let us review briefly what we have learned about DIC.

First—It is a circumstance in which **localization** of clotting and lysis has **failed**.

Second—It is **not** primarily a lytic disease. Lysis is a subsequent resulting phenomenon.

Third—The result of fibrinolysis is the production of fibrin split products (FSP). FSP produce platelet dysfunction and inhibit the cross-linking of fibrin.

Fourth—DIC has **causes** which usually can be discovered, and which require **treatment** for a successful outcome. These causes can be separated adequately into the "four components of hemostasis" categories for ease of memory, and for providing a logical approach to treatment.

Fifth—Evaluation of the consumptive process (platelets, factors V, VIII, and fibrinogen (I) most importantly), and treatment with components to replace consumed constituents, buys time to treat the primary cause, and stabilizes the patient's hemostatic mechanism.

Sixth—Heparin and epsilon aminocaproic acid (EACA) have limited use, and **may** benefit **selected** patients who are refractory to other more basic therapy, or who have unique circumstances. Those circumstances require sophisticated consultative assistance from a hematologist.

Chapter 7
ANALYSIS OF A BLEEDING PATIENT

Uncontrolled bleeding is a frustrating problem with which to deal, and requires systematic analysis and treatment. In this chapter we will present a systematic analysis, using real patient case examples. While we will touch upon treatment, the specific therapy for various disorders will be presented in the next two chapters.

1. VASCULAR INTEGRITY
2. PLATELETS
3. COAGULATION CASCADE
4. CLOT LYSIS

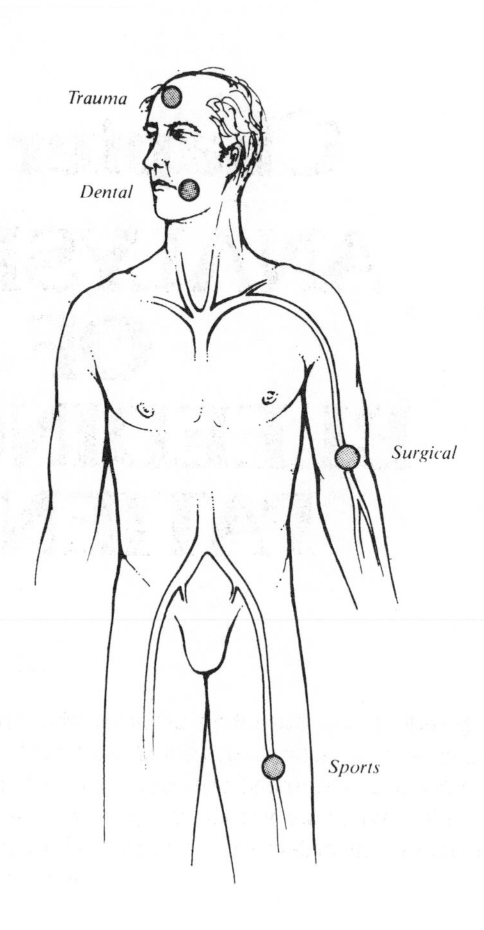

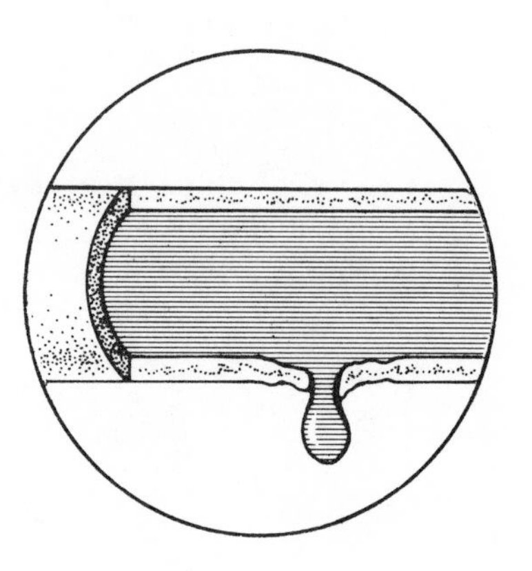

History of Bleeding?

Vascular Integrity is evaluated best by a good history. This applies not only to the preoperative patient, but to the postoperative bleeding patient as well. In the preoperative period, the following bleeding history is informative:

Neonatal period:	circumcision birth trauma
Childhood period:	dental procedures surgical procedures trauma during play
Teenage period:	sports injuries
Adulthood:	bleeding during childbirth bleeding during surgery bleeding from trauma

1. VASCULAR INTEGRITY
2. PLATELETS
3. COAGULATION CASCADE
4. CLOT LYSIS

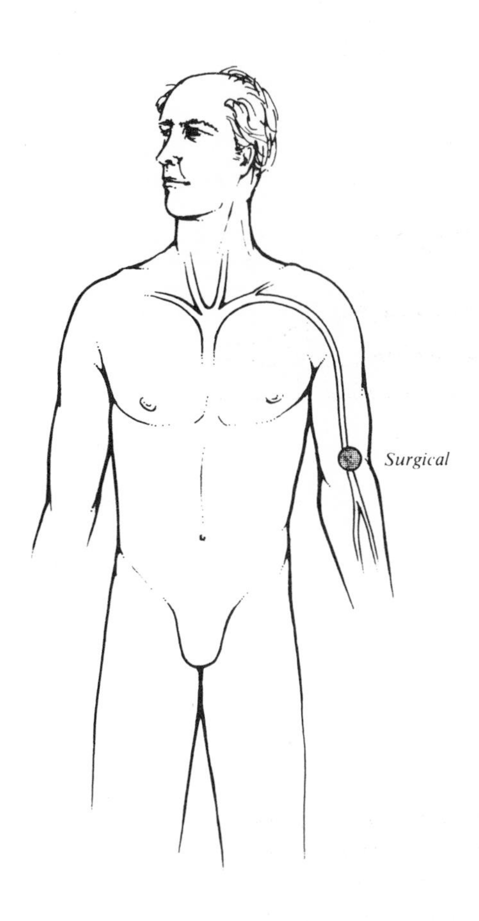

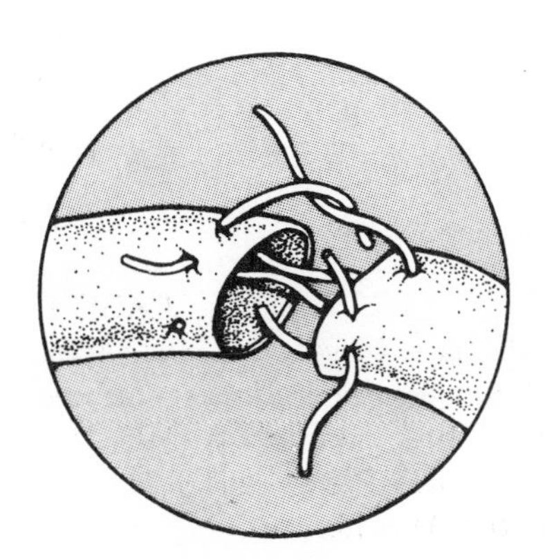

In the postoperative period, the history of inadequate suture placement, or inadequate inspection may be important. **Suspicion** is the key to success. The diagnosis also may be one of exclusion. That is—if platelet or factor deficiencies are ruled out by appropriate testing, the patient has a **suture deficiency**.

Various diagnostic tests may aid in the confirmation of inadequacies of vascular integrity. Certainly, direct inspection serves the anesthesiologist or surgeon well. Additional studies, such as angiography, "CAT" scanning, ultrasound, endoscopy, etc. may hasten a correct diagnosis of inadequate vascular integrity.

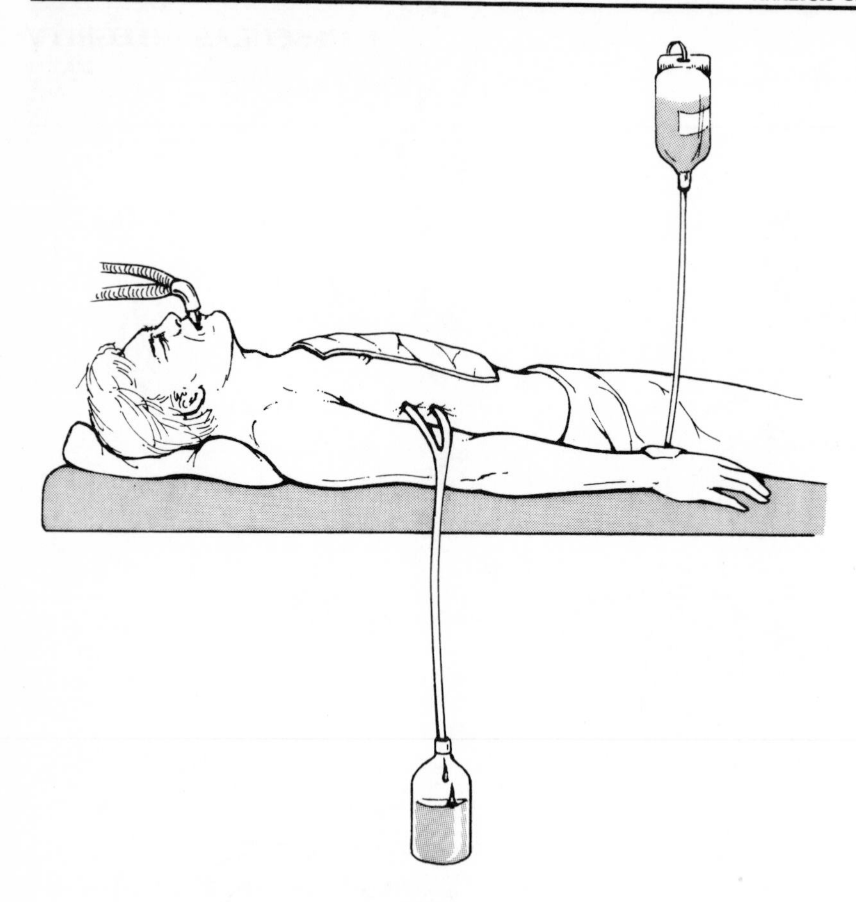

CASE 1

C.P.B. is a 44 year old white male with coronary artery disease. Three hours ago, he underwent an uneventful coronary artery bypass grafting of three coronary vessels. The cardiopulmonary bypass time was 52 minutes. Preoperatively he was receiving only propranolol. He has no bleeding history.

Postoperatively his chest tube output continues at 450 ml/hour, and is showing no signs of decreasing. His vital signs are stable, with continuing transfusions of blood to match his losses.

Preop: Hct 47%
Platelet count 280,000/mm^3
aPTT and PT—normal

Postop: Hct 36%
Platelet count 210,000/mm^3
Bleeding time 5.1 minutes
aPTT 34.1 seconds (normal)
PT 72% (normal)

Where is the bleeding defect?

____

1. VASCULAR INTEGRITY
2. PLATELETS
3. COAGULATION CASCADE
4. CLOT LYSIS

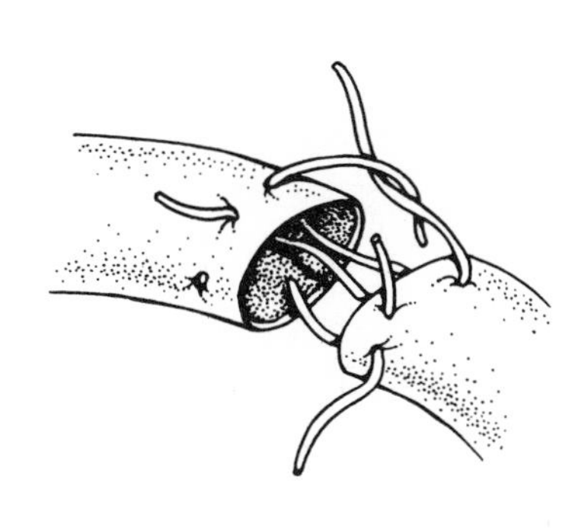

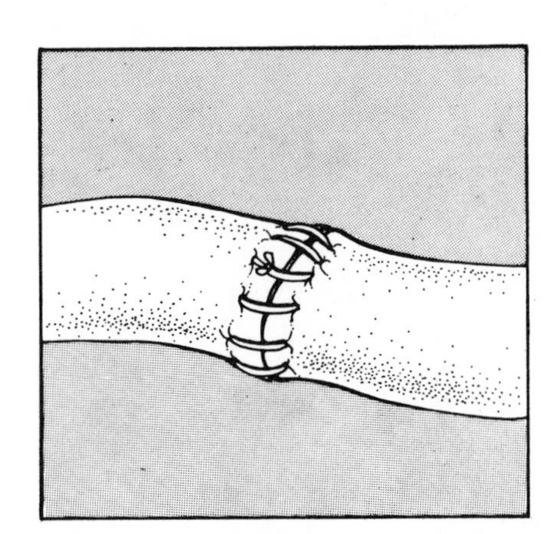

CASE 1 (continued)

Vascular integrity?	Losses are high, suspicion should be high. No other bleeding sites are seen. Preoperative history is normal.
Platelets?	Qualitatively and quantitatively normal.
Coagulation cascade?	Normal aPTT (intrinsic) Normal PT (extrinsic) (no heparin effect)
Clot lysis?	No signs of consumption of platelets nor factors, nor generalized lysis.

The defect is in vascular integrity. (C.P.B. was taken to the operating room, where a bleeding bypass graft was sutured, and his recovery was thereafter uneventful.)

1. VASCULAR INTEGRITY
2. PLATELETS
3. COAGULATION CASCADE
4. CLOT LYSIS

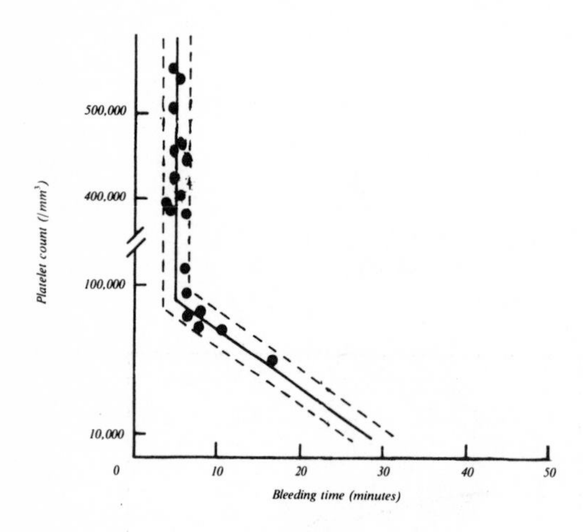

BLEEDING TIME

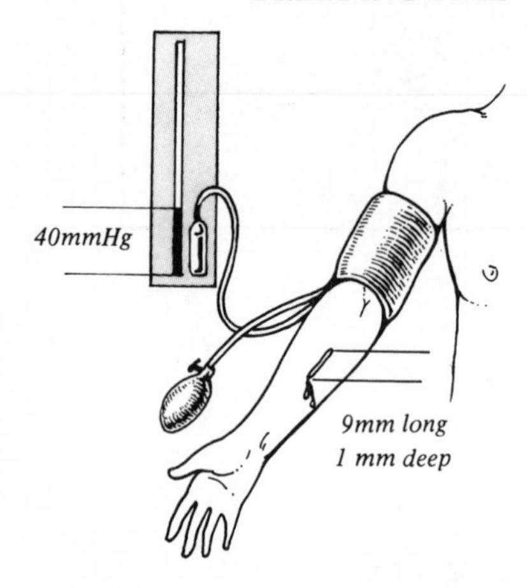

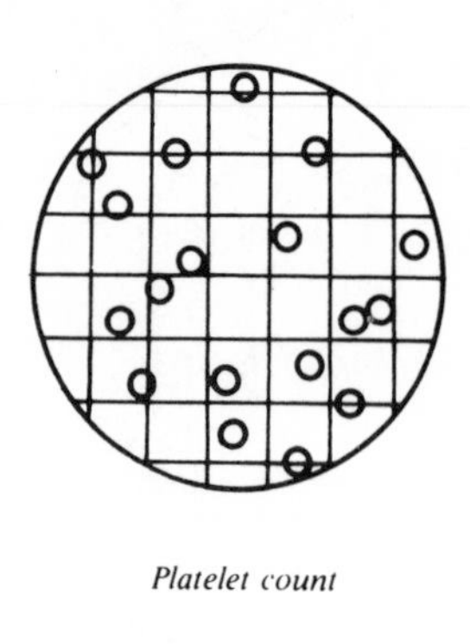

Platelet count

Platelets are assessed in the operative or perioperative period by two evaluations—quantitatively by the platelet count, and qualitatively by the bleeding time. Platelets can be deficient in number, or quality, or both.

The bleeding time can be difficult to perform in the operative setting, but a **crude index** to the bleeding time may be seen in the surgical wound. The platelet count can be performed by the laboratory in a few minutes. A platelet count of greater than 100,000/mm³, **if of reasonable quality**, is usually sufficient for hemostasis. Remember that drugs, such as aspirin can substantially impair platelet quality, even if platelets are available in sufficient number.

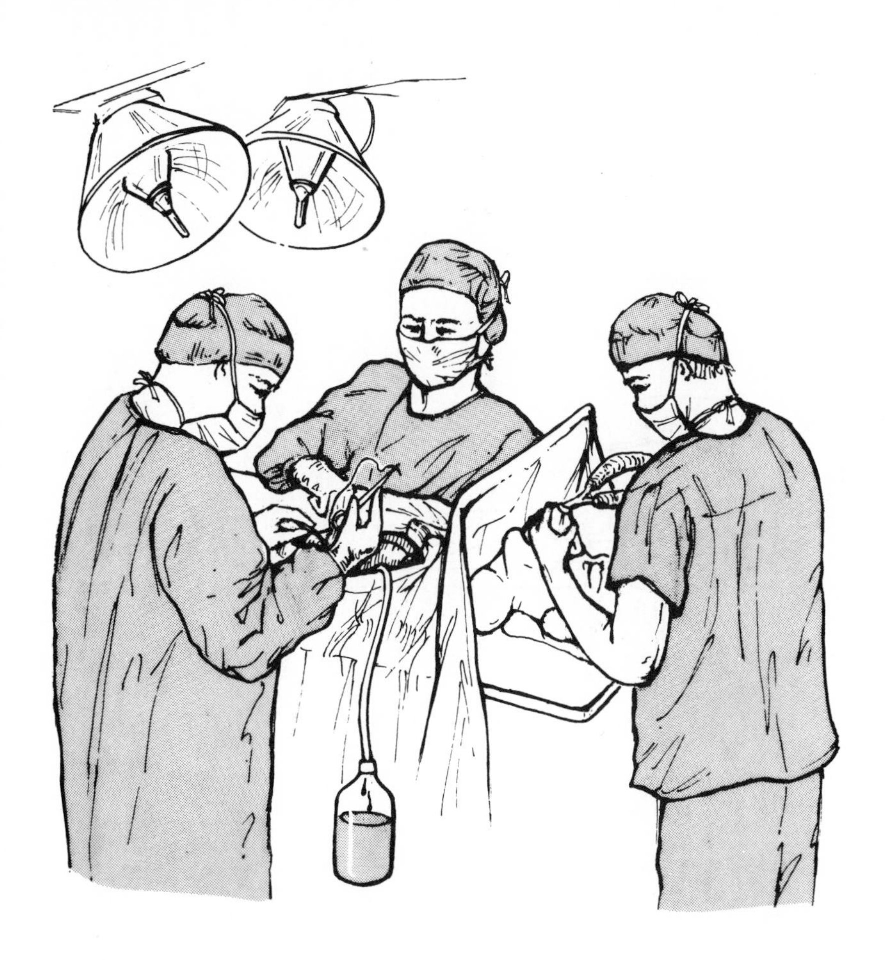

CASE 2

P.L. is a 58 year old woman admitted to the hospital for a left mastectomy two years previously without problems. She has no other abnormal history.

Preop:	Hct 32%
	Platelet count 45,000/mm^3
	aPTT 32 seconds (normal)
	PT 90% (normal)

At her second operation, bleeding is a major problem.

Intraoperative:	Hct 26%
	Platelet count 35,000/mm^3
	aPTT 34 seconds
	PT 86%

Where is the bleeding defect?

____

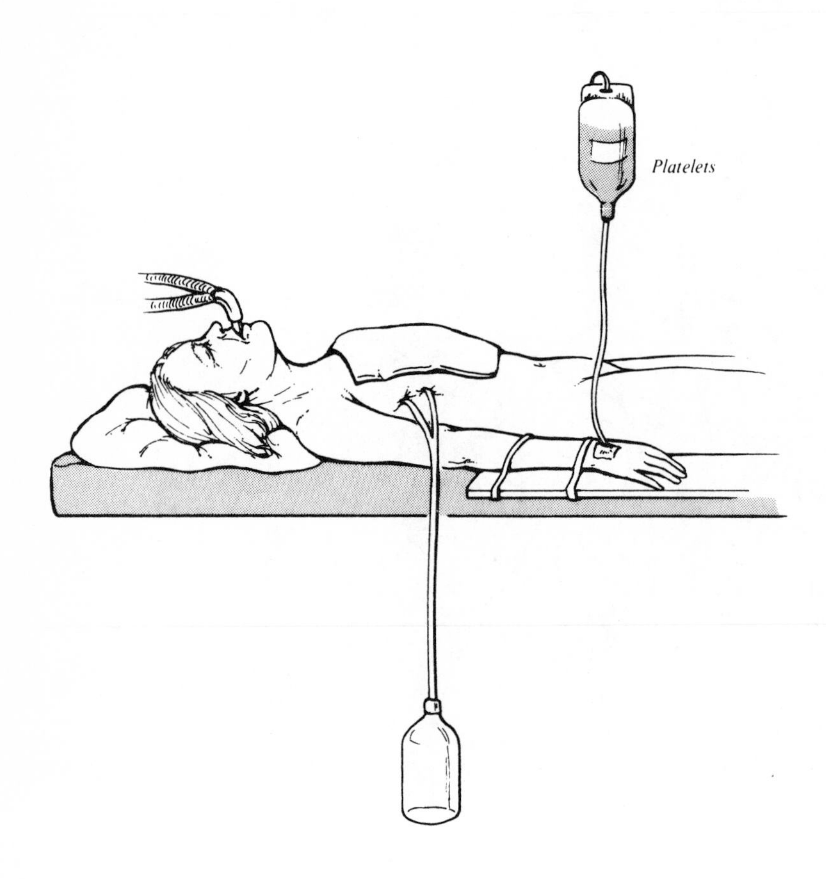

CASE 2 (continued)

Vascular integrity?	No obvious surgical holes nor open vessels at operation.
Platelets?	Count is low (confirming preoperative platelet deficit).
Coagulation cascade?	aPTT normal (intrinsic) PT normal (extrinsic)
Clot lysis?	No oozing from other sites. No consumption evident in coagulation proteins.

(P.L. had a deficient **number** of platelets. She was given six platelet packs intraoperatively, and the bleeding stopped. She should have had them preoperatively.)

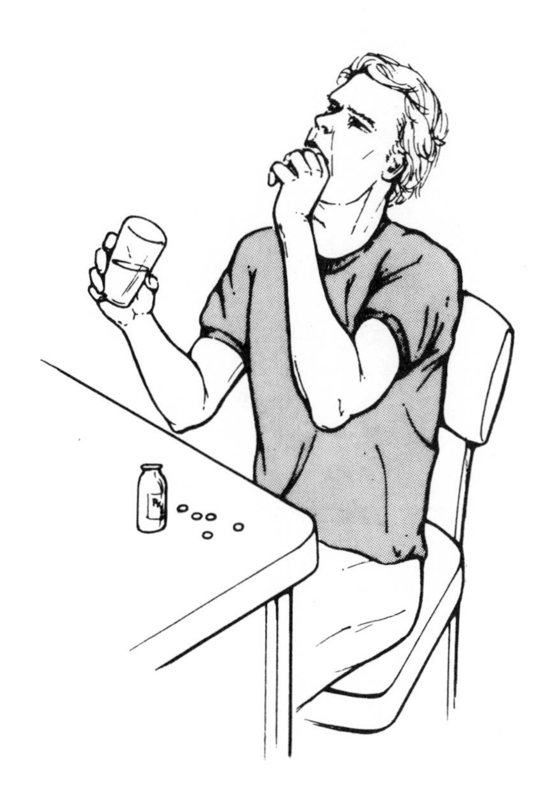

CASE 3

A.S.A. is a 42 year old male with a compressed lumbar disc, scheduled for lumbar laminectomy and discectomy. His only significant history is that of tension headaches occurring every few days, for which he ingests six Excedrin® tablets for relief on the days of headache.

His preoperative laboratory examinations disclose:

Hct	47%
Platelet count	310,000/mm^3
Bleeding time	14 minutes
aPTT	33 seconds
PT	90%

Where is his (potential) bleeding defect?

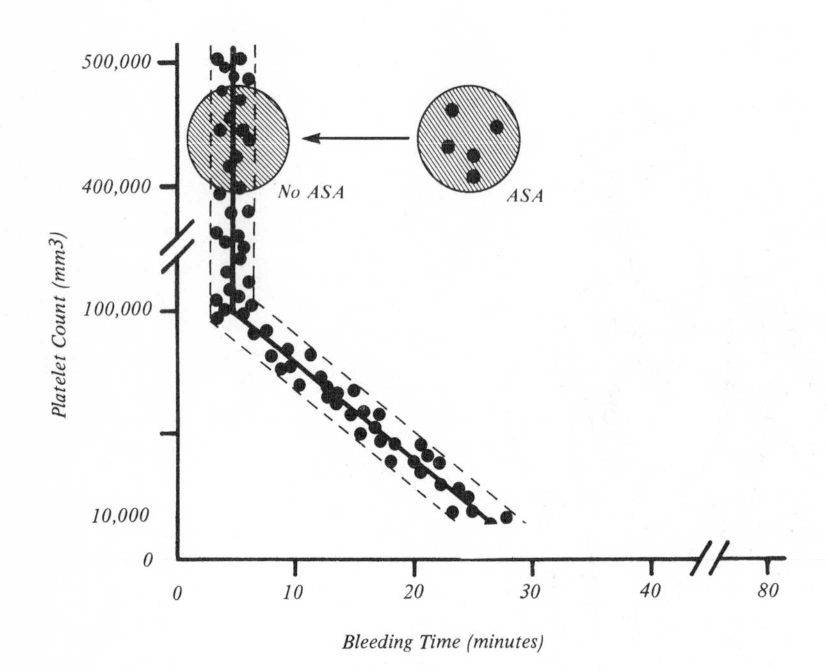

CASE 3 (continued)

Vascular integrity?	No obvious problems seen.
Platelets?	Count is normal. Bleeding time is prolonged (why?)
Coagulation cascade?	aPTT normal (intrinsic) PT normal (extrinsic)
Clot lysis?	(no tests ordered)

Should surgery be delayed? Yes—A.S.A. was sent home, and requested to take no more medications containing aspirin. He complied, and two weeks later, he had an uneventful laminectomy and discectomy (with a preoperative bleeding time of 5.1 minutes).

[Note—In an emergency, with a prolonged bleeding time due to aspirin ingestion, several platelet units can be administered to assist in the platelet aggregation process. Not ideal, nor inexpensive, but sufficient for **emergency** conditions.]

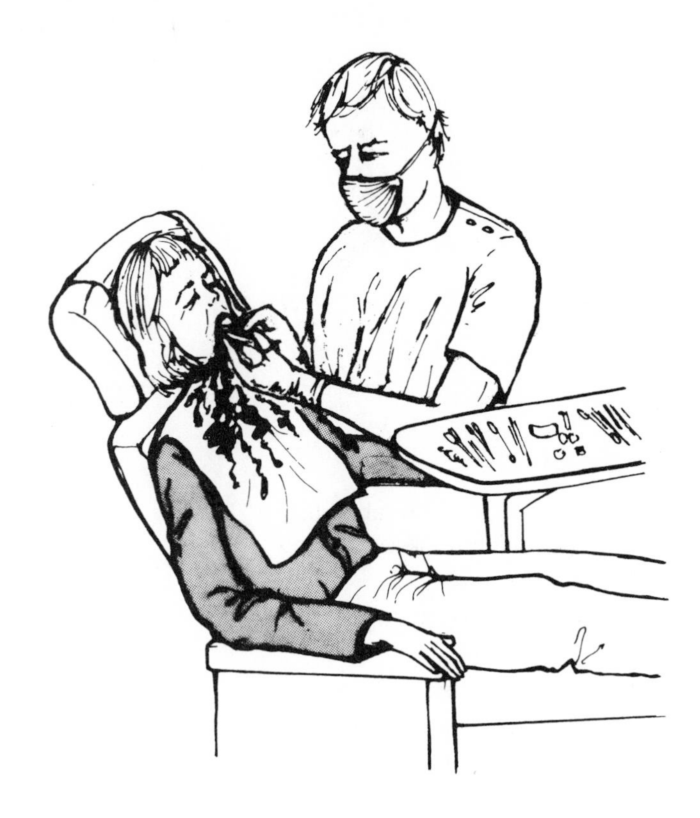

CASE 4

V.W. is a 39 year old female, who presents to the hospital emergency room with fever and right lower quadrant abdominal pain. She is not pregnant and takes no drugs. Her surgeon desires to perform an emergency appendectomy.

She has an unusual history, however. During tonsillectomy at age 8, she bled excessively, and required some type of blood transfusion. Excessive bleeding occurred again at age 17, during extraction of wisdom teeth. Preoperative laboratory work at this hospitalization demonstrates the following:

Hct	41%
Platelet count	190,000/mm^3
Bleeding time	18 minutes
aPTT	38.7 seconds/control 37.9 seconds
PT	74%

Where is the (potential) defect, and why? Should surgery commence immediately?

1. VASCULAR INTEGRITY
2. PLATELETS
3. COAGULATION CASCADE
4. CLOT LYSIS

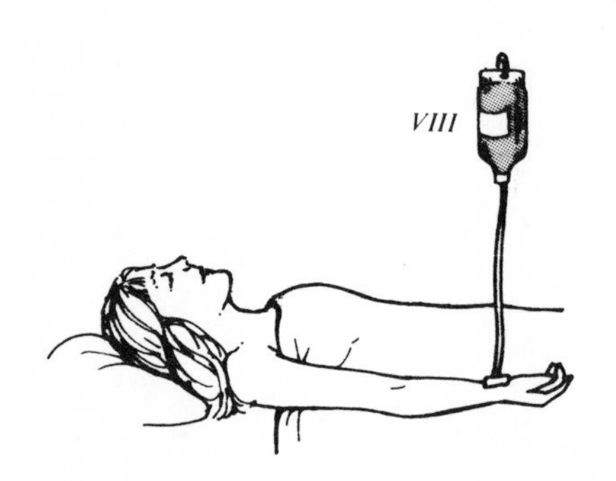

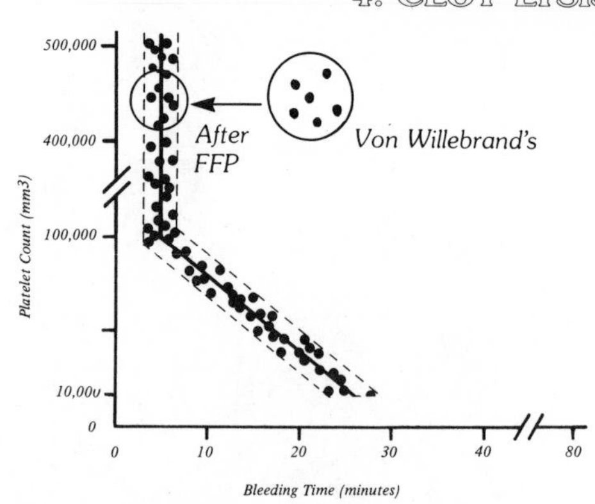

CASE 4 (continued)

This patient is more tricky than patient A.S.A. The laboratory work appears similar, but with a significantly different history. [Keep your guard up—the history is important!]

Vascular integrity?	No obvious large vessels damaged, nor trauma history.
Platelets?	Count is normal BUT bleeding time is greatly prolonged, and she is taking no drugs.
Coagulation cascade?	aPTT is normal (intrinsic). PT is normal (extrinsic). BUT could there still be a coagulation protein problem?
Clot lysis?	(No tests ordered; consumption of factors or platelets appears unlikely.)

On the basis of a hunch, and a similar patient eight years previously, the anesthesiologist requested a factor VIII level. It was returned as 20% of normal. The patient had Von Willebrand's disease, a **qualitative**, functional platelet deficit occurring with a concomitant reduction in factor VIII activity. The stress of surgery, and some bleeding could have easily further reduced the factor VIII activity into the bleeding range.

She was given cryoprecipitate and fresh frozen plasma, and received an uneventful appendectomy. The administration of the factor VIII in cryoprecipitate or fresh frozen plasma is sufficient for hemostasis, including the qualitative platelet deficit, as it contains "stimulating agents" for platelet aggregation. Platelet administration is not usually necessary. [As you can see, not all patients have single, isolated deficits, but most do.]

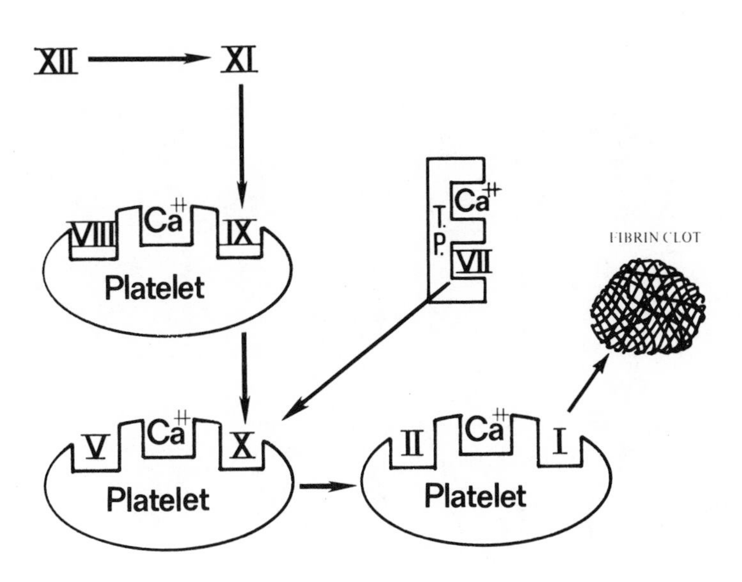

The coagulation cascade can be abnormal because of a variety of conditions. Phospholipids may not be present, factors may be deficient, and inhibitors (natural or otherwise) may alter the cascade. We'll remind you of the information learned under disorders of the coagulation cascade:

Inactive Factor Disorders

Hereditary — factors VIII, IX, or XI

Acquired — Antibodies to various factors

- — coumadin therapy
- — vitamin K deficiency
- — liver disease

} factors II, VII, IX, and X

- — consumptive or dilutional processes

} factors V, VIII and fibrinogen

Active Factor Deficiencies

Inhibition by heparin (working via AT-3 to "tie up" thrombin and other activated serine proteases)

Inhibition by fibrin split products

Remember that the intrinsic pathway is tested by the aPTT or ACT. The extrinsic pathway is tested by the PT. And the final stages are tested by the fibrinogen level, thrombin time, and occasionally the reptilase time.

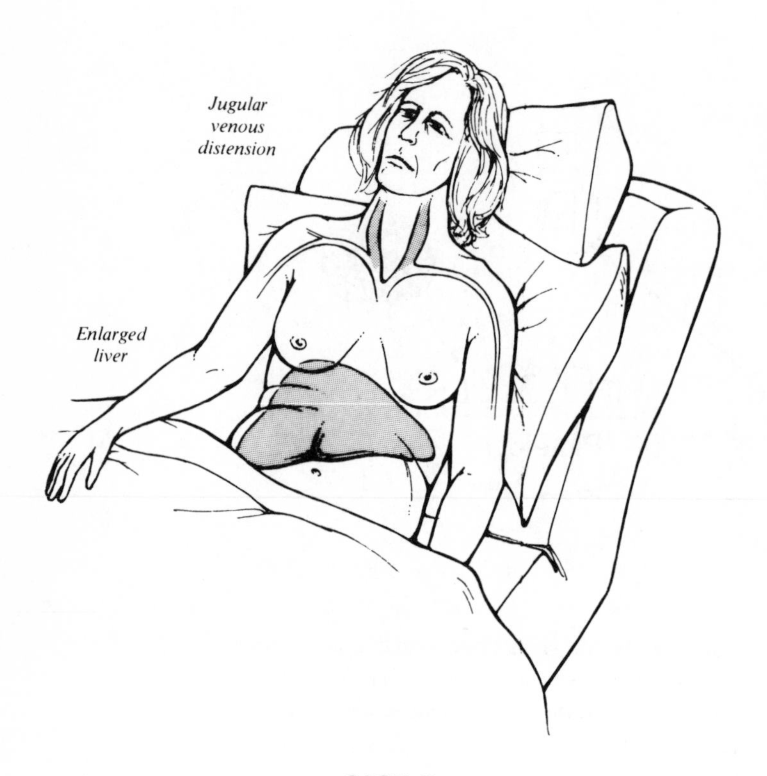

CASE 5

M.R. is a 48 year old woman admitted to the hospital for surgical correction of severe mitral valve insufficiency (regurgitation). Exercise intolerance is present, and signs of biventricular cardiac failure are evident. She displays an enlarged liver, and jugular venous distension. She has no history of a bleeding disorder. Medications being taken are digoxin and diuretics.

Her preoperative laboratory work demonstrates:

Hct	36%
Platelet count	210,000/mm^3
aPTT	33 seconds (control 35 sec)
PT	37%

She is taken to the operating room, and a mitral valve replacement performed. Do you think the timing of her surgery is wise?

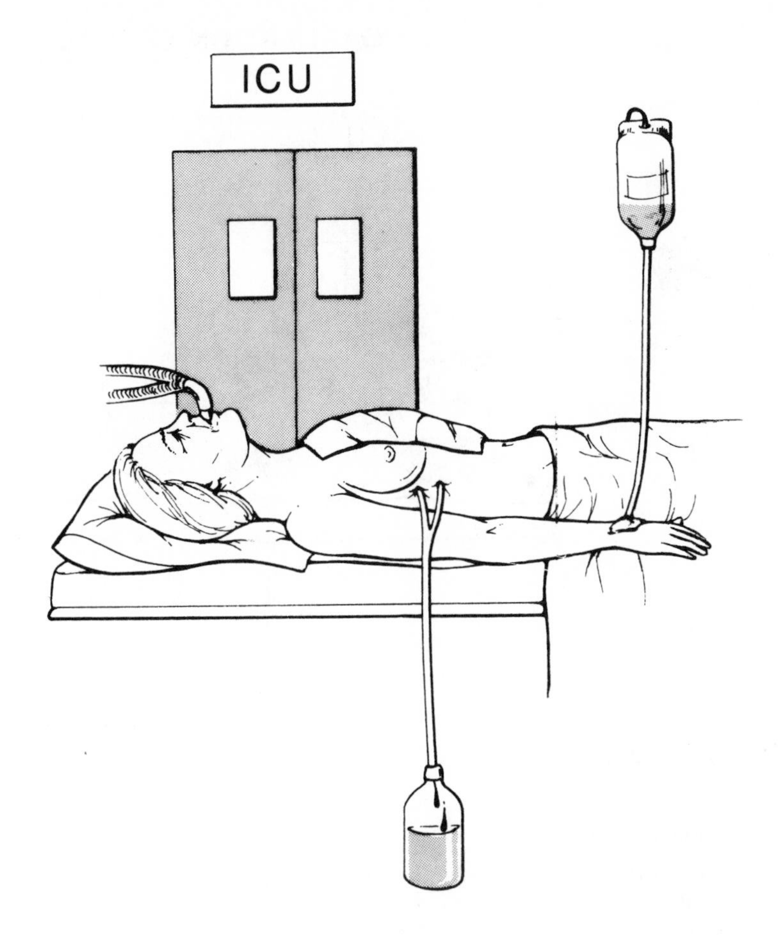

CASE 5 (continued)

M.R. received large doses of protamine in the operating room to stop bleeding, but to no avail. She continued to ooze from every surgical site in the I.C.U. Two hour postoperative laboratory values were as follows:

Hct	28%
Platelet count	145,000/mm^3
Bleeding time	6.2 minutes
aPTT	46 seconds (control 33.5 seconds)
PT	21%
Thrombin time	normal
Fibrinogen level	225%

Where is the defect? Why is she continuing to bleed? What can be done?

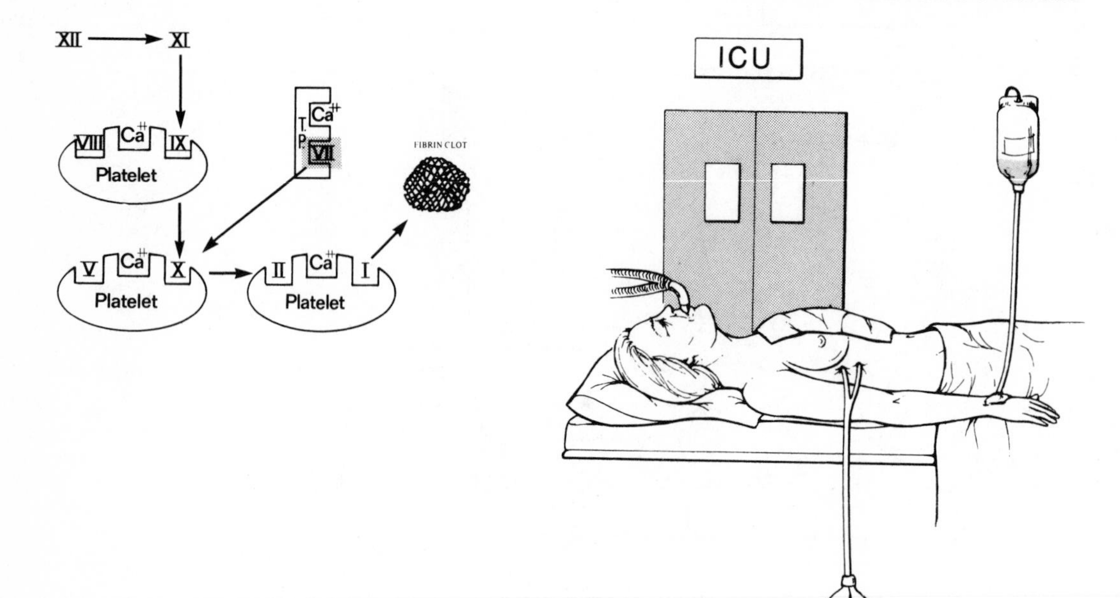

CASE 5 (continued)

Vascular integrity?	No obvious surgical holes. And multiple wounds are bleeding.
Platelets?	Platelet count is normal. Bleeding time is normal.
Coagulation cascade?	aPTT is slightly abnormal (intrinsic) PT is abnormal (extrinsic) Thrombin time is normal
Clot lysis?	No consumption of platelets nor fibrinogen.

The defect is basically in the extrinsic system. Factor VII is reduced by her liver disease to a level consistent with clinical bleeding. A further prolongation of the PT has occurred intraoperatively during banked blood transfusion, since bank blood is dificient in the labile factors VIII and V. This accounts for the slightly abnormal aPTT as well. The thrombin time is normal, ruling out heparin effect as a cause of bleeding or a cause for the abnormal aPTT and PT. (Because of the vascular congestion in her liver, from cardiac failure, the administration of Vitamin K will be of little value. She was given fresh frozen plasma, along with vasodilators to allow for the volume of fresh frozen plasma, and had an uneventful postoperative course. Her aPTT and PT returned to normal.)

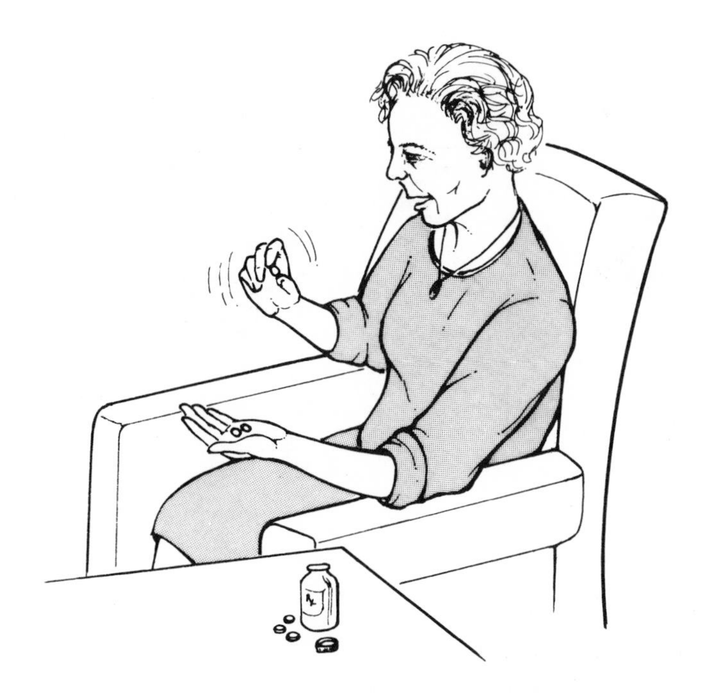

CASE 6

M.S. is a 69 year old woman admitted to the hospital for semi-elective mitral valve replacement. She has had a long-standing mitral stenosis, complicated recently by two apparently embolic strokes. She received a mitral commissurotomy 10 years ago. She is now receiving coumadin therapy, and has no residual central nervous system problems. She has no present bleeding history. She also receives digoxin, but has no signs of congestive failure. Her preoperative laboratory values are as follows:

Hct	35%
Platelet count	185,000/mm^3
Bleeding time	5.6 minutes
aPTT	43 seconds (control 33 seconds)
PT	11%
Thrombin time	normal

Is M.S. ready to receive her mitral valve replacement?

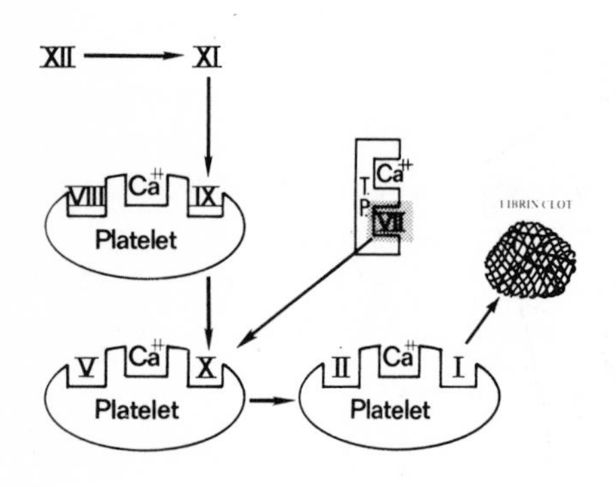

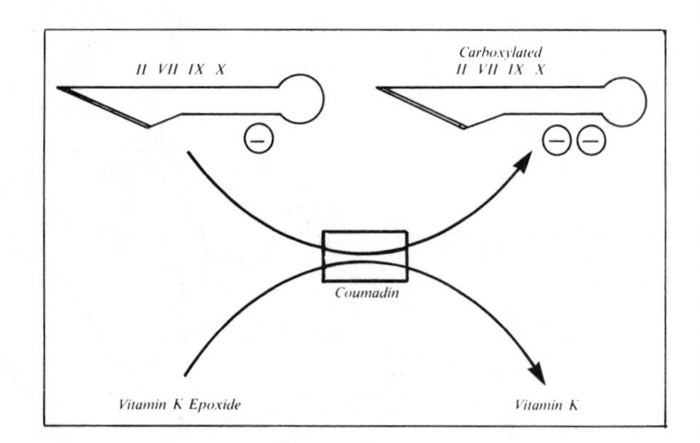

CASE 6 (continued)

No. Let us evaluate her coagulation status:

Vascular integrity?	No obvious problems. No carotid bruits are heard. Emboli appear to come from the heart.
Platelets?	Normal platelet count. Normal bleeding time.
Coagulation cascade?	aPTT is slightly abnormal PT is markedly abnormal Thrombin time is normal
Clot lysis?	No tests ordered (No abnormalities suspected.)

The problem is her coumadin therapy. The markedly abnormal PT is caused by a profound Factor VII deficiency. Other factor decreases are seen in the slightly abnormal aPTT. But anticoagulation is necessary in hopes of preventing additional emboli from the heart. On the other hand, she'll have a fairly prolonged surgery (because of her "re-do" status), and bleeding will be greatly increased. Correction of the PT intraoperatively will be frought with difficulty. What is the proper approach?

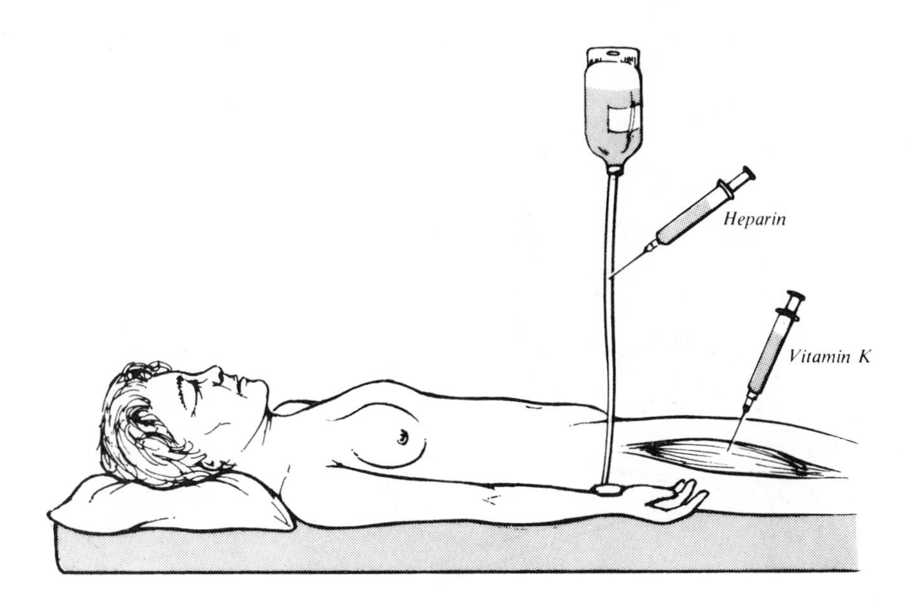

CASE 6 (continued)

Clearly she needs to be anticoagulated for embolic protection. But she also needs to have her inactive (liver-produced) factors nearer to normal concentration.

The correct approach is to switch her coumadin therapy to heparin therapy, thereby continuing her "embolic protection", but giving her liver a chance to produce factors II, VII, IX, and X. **Judicious** use of vitamin K facilitates the process of factor production.

M.S. was maintained on intravenous heparin therapy for three days, without coumadin administration. Heparin dosage was adjusted so that her aPTT was maintained at 2-2½ times control, each specimen being drawn for testing just prior to her next heparin dose. This required a heparin dosage of 7500 units each four hours.

The PT returned to her normal value of 74%, (this dosage of heparin producing a two-fold increase in the aPTT does not affect appreciably the PT.) She then underwent an uneventful mitral valve replacement, with removal of left atrial clot. Her post-bypass course required the administration of three units of fresh frozen plasma, and four platelet packs.

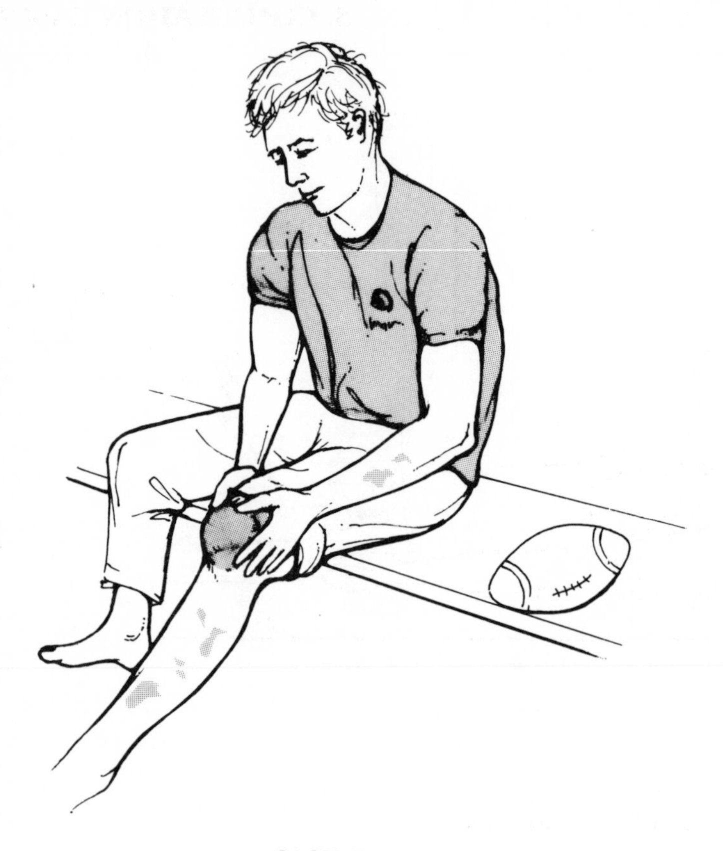

CASE 7

H.A. is an 18 year old college student who presents to the emergency room with a swollen left knee. He was recently playing touch football. He is in excellent health, and takes no medications. Upon questioning, he recalls heavy bleeding during a tooth extraction several months ago. His maternal uncle died mysteriously after a surgical procedure at age 20, said to be from bleeding.

Upon examination, numerous bruises over his legs and torso are evident. The left knee is warm, swollen, tender, and held in a fixed position.

His laboratory examinations demonstrate:

Hct	41%
Platelets	310,000/mm^3
Bleeding time	4.5 minutes
aPTT	50 seconds (control 32 seconds)
PT	100%

What defect do you suspect is present?

1. VASCULAR INTEGRITY
2. PLATELETS
3. COAGULATION CASCADE
4. CLOT LYSIS

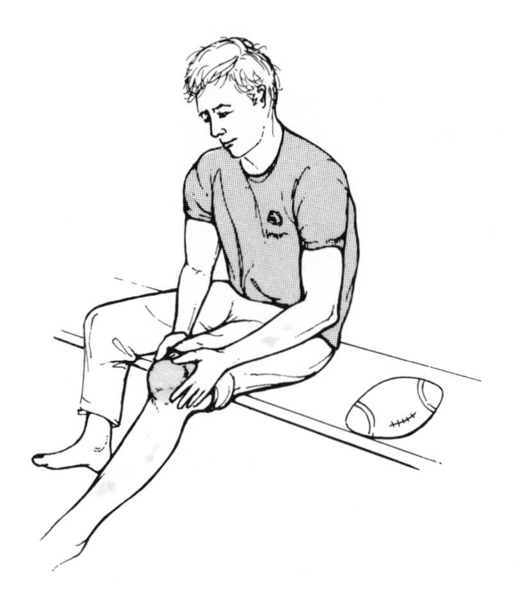

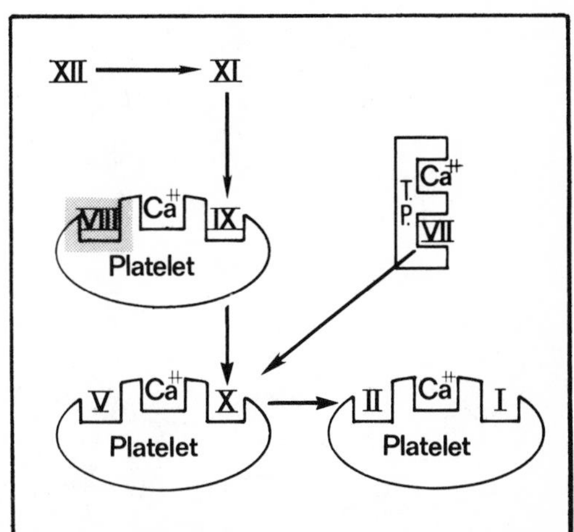

CASE 7 (continued)

Vascular integrity?	Perhaps. A broken major blood vessel in the knee could produce some of the physical signs, but **not** the abnormal laboratory values.
Platelets?	Normal platelet count. Normal bleeding time.
Coagulation cascade?	aPTT abnormal (why?). PT normal (extrinsic).
Clot lysis?	Perhaps on physical signs. However, no consumption of platelets or fibrinogen is evident (normal PT).

The defect is an isolated one.

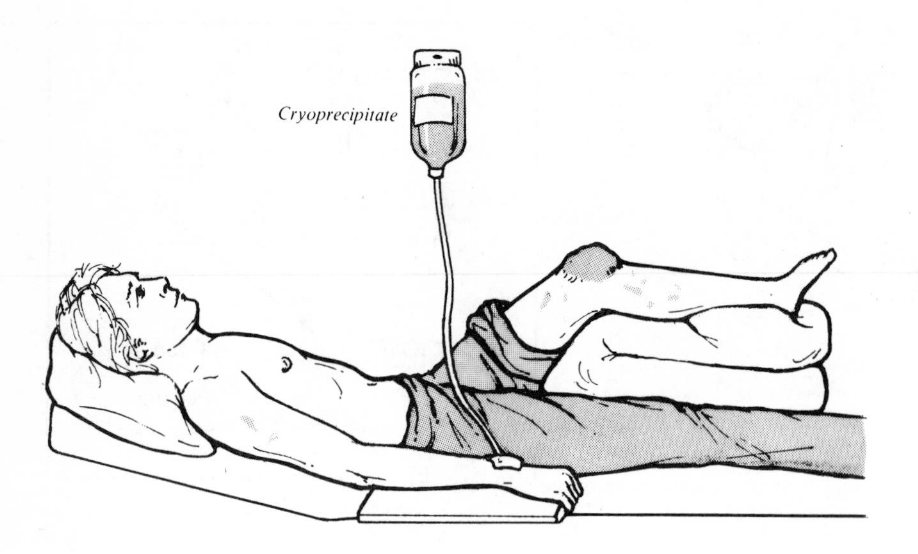

CASE 7 (continued)

H.A. clearly has a defect upon testing of the intrinsic system. His extrinsic and final common pathways are normal. Platelet quantity and quality are normal. Where exactly is the deficiency?

Without further testing, the exact cause of the deficiency can only be guessed. H.A.'s physician requested factor VIII and IX levels. Factor IX was normal, but factor VIII was 8% of normal. He has **hemophilia A**. Therapy with 4500 units of factor VIII via cryoprecipitate, plus orthopedic care of his knee, provided control of his injury. Continuity of care was provided by a hematologist.

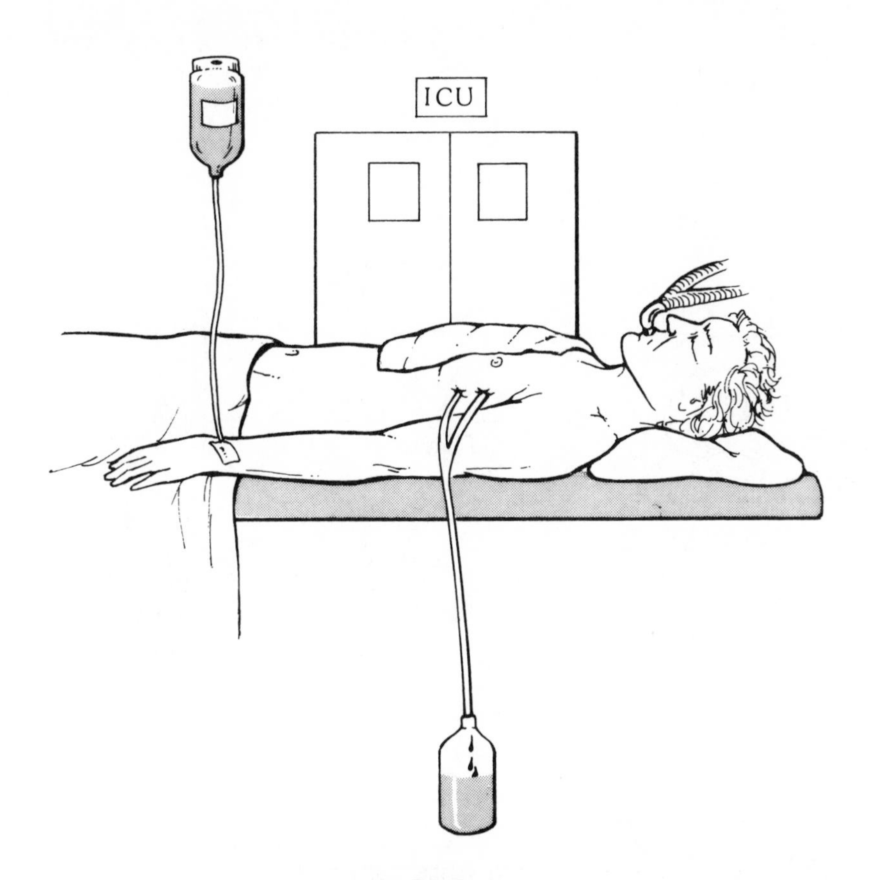

CASE 8

N.E.P. is a 38 year old male with aortic valvular insufficiency. He takes no routine medications, and has no history of bleeding. He exhibits no present signs of congestive heart failure, and has never been previously hospitalized.

After an uneventful aortic valve replacement with 28 minutes of cardiopulmonary bypass, he is transported to an intensive care unit (I.C.U.). The oozing seen during closure of the sternotomy is still evident in the I.C.U. His postoperative laboratory values demonstrate:

Hct	36%
Platelets	155,000/mm^3
Bleeding time	4.8 minutes
aPTT	78 seconds (control 34 seconds)
ACT	180 seconds (control 96 seconds)
PT	68%
Fibrinogen	290 mg%

Where is the defect?

1. VASCULAR INTEGRITY
2. PLATELETS
3. COAGULATION CASCADE
4. CLOT LYSIS

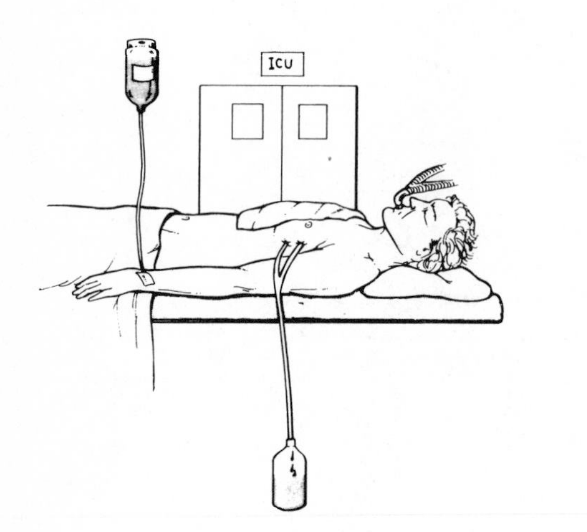

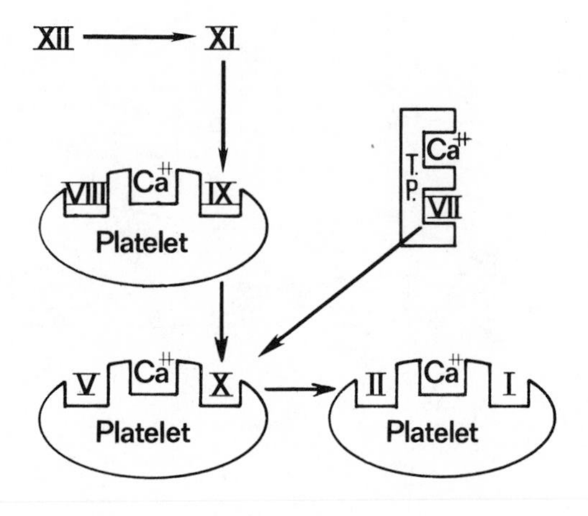

CASE 8 (continued)

Vascular integrity?	Perhaps. A loose suture, vessel damaged during closure, or aortic hole might cause the bleeding. (Keep this one as second chioce.)
Platelets?	Normal platelet count. Normal bleeding time.
Coagulation cascade?	aPTT, ACT — Intrinsic, abnormal PT (extrinsic, normal) Thrombin time ordered: 60 seconds (control, 15 seconds)
Clot lysis?	(No tests ordered.) Fibrinogen and platelets normal.

The addition of the thrombin time to testing in this patient pinpoints the problem in the last stage of fibrin formation, or in the intrinsic pathway as well. However, what is the most common intrinsic deficit in this group of surgical patients postoperatively, especially one which prolongs the thrombin time in the absence of obvious clot lysis?

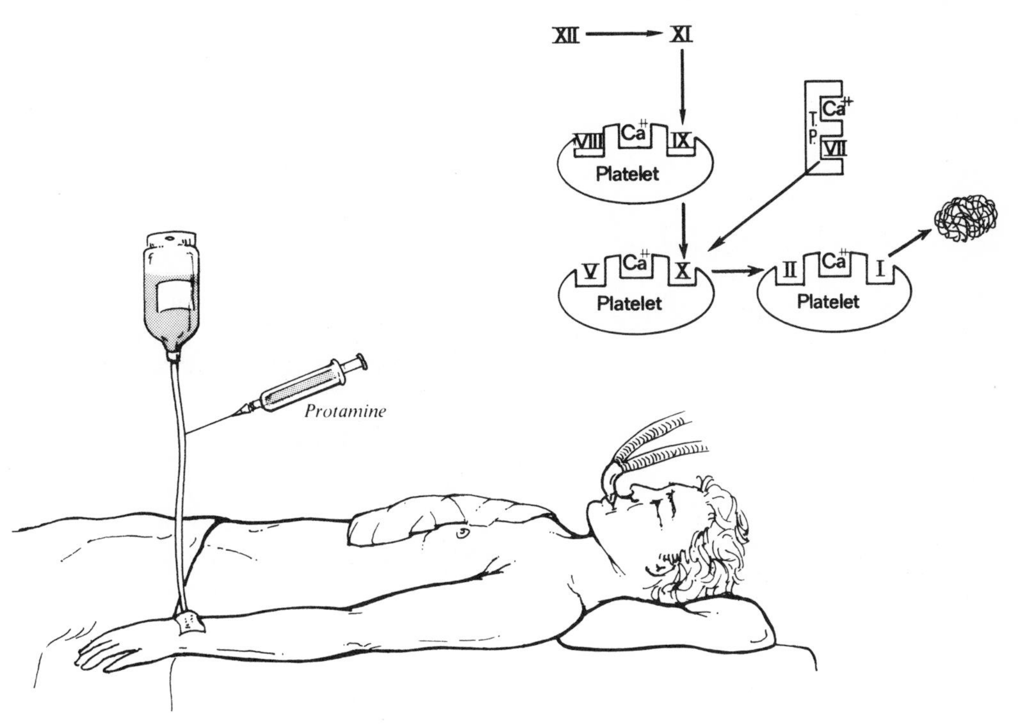

CASE 8 (continued)

Again, the history is important. In this hospital, heparin and protamine are administered in the operating room by a predetermined formula, not taking into account the individual requirements for these two drugs. This patient demonstrates all of the signs of **heparin** effect. Heparin's effect would prolong the aPTT and ACT. Heparin's effect on the thrombin time is consistent with the laboratory values. This case clearly demonstrates the value of the thrombin time in separating the effects of heparin from factor deficiencies. (A reptilase time, if performed for additional confirmation, would be normal, since heparin does not affect reptilase-R's ability to split fibrinogen.)

In the I.C.U., N.E.P. received a titration of protamine until the ACT was normal. The aPTT and thrombin time also returned to normal, and the patient's bleeding ceased. Failure to correctly use heparin and protamine scientifically in the operating room cost N.E.P. three extra units of blood, administered to cover bleeding losses. A plot of heparin and protamine versus the ACT, performed in the operating room would have prevented this from happening. (See Appendix on ACT and heparin plotting.)

1. VASCULAR INTEGRITY
2. PLATELETS
3. COAGULATION CASCADE
4. CLOT LYSIS

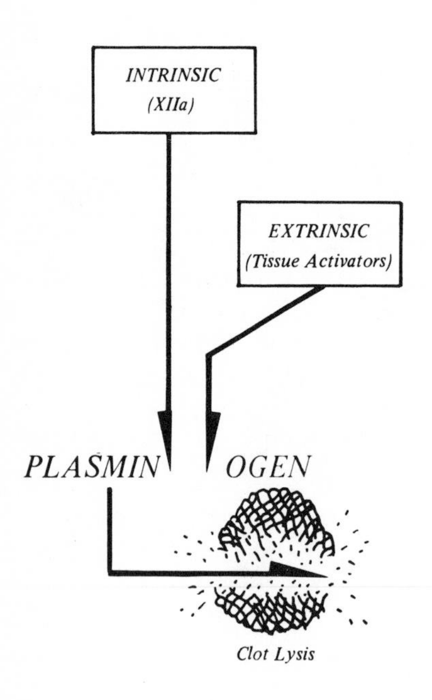

Clot Lysis

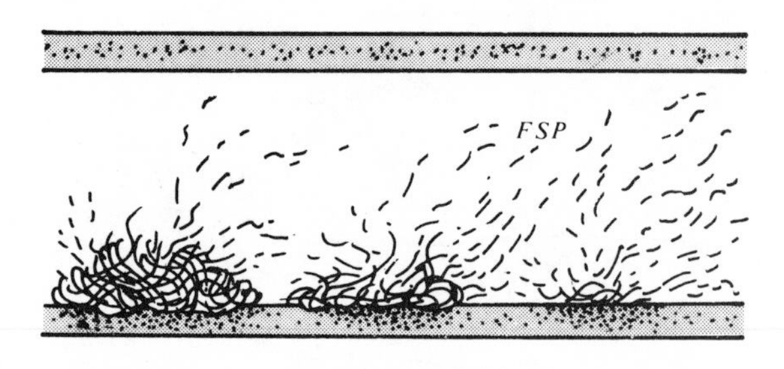

Clot Lysis

You will recall that clot lysis is necessary for the effective reestablishment of circulation in an injured area, occurring concomitantly with vascular healing. It is a parallel system to the coagulation cascade, but more simple. It has an intrinsic activator (XIIa), and extrinsic activators (tissue activators such as urokinase and streptokinase). When functioning normally, it is a routine, beneficial system.

The end product of the lytic system is plasmin, which may degrade either fibrin or fibrinogen into fibrin split products (FSP). These FSP are removed by hepatic Kupffer cells, and in high concentration may produce platelet dysfunction and inhibit fibrin cross-linking. The problem in clot lysis is when the system becomes excessively activated either by fibrinolytic activators, or by the excessive formation of fibrin, such as in DIC. If anti-plasmin is ineffective in controlling plasmin, and high concentrations of FSP are produced, coagulation disorders may result. These may include platelet dysfunction, platelet consumption, factor V, VIII, fibrinogen consumption, and inhibition of fibrin cross-linking.

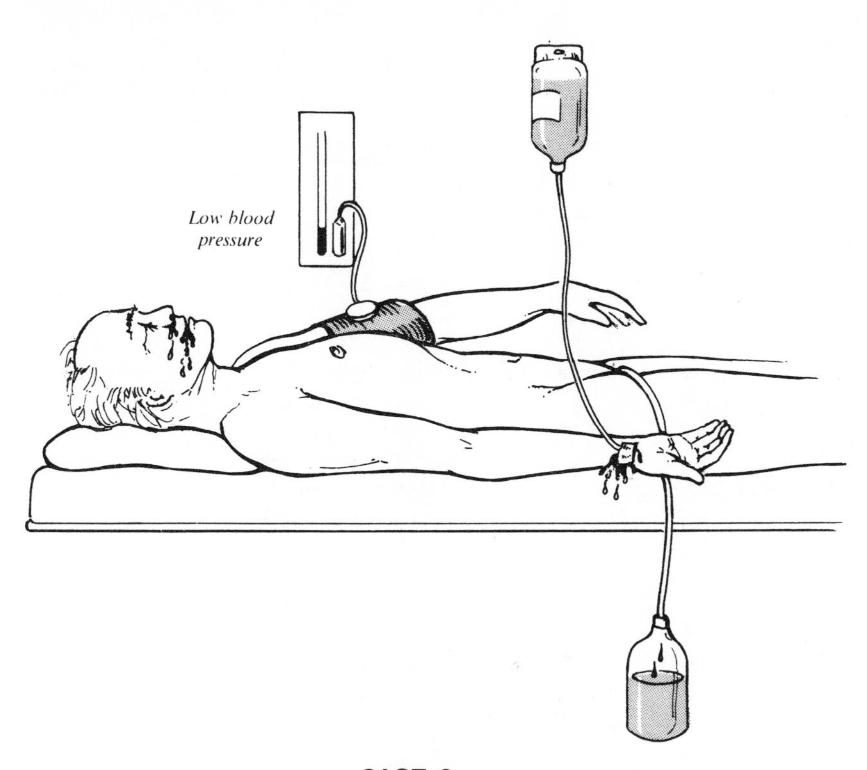

CASE 9

P.S. is a 78 year old male admitted for trans-urethral resection of the prostate (TURP). He has never been hospitalized, and takes no medications. Other than his age, he exhibits no signs of health problems. His routine preoperative laboratory results are:

PVCS	43%
Platelet count	360,000/mm^3
aPTT	34 seconds (control 35 seconds)
PT	92%

He received a TURP of 50 minutes duration, under uneventful spinal anesthesia. However the urologist commented at the conclusion of the procedure that there appeared to be much bleeding within the bladder and urethra. In the recovery room, the urine collecting bag was dark red, and the patient's arterial blood pressure lower than his normal. The patient was noted also to be oozing from his intravenous cannula site. Recovery room laboratory work demonstrates:

PCV	30%
Platelet count	240,000/mm^3
aPTT	60 seconds
PT	45%

What coagulation defect is present?

1. VASCULAR INTEGRITY
2. PLATELETS
3. COAGULATION CASCADE
4. CLOT LYSIS

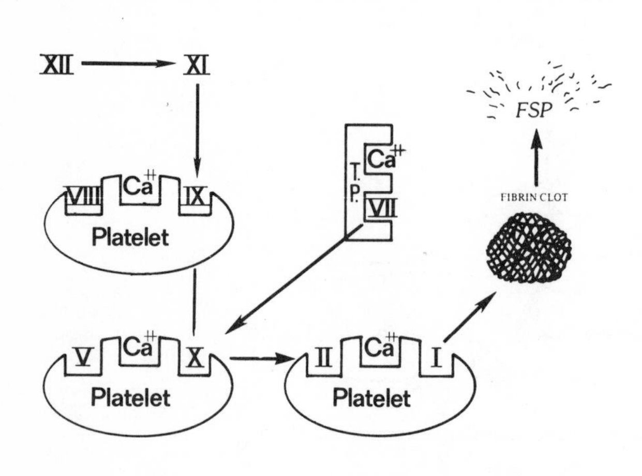

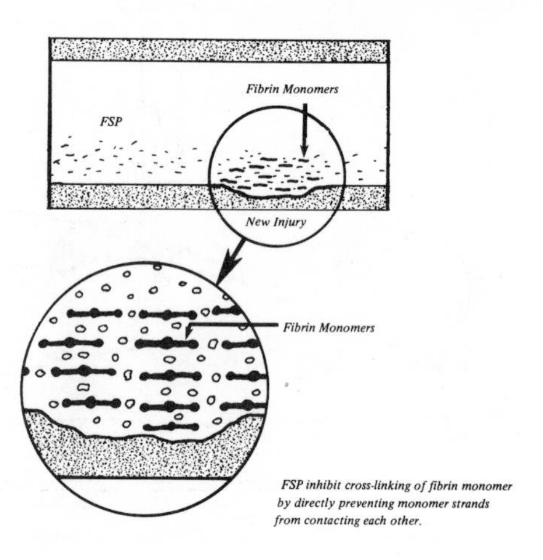

FSP inhibit cross-linking of fibrin monomer by directly preventing monomer strands from contacting each other.

CASE 9 (continued)

Vascular integrity?	Perhaps a number of open vessels in the surgical area, but this wouldn't alter the laboratory results.
Platelets?	Platelet count decreased, but not markedly. (Bleeding time performed—10.3 minutes).
Coagulation cascade?	aPTT prolonged. PT prolonged. (Thrombin time performed—prolonged twice normal.) (Reptilase time performed—normal)
Clot lysis?	Fibrin split products at 1:160 dilution

P.S. has developed the presence of fibrin split products (FSP). In addition, the intrinsic and extrinsic pathways, as well as the last step to fibrin formation, are impaired. There is platelet dysfunction despite adequate numbers. If the problem were consumption of factors V, VIII, and I, the aPTT, PT, and TT would all be abnormal, but the reptilase time would be abnormal as well. The reptilase time is **normal**, which is the usual case in the presence of FSP. Thus the reptilase time is a valuable addition in the analysis of disorders of the final step to fibrin formation.

P.S. developed a fibrinolytic state because of the release of urokinase during prostatic surgery. A hematologist was consulted in his care, and P.S. was treated with epsilon amino caproic acid (EACA) and blood transfusions. As the concentration of FSP decreased, his coagulation status normalized and the bleeding ceased.

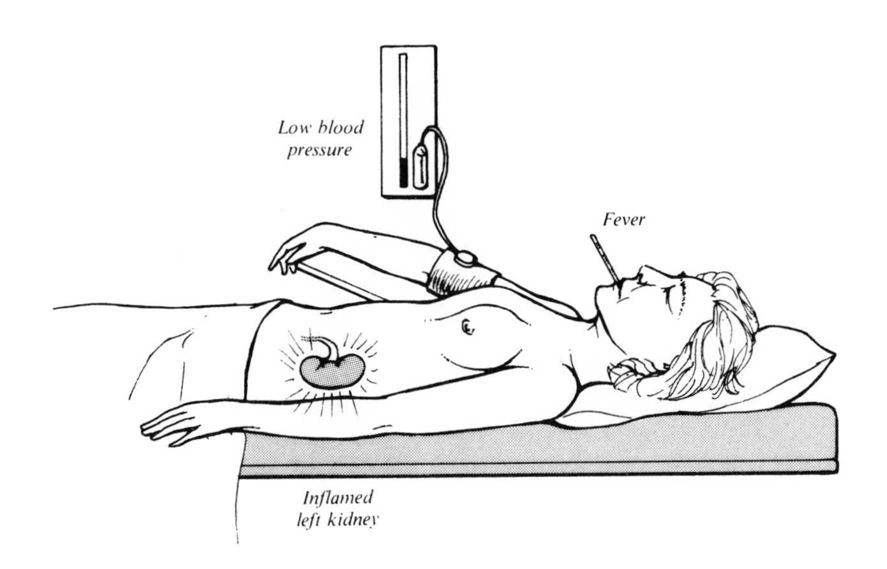

CASE 10

S.E.P. is a 47 year old woman admitted with a diagnosis of "fever of unknown origin". She was perfectly well until three days previously, when she noticed malaise, mild fever, abdominal pain, and midback pain. She has never been hospitalized and is taking no medications. The first night in the hospital the nurses note that she is diaphoretic, hypotensive, dyspneic, and has a temperature of 40°C. There is no urine output. She is treated with fluids, morphine, alcohol rubs, and oxygen. Her laboratory results demonstrate:

PCV	48%
Platelet count	80,000/mm^3
aPTT	56 seconds (control 34 seconds)
PT	38%
Fibrinogen level	95 mg%

She continues to deteriorate.

What is your further laboratory work, diagnosis, and treatment?

1. VASCULAR INTEGRITY
2. PLATELETS
3. COAGULATION CASCADE
4. CLOT LYSIS

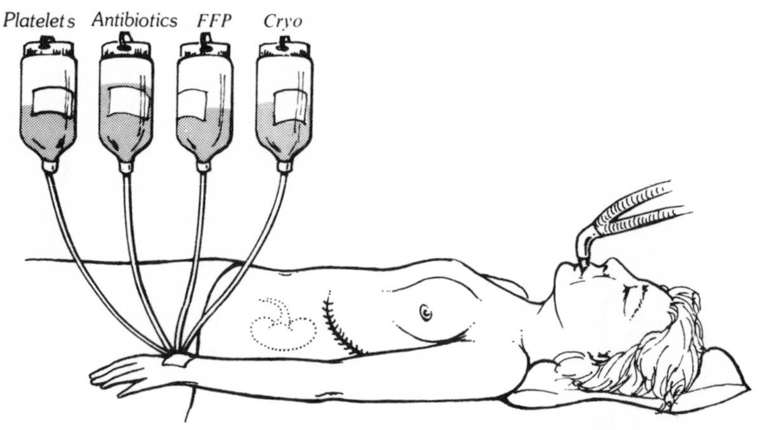

CASE 10 (continued)

Vascular integrity?	Abdomen not enlarging, but tender. ECG within normal limits. Chest x-ray within normal limits.
Platelets?	Platelet count decreased (repeat study 55,000/mm^3). Bleeding time performed: 25 minutes
Coagulation cascade?	aPTT abnormal (intrinsic) PT abnormal (extrinsic) Fibrinogen decreased (repeated at 80 mg%) (Thrombin time performed: three times normal)
Clot lysis?	Fibrin split products 1:320
Urinalysis?	Cloudy, with gram negative rods on smear

This patient is in septic shock of renal origin. All studies indicate a consumptive process (factors V, VIII, fibrinogen, and platelets). The cause of this disseminated process has been located. S.E.P. is treated with antibiotics, fluids, surgical removal of an infected left kidney, and the administration of platelets, fresh frozen plasma, and cryoprecipitate. She makes a full recovery.

This case demonstrates the necessity of locating and treating vigorously the underlying cause of the process of DIC, as well as supportive and replacement therapy.

The flow sheet on the previous two pages summarizes an analytical approach to the bleeding patient. If these steps are followed in order, a clear picture should emerge demonstrating the disorder(s), and suggesting treatment. A word of caution regarding interpretation is warranted.

If the bleeding time, ACT or aPTT, and PT are all **normal**, and the patient is still bleeding, one (or more) of three circumstances is usually present:

1. There are surgical holes! (That is, a defect in vascular integrity exists, occasionally the diagnosis by exclusion.) This will require surgical repair, and no amount of "coagulation therapy" will solve this problem.
2. The patient is hypothermic, and the tests such as the ACT, aPTT, and PT (run **in vitro** at 37°C) do **not** represent the **in vivo** conditions. Either warm the patient, and/or retest the patient with the tests run at the patient's lower temperature, to confirm a hypothermic coagulopathy.
3. The laboratory tests are in error.

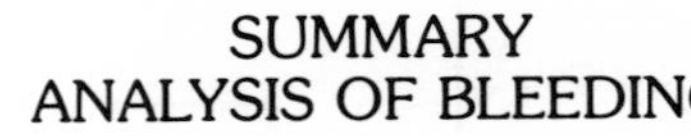
SUMMARY
ANALYSIS OF BLEEDING

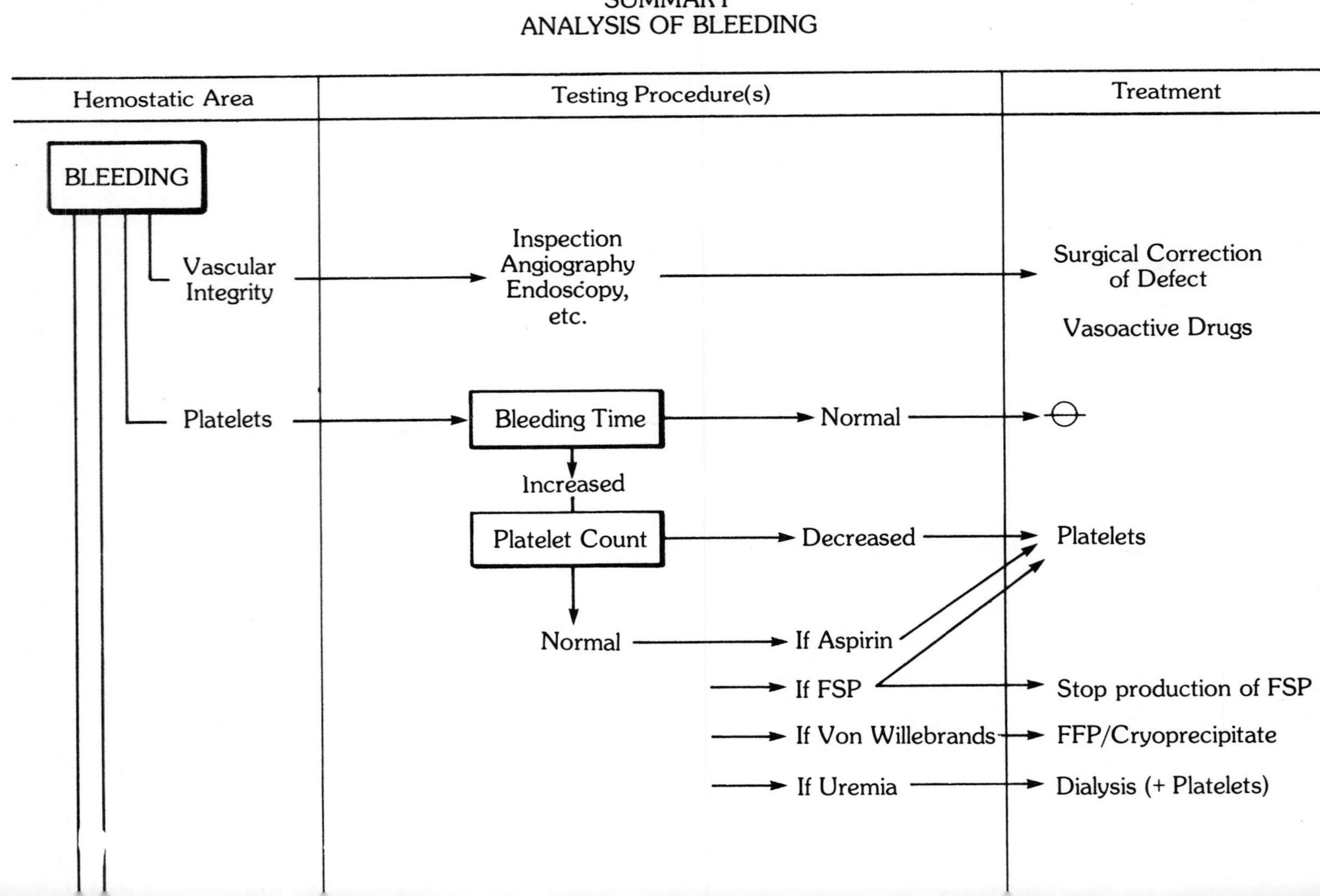
Hemostatic Area
Testing Procedure(s)
Treatment
BLEEDING
Vascular Integrity
Inspection
Angiography
Endoscopy,
etc.
Surgical Correction of Defect
Vasoactive Drugs
Platelets
Bleeding Time
Normal
Increased
Platelet Count
Decreased
Platelets
Normal
If Aspirin
If FSP
Stop production of FSP
If Von Willebrands
FFP/Cryoprecipitate
If Uremia
Dialysis (+ Platelets)

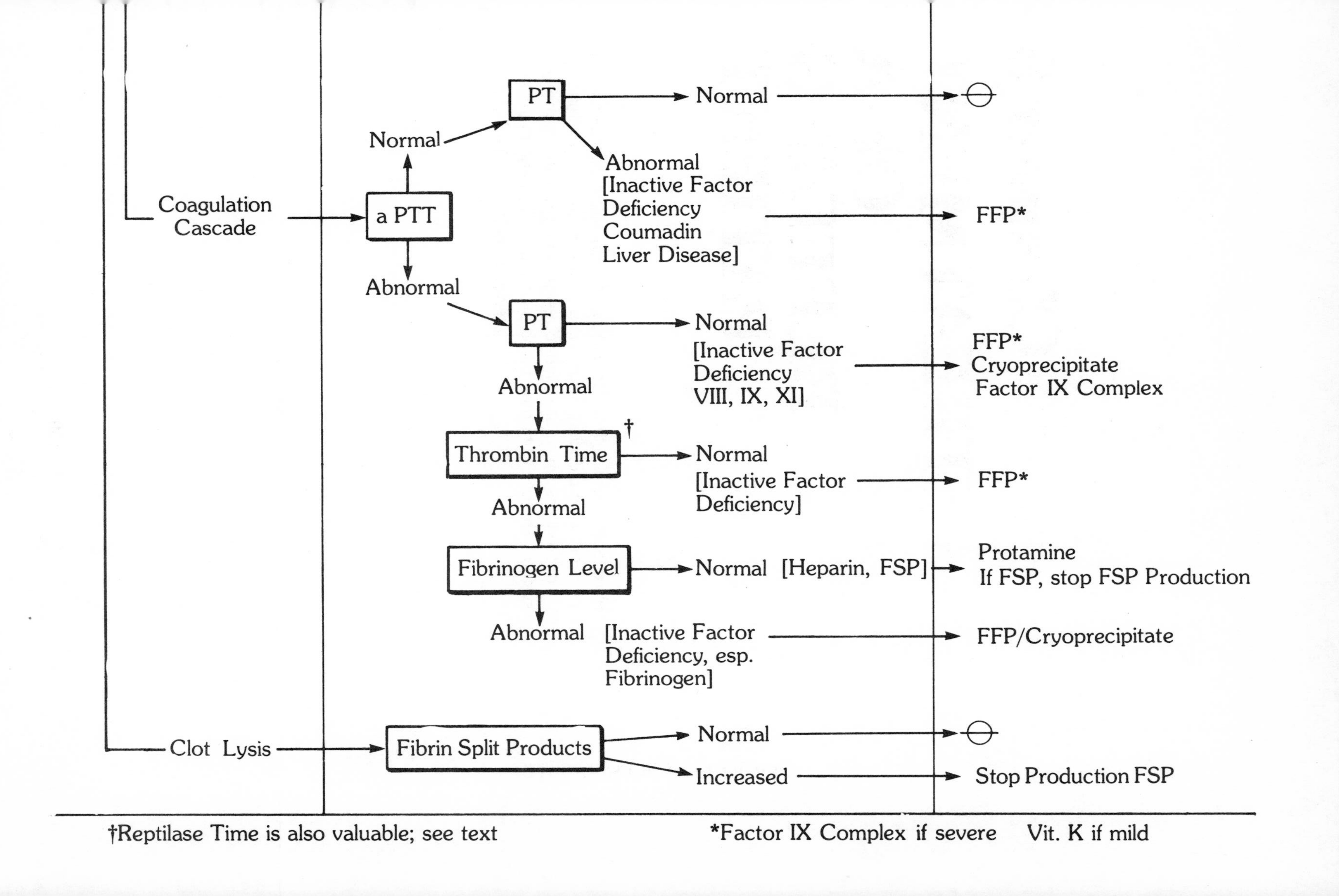

†Reptilase Time is also valuable; see text

*Factor IX Complex if severe Vit. K if mild

Chapter 8
TREATMENT OF A BLEEDING PATIENT

This chapter deals with the treatment of hemostatic disorders which produce bleeding. Thus it is a summary of the "patching-up" procedures which are used to restore to normal the hemostatic system. The use of human blood products, drugs, and therapeutic interventions is presented in detail.

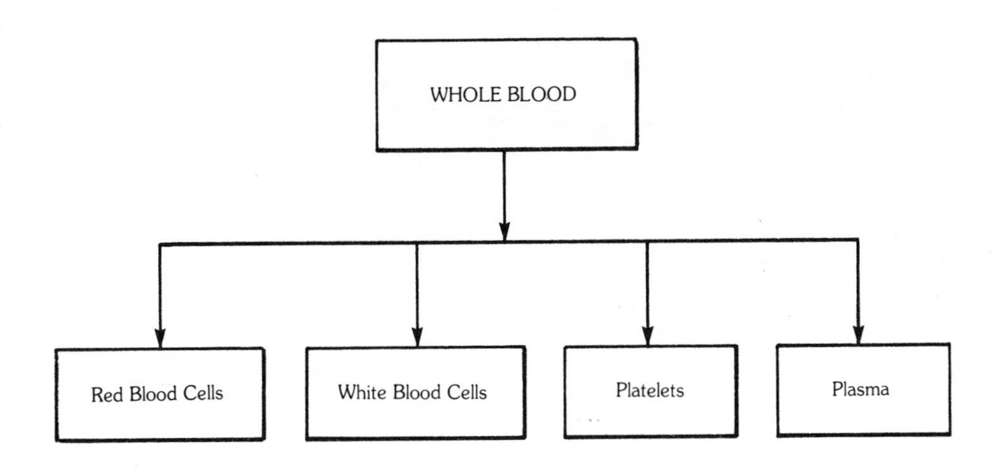

The use of human blood products for replacement of consumed, diluted, destroyed, or lost blood components is rapidly evolving. New methods of collection, storage, preparation, and utilization are being discovered, which may significantly increase shelf life and enhance the "quality" of the transfused unit.

The old concept "whole blood for everything" has vanished. Human blood products are scarce, and component therapy maximally utilizes each donated unit for multiple recipients—each component for a specific therapy. This also means that each patient will be exposed only to those components needed, and reduces risks from transfusion of blood products.

---

1. *Human blood products are ____________.* — ***scarce***
2. *____________ therapy is used for specific treatment.* — ***component***
3. *Component therapy minimizes the risk of ____________ from blood product use.* — ***complications***

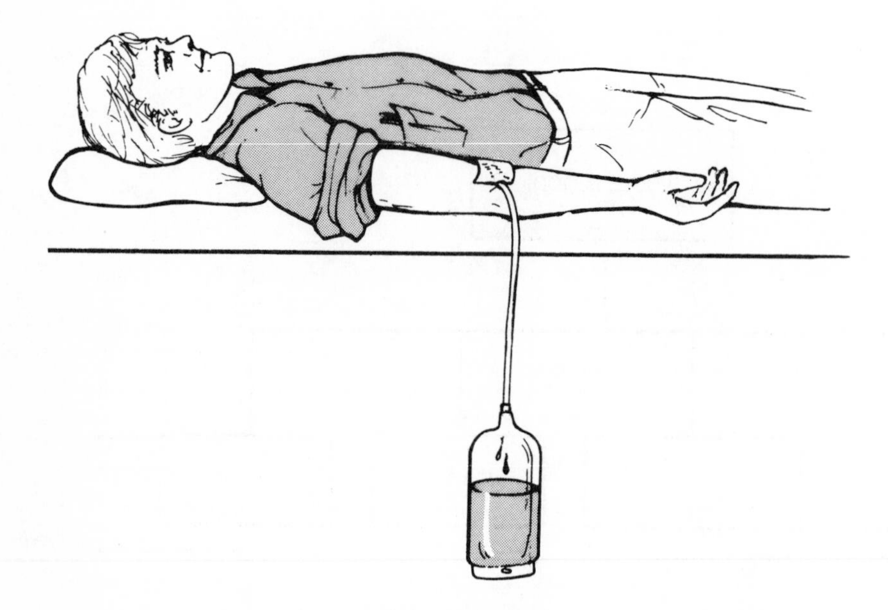

We discuss treatment in the same order as we discuss disorders. Each therapeutic modality will be presented, with various options discussed.

Details of each component will be presented separately in this chapter. Components are derived from fresh whole blood. A unit of whole blood is collected into a bag containing CPD solution (citrate, phosphate, dextrose), used as preservative and anticoagulant. The citrate binds all available calcium (Ca++). Under storage conditions the unit may be used during the next 28 days, and/or components harvested. It is important to realize, however, that several changes occur in the storage of **CPD whole blood**:

Granulocytes	—become non-viable
Platelets	—become non-viable
Factors V, VIII	—are labile and are made useless
Calcium	—is bound
Citrate	—is present in high concentration

Banked whole blood is deficient in

______________,	*platelets*
______________,	*factor V*
______________, *and*	*factor VIII*
______________.	*available Ca++*

What Happens to a Unit of Donated Whole Blood?

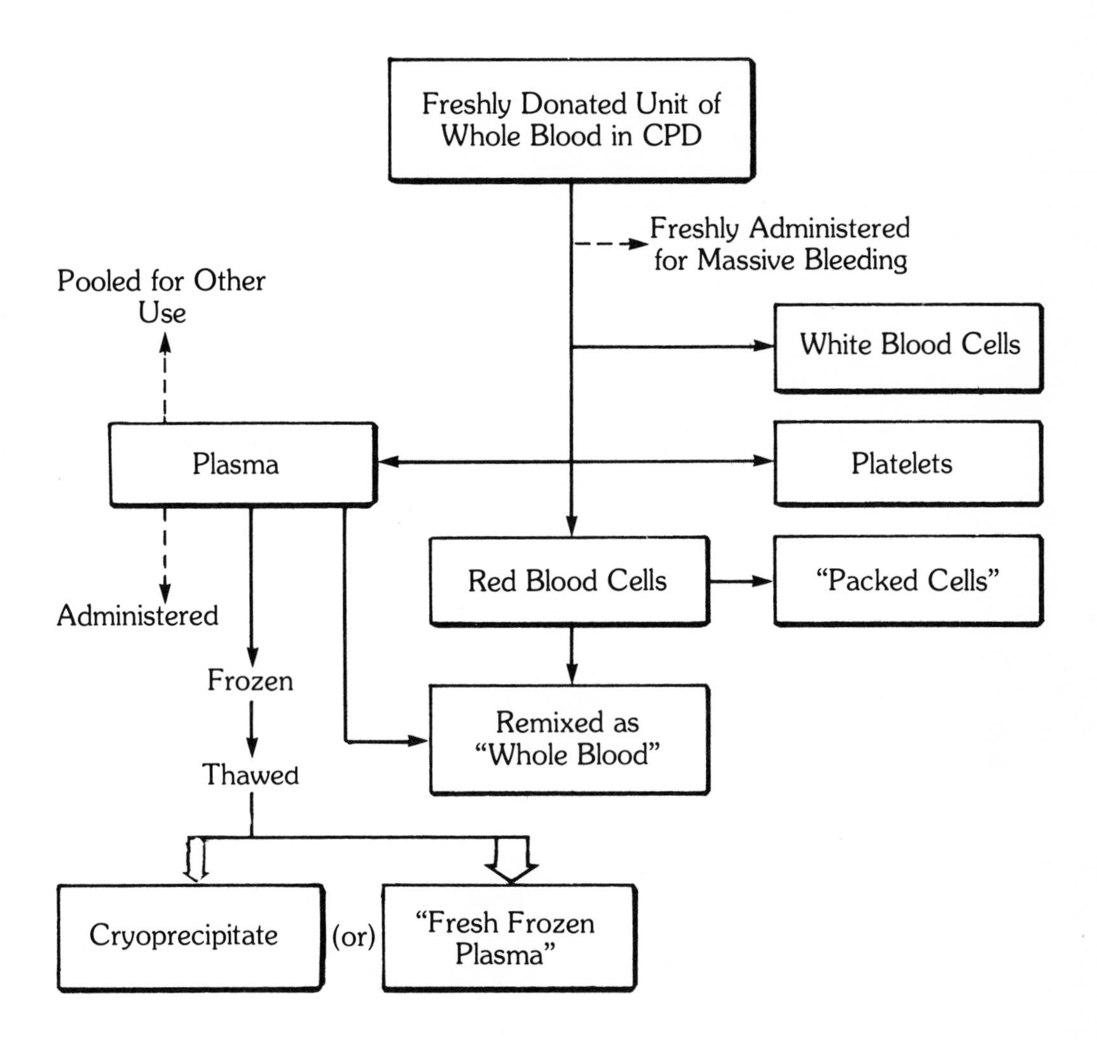

Let us then analyze systematically how these components might be used effectively.

1. VASCULAR INTEGRITY
2. PLATELETS
3. COAGULATION CASCADE
4. CLOT LYSIS

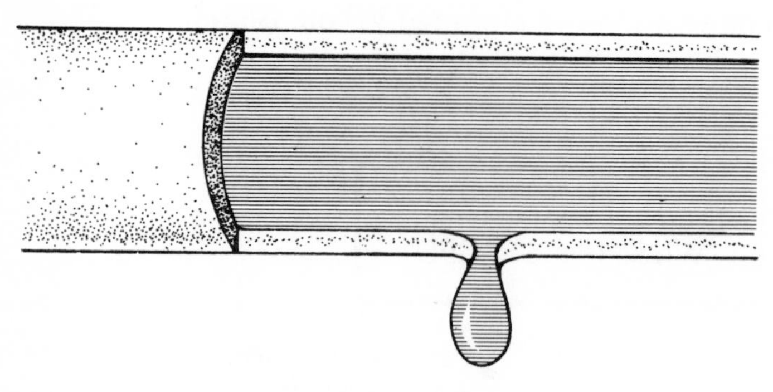

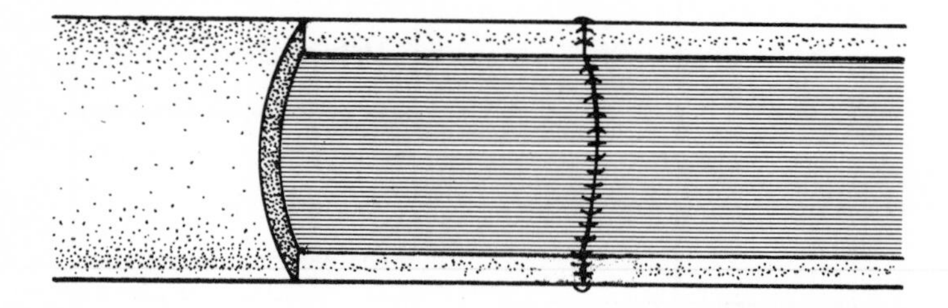

A defect in vascular integrity will produce bleeding by many mechanisms already discussed. Treatment is aimed at the cause:

Open vessels require surgical correction (suture, cauterization, packing, etc.)

Open vessels also may respond to selective vasoconstriction:
- iced saline (gastric bleeding)
- systemic drugs
- regional drugs (selective gastric artery vasoconstrictors)
- prostaglandins (treatment of patent ductus arteriosus)

Open vessels also may respond to controlled hypotension produced by:

- vasodilators
- beta-blocking agents
- positioning of the patient
- anesthetic agents

---

1. *Open vessels require ______________.* — ***surgical correction***
2. *Open vessels may respond to ______________.* — ***vasoconstriction***
3. *Open vessels may respond to controlled ______________.* — ***hypotension***

1. VASCULAR INTEGRITY
2. PLATELETS
3. COAGULATION CASCADE
4. CLOT LYSIS

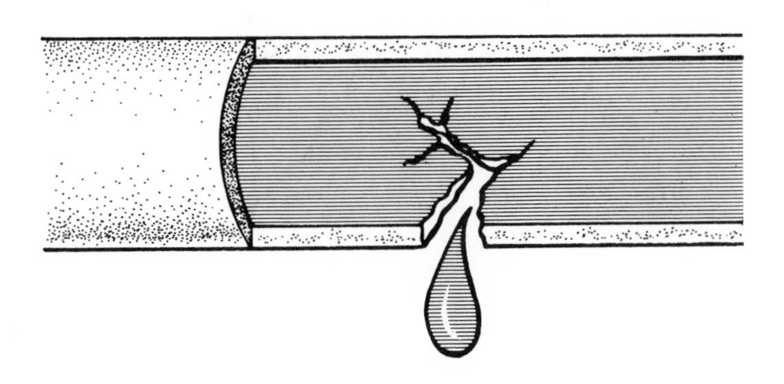

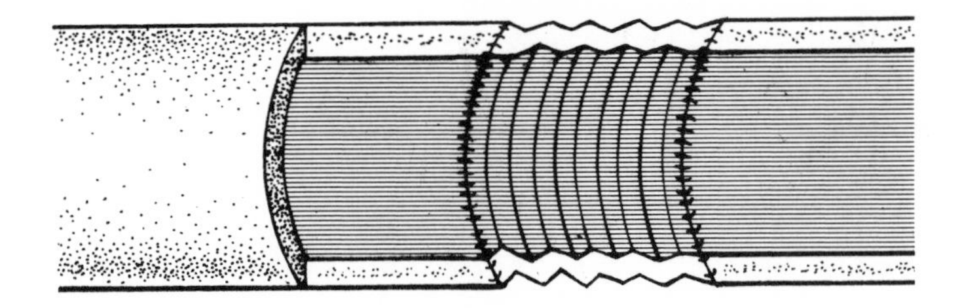

Abnormal vessels may require treatment with steroids or antibiotics to stabilize the endothelium (burns, vasculitis, sepsis, etc.). Abnormal vascular endothelium may require replacement, such as with new cardiac valves or vascular grafts to restore a semblance of normalcy.

In any event, bleeding from a loss of vascular integrity requires attention to restoration of vascular integrity. Administration of blood components, drugs, whole blood, etc. into a patient who is bleeding from open vessels is wasteful, ineffective, and expensive. However it may be necessary to provide time for definitive therapy. Open or damaged vessels require correction.

---

1. *Abnormal vessels may require treatment to stabilize the ______________.* — ***endothelium***
2. *Abnormal vessels may require artificial ______________.* — ***grafts***
3. *A defect in vascular integrity must be ______________ in order to stop bleeding.* — ***corrected***

1. VASCULAR INTEGRITY
2. PLATELETS
3. COAGULATION CASCADE
4. CLOT LYSIS

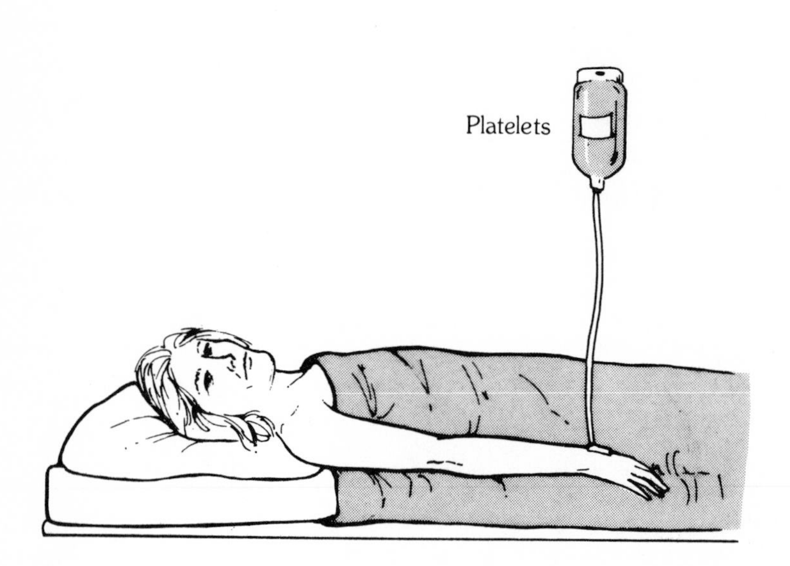

Treatment of quantitative platelet disorders involves the administration of viable platelets. Concomitant prevention or correction of platelet dilution, destruction, consumption, or loss should be accomplished. For acute thrombocytopenia (less than 60,000 platelets/mm^3) one platelet unit should be administered for each 10,000/mm^3 increase desired in the adult. Each platelet unit administered will provide an increase in platelet count depending upon vascular volume, number of platelets in the transfused unit, intravascular platelet viability, filtration during administration, etc. The goal is to provide a maintained platelet count of at least 100,000/mm^3 of functionally normal platelets.

---

1. *The treatment for a decreased platelet count is __________.* — ***platelets***
2. *One platelet unit should increase the platelet count by approximately __________.* — ***10,000/mm^3***
3. *The goal in platelet therapy is a minimum count of normal platelets of __________.* — ***100,000/mm^3***

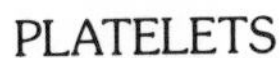

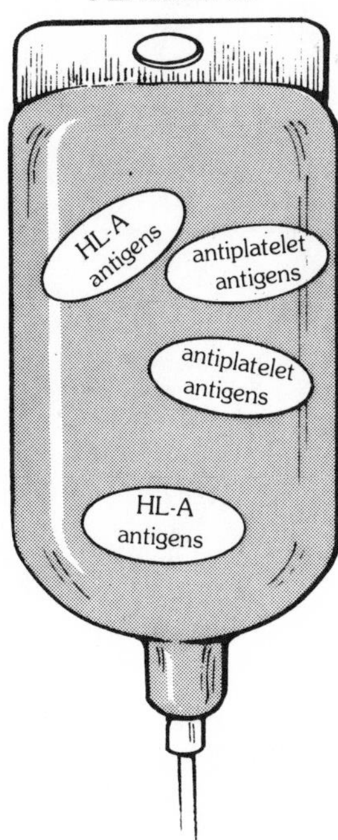

Platelets are separated and prepared from freshly donated blood, and by plateletpheresis techniques. Each concentrated platelet unit should contain a minimum of 5.5×10^{10} platelets in 30-50 ml of plasma, enough to increase the platelet count by $10{,}000/mm^3$. There should be a minimum of red blood cell contamination of the platelet unit, thus ABO cross-matching is rarely required.

Administered platelets may contain many antigens. Among them are antiplatelet antigens, and HL-A antigens. The $Rh_o(D)$ antigen also may be present, if there is red cell contamination, but is uncommon. The platelet antigens PL-1 and PL-2 are of little consequence for our purposes. If antibodies against platelets are present, HLA-matched platelets should be used. Platelets from Rh negative donors should be used if Rh immunization is a potential problem.

---

1. *In platelet therapy, ABO ______________ is rarely performed.* — ***crossmatching***
2. *If anti-platelet antigens are present, use ______________-matched platelets.* — ***HLA***
3. *If Rh problems are expected, use platelets from ______________ donors.* — ***Rh negative***

1. VASCULAR INTEGRITY
2. PLATELETS
3. COAGULATION CASCADE
4. CLOT LYSIS

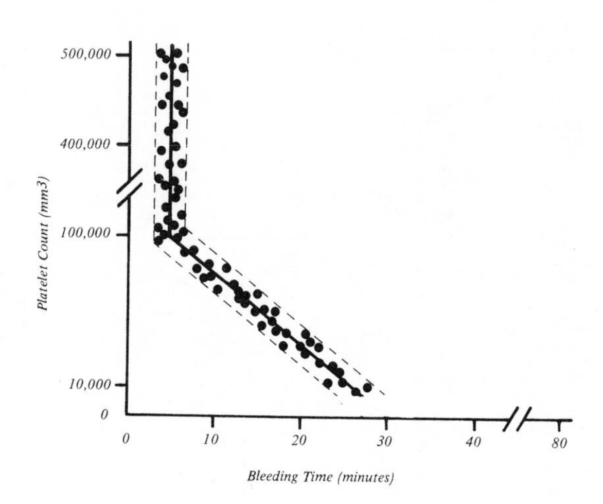

Treatment of qualitative platelet disorders must involve the diagnosis of the cause of the disorder, and then appropriate therapy:

If drug inhibition (ASA, sulfinpyrazone protamine, etc.)	stop the drug
If inhibition by fibrin split products (FSP)	Stop production of FSP
If von Willebrand's disease	Correct the plasma defect with fresh frozen plasma
If uremic patient	Provide hemodialysis
If platelet storage defect	Provide time, and use freshest available platelets

In addition, one or two platelet units from normal donors can be utilized to assist in recruitment (aggregation) of any dysfunctional platelets. The goal here is to have a sufficient number of functionally normal platelets to produce a normal bleeding time.

---

1. If aspirin inhibition of platelets, ______________. — ***stop aspirin***

2. If aspirin inhibition of platelets, also administer ______________. — ***platelets***

3. If von Willebrand's disease, administer ______________ ______________. — ***fresh frozen plasma***

4. The goal isa normal ______________. — ***bleeding time***

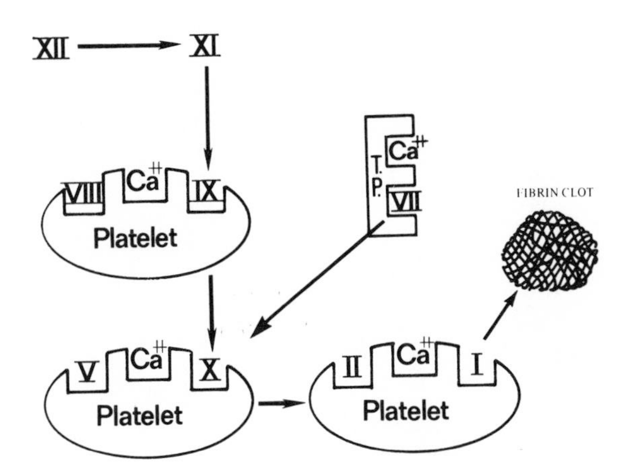

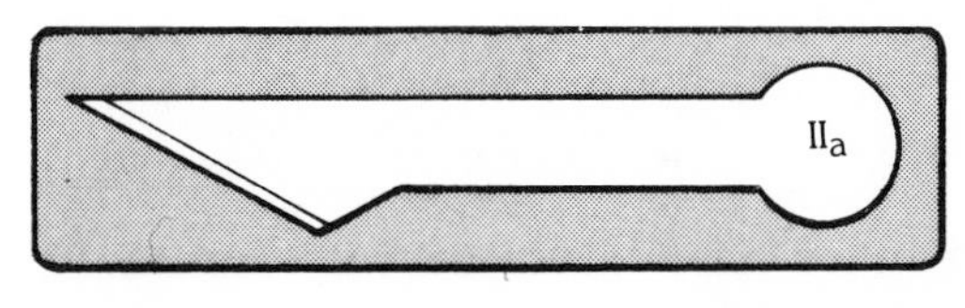

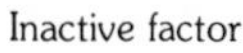
Inactive factor

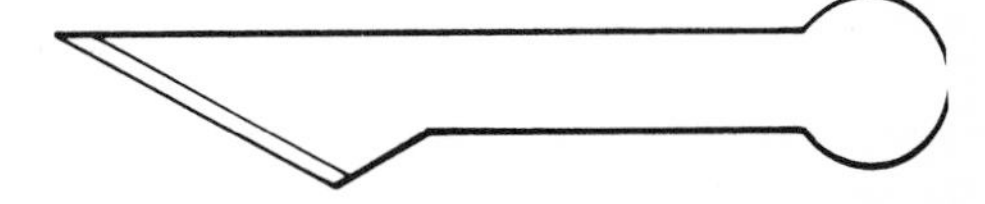
Active factor

Abnormalities or disorders of the coagulation cascade involve both inactive factor abnormalities and active factor disorders. These can be of a chronic nature, either hereditary or acquired; or of an acutely acquired nature. Correct, specific diagnosis of etiology provides a basis for definitive treatment.

We present first the treatment of inactive factor disorders (hereditary and acquired), and then the treatment of active factor abnormalities. Inactive disorders are treated with blood products. Active disorders are treated by removal of the inhibitor.

The therapeutic modalities available are not that many. They are presented in the order of use, according to diagnosis. They are summarized, with an accompanying flow sheet, at the chapter's end.

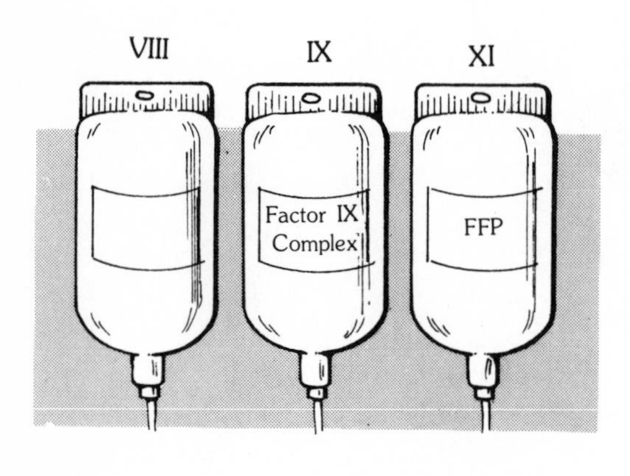

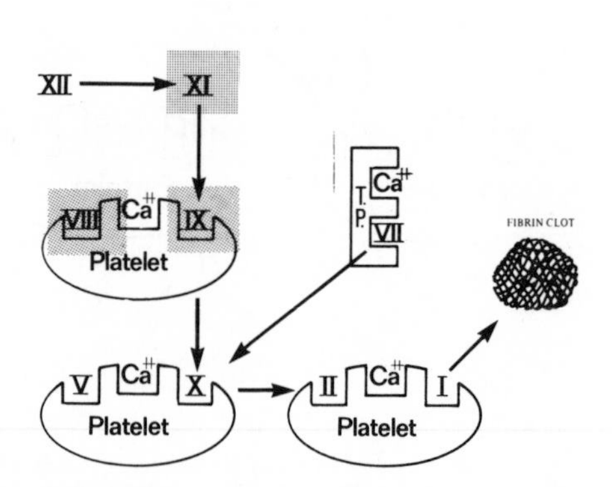

Disorders of hereditary inactive factor deficiencies are those of the three hemophiliac diseases. Therapy should be based upon known factor activities of deficient factors VIII, IX, or XI, from factor assays.

factors VIII, IX, XI	all present in Fresh Frozen Plasma (FFP), in concentrations usually found in normal donor plasma
factor VIII	FFP and cryoprecipitate
factor IX	FFP and factor IX complex preparations (Proplex®, Konyne®)

FFP, cryoprecipitate, and factor IX complex are distinctly different with respect to constituents, indications, contraindications, and risks. (They will be discussed in detail later.)

---

1. *Factor VIII replacement may be obtained with ______________ or ______________.* — ***fresh frozen plasma cryoprecipitate***

2. *Factor IX replacement requires the use of ______________ or ______________.* — ***fresh frozen plasma factor IX complex***

3. *______________ may be used for **all** inactive factor deficiencies.* — ***fresh frozen plasma***

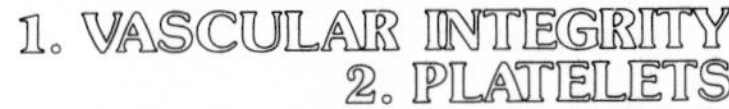

3. COAGULATION CASCADE

4. CLOT LYSIS

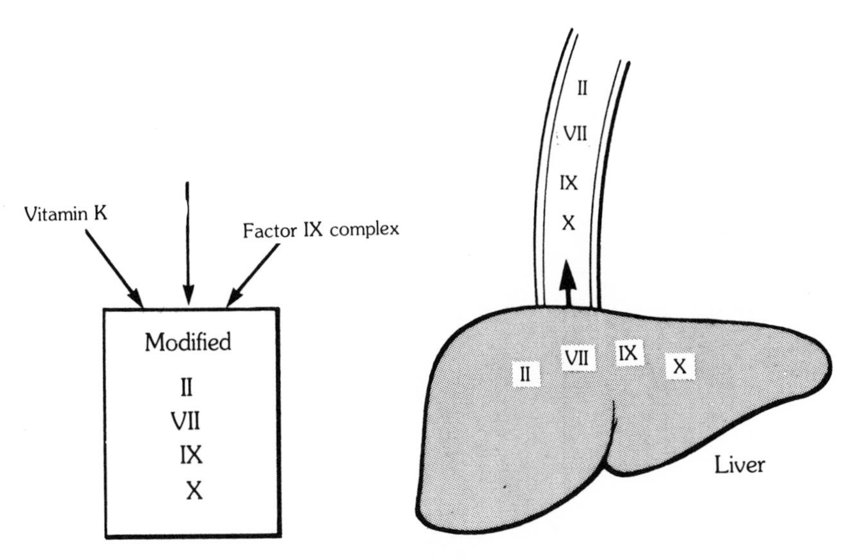

Acquired inactive factor disorders may be due to inadequate hepatic production of the vitamin K modified factors II, VII, IX, and X. This may be secondary to liver disease, vitamin K deficiency, or coumadin therapy. Treatment is based upon the severity of bleeding, and the degree of prolongation of the aPTT or PT. Treatment can be divided into three categories:

A. Bleeding is not severe, hepatic function is adequate, and time is of no special concern	Vitamin K (and discontinue coumadin if present)
B. Bleeding is moderate and/or function is poor, and/or time may be critical	Fresh Frozen Plasma (FFP)
C. Severe life-threatening bleeding is present, and FFP is either ineffective or the volume to be administered must be very small	Factor IX Complex

The endpoint is the normalizing both of the aPTT (IX, X, II) and the PT (VII, X, II), in the absence of other causes of abnormal intrinsic and extrinsic testing.

Deficiencies of factors II, VIII, IX, and X may be treated with

____

____

____

vitamin K

fresh frozen plasma

factor IX complex

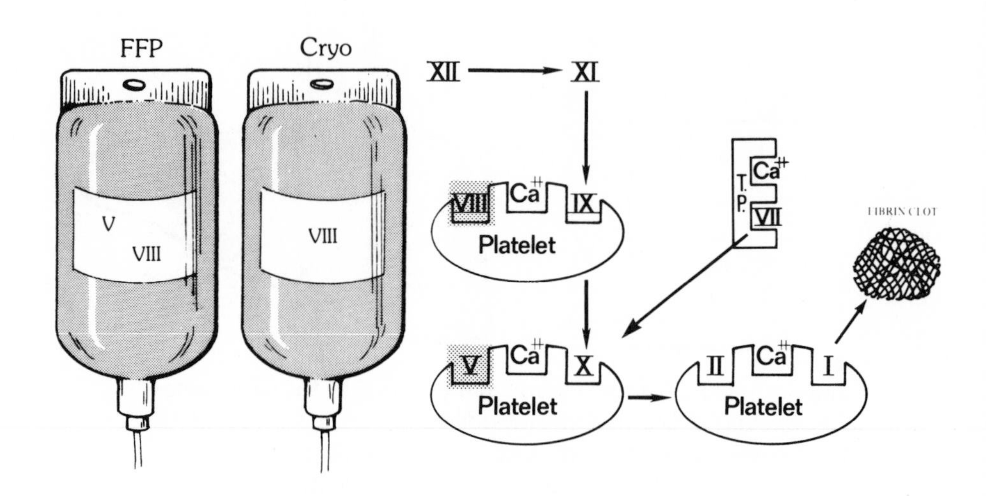

Acquired inactive factor deficiencies of **labile** factors V and VIII may be due to dilution, destruction, consumption, or loss. This occurs in DIC, cardiopulmonary bypass, massive bank blood transfusion, antibodies, etc. This does not represent a "production problem". Replacement is provided as outlined below:

factor V —fresh frozen plasma until the PT or aPTT (or both) is normal

factor VIII —fresh frozen plasma or cryoprecipitate until the aPTT is normal

---

1. Acquired factor V deficiency is treated with ________.	***fresh frozen plasma***
2. Acquired factor VIII deficiency is treated with ________, or ________.	***fresh frozen plasma*** *cryoprecipitate*
3. The goal in factor V or VIII therapy is a normal ________, and cessation of bleeding.	*aPTT*

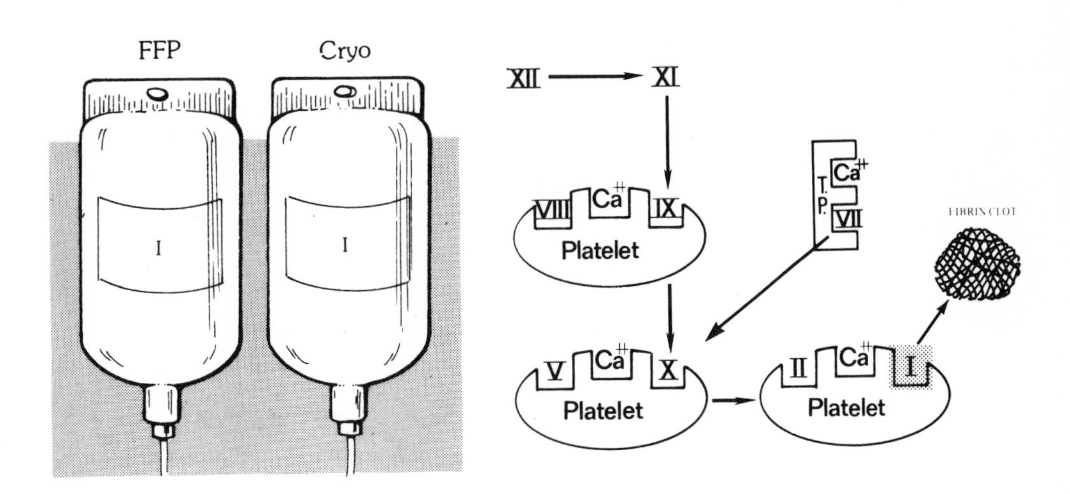

Disorders of fibrinogen (I), either by deficiency or abnormal type of fibrinogen, require the administration of fibrinogen:

fresh frozen plasma —Factor I concentration identical to a similar volume of normal plasma. One unit FFP = 8% of factor I normally circulating. 12 units FFP **theoretically** replaces all factor I

cryoprecipitate —1/4 of original plasma content of factor I recovered, but contained in a smaller volume

The goal should be a fibrinogen level greater than 200 mg%, and a normal thrombin time in the absence of other coagulation abnormalities.

---

1. *Fibrinogen disorders require administration of fibrinogen with either ______________ or ______________.* — ***fresh frozen plasma cryoprecipitate***

2. *The goal in fibrinogen therapy is a fibrinogen level of greater than ______________.* — ***200 mg%***

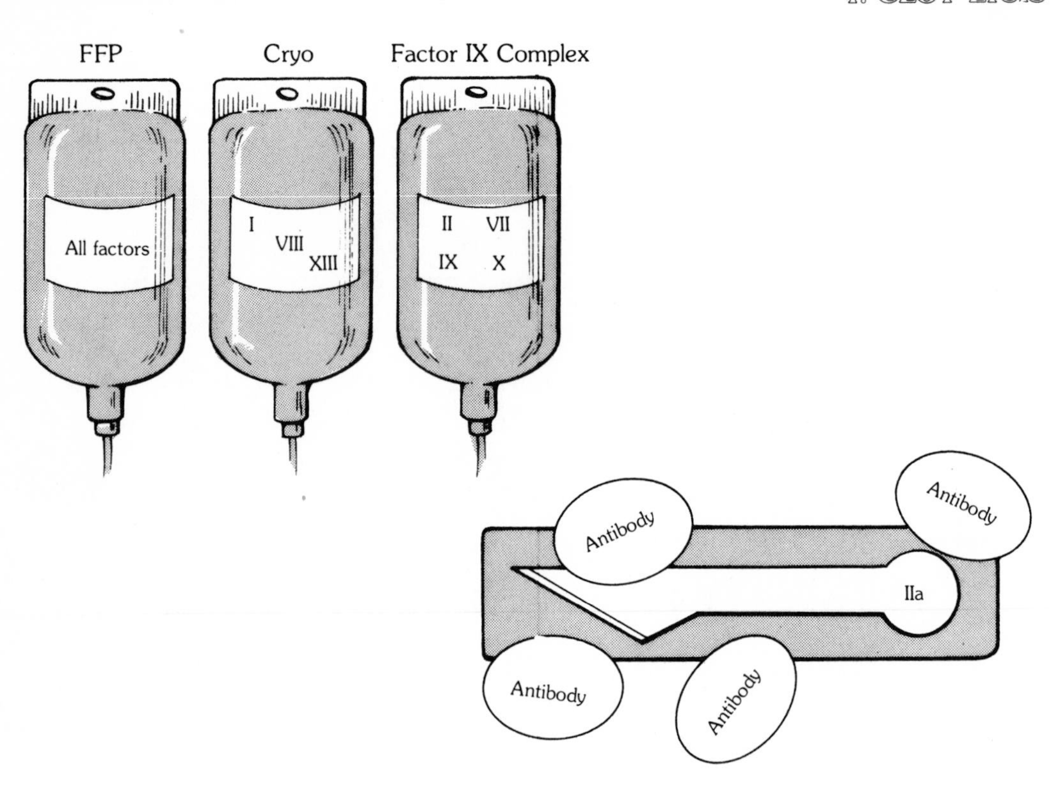

Antibodies acquired against inactive factors may produce a deficiency of that factor's activity. A common antibody problem is seen with factor VIII antibodies produced by the host against administered factor VIII in hemophilia A. The treatment involves the administration of new factors, in as "pure" a form as possible:

fresh frozen plasma	—all factors
cryoprecipitate	—VIII, I, XIII
factor IX complex	—II, VII, IX, X

Plasmapheresis techniques may be employed to reduce the antibody titers in selected patients. The goals may be variable, but involve the normalization of either the aPTT or PT (or both), depending upon which factor is altered by the antibody.

---

1. Fresh frozen plasma provides __________. — ***all factors***

2. Cryoprecipitate provides factors __________. — ***VIII, I, XIII***

3. Factor IX complex provides factors __________. — ***II, VII, IX, X***

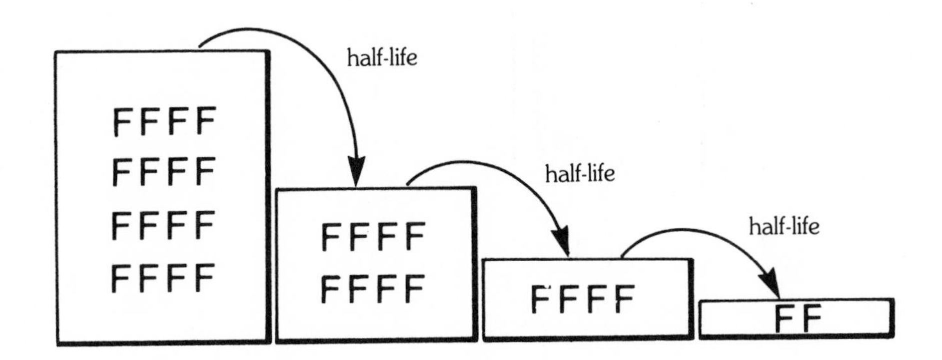

Let us examine the half-life of each factor, and the approximate concentrations necessary for surgical bleeding in isolated eficiencies:

Factor	In-vivo 1/2 Life	Minimum Concentration for Surgical Hemostasis (% of normal)
I	4-6 days	35-50
II	3-4 days	20-40
V	15-24 hours	10-20
VII	4-6 hours	10-20
VIII	12-18 hours	25-30
von Willebrand's Factor	?	20-40
IX	18-30 hours	20-25
X	48-60 hours	10-20
XI	60 hours	20-30
XII	50-70 hours	0
XIII	3 days	1-3
AT-3	?	?

(Modified from Ellison[3] and Biggs[1].)

1. VASCULAR INTEGRITY
2. PLATELETS
3. COAGULATION CASCADE
4. CLOT LYSIS

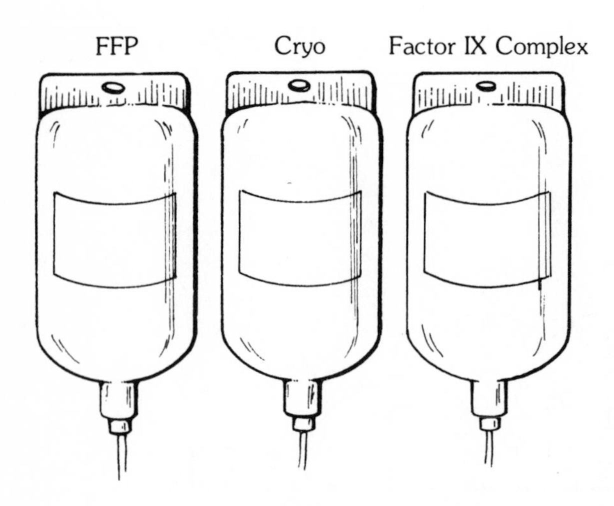

The following therapeutic materials are available. The approximate recovery of each factor which may be expected during administraion of these materials is as follows:

Factor	Therapeutic Materials Available	Approximate recovery in vivo as % of infused dose
I	FFP, cryoprecipitate	50;
II	FFP, factor IX complex	50-100
V	FFP	50
VII	FFP, factor IX complex	?
VIII	FFP, cryoprecipitate, other VIII preparations	50-80
von Willebrand's Disease	FFP, cryoprecipitate	?
IX	FFP, cryosupernate, factor IX complex	25-50
X	FFP, factor IX complex	50-100
XI	FFP	100
XII	(not needed)	—
XIII	FFP	50-100
AT-3	FFP	(100?)

(Modified from Ellison[3] and Biggs[1].)

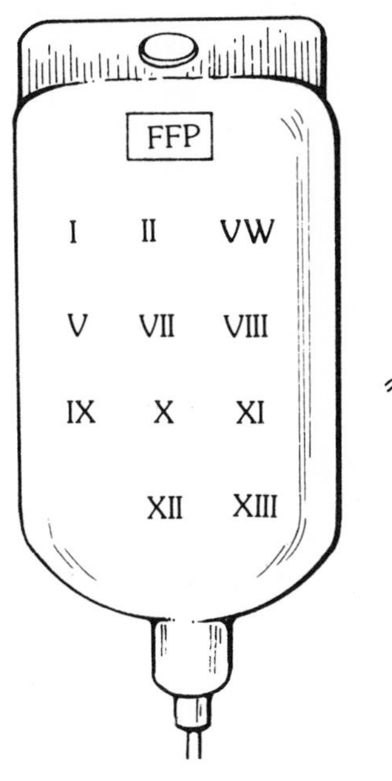

≈8% Plasma volume

Fresh frozen plasma (FFP) contains all of the factors and activity normally found in a similar volume of plasma circulating in a normal person (unless any constituent has been removed by the blood bank). Of course, there is a distribution of "normal" values for all donors, and thus some variability for each factor from donor-to-donor. Since each FFP unit is prepared from one donor, it carries the same risks of hepatitis as a unit of fresh whole blood. Red cell "contamination" of an FFP unit should be minimal, but is possible. FFP should be administered within the recipient's ABO compatible blood group, and used within two hours of thawing. Since none of the factors are concentrated, the volume of infusion may be limited by the available vascular space.

Each unit of FFP represents approximately 8% of a normal person's plasma volume (250 ml/3000 ml x 100). Three units of FFP (approximately 10 ml/kg) thus will replace 1/4 (24%) of a patient's factors. (This ignores concomitant dilution, destruction, loss, or consumption of infused factors.)

---

1. *Fresh frozen plasma contains ______________.* — ***all factors***

2. *Fresh frozen plasma should be used within ______________ of thawing.* — ***two hours***

3. *Each unit of fresh frozen plasma will replace approximately ______________ of an adult's factors.* — ***8%***

Cryo

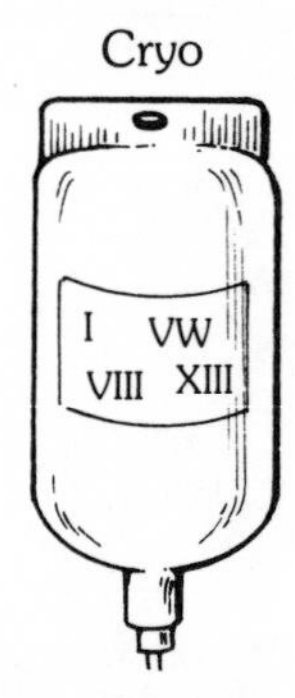

Cryoprecipitate is produced from a single donor of blood, by a freeze-and-thaw process. It is then pooled with other cryoprecipitate preparations from other donors to provide enough factor VIII for treatment. Each donor blood unit provides approximately 80-100 units of factor VIII. The percentage of original plasma content of clotting factors recovered in cryoprecipitate can be summarized as follows:

Factor	Percent*
I	23
II	1
V	1
VII	2
VIII	30-50
von Willebrand's factor	40-75
IX	5
X	1
XI	1
XII	2
XIII	30

Thus cryoprecipitate is used for four basic indications—factor VIII deficiencies in hemophilia A, fibrinogen deficiencies from many causes, the need for the platelet aggregation factor in von Willebrand's disease, and factor XIII deficiency.

(*American Association of Blood Banks: **Blood Component Therapy.**)

Cryoprecipitate is used for replacement of factors

______________ *I*

______________ *VIII*

______________ *von Willebrand's*

______________ *XIII*

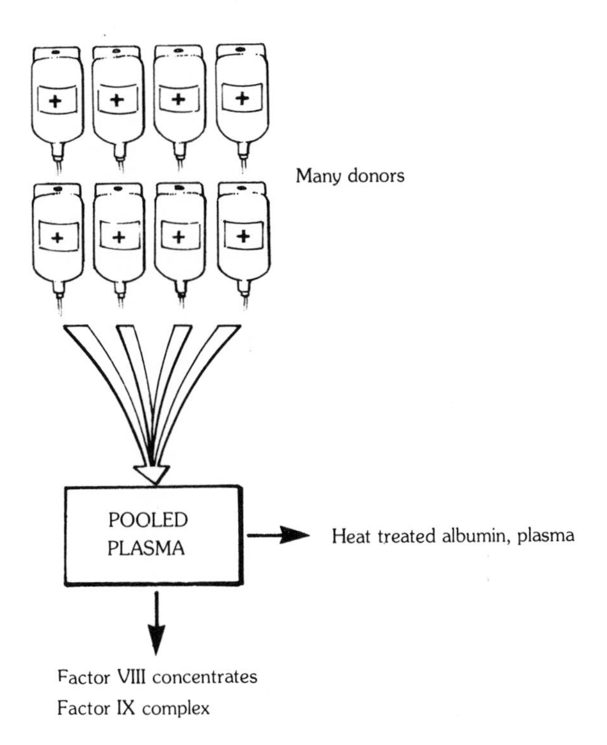

Pooled plasma is no longer directly administered. The high incidence of hepatitis has made its direct use of little value when components are available. Pooled plasma is utilized in the process of preparing other materials by fractionation, such as albumin, plasma protein fraction, anti-hemophiliac factor (AHF lyophilized concentrates), and factor IX complex.

Thus pooled plasma serves as a beginning material for manufactured protein products used for intravascular volume expansion, treatment of burns, treatment of hypoproteinemia, treatment of hyperbilirubinemia, chronic administration of AHF in hemophilia A, and factor IX complex administration. With the exception of AHF concentrate and factor IX complex, these products are heat treated to inactivate hepatitis virus(es), and are devoid of coagulation factors.

---

1. Pooled plasma is used for ______. — ***preparing other products***

2. Pooled plasma administered directly carries a high risk of ______. — ***hepatitis***

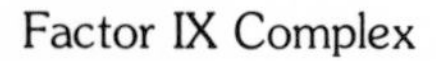

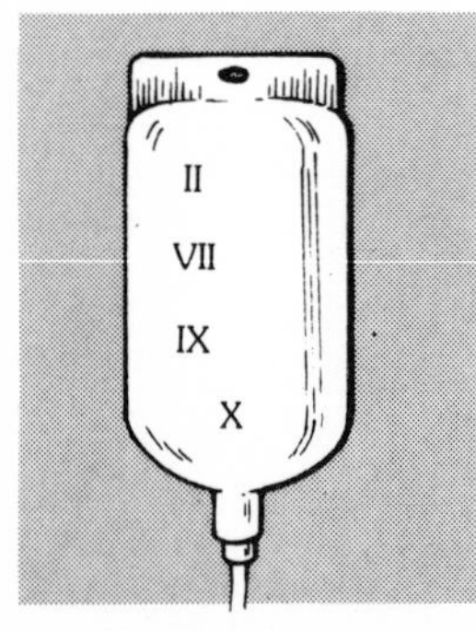

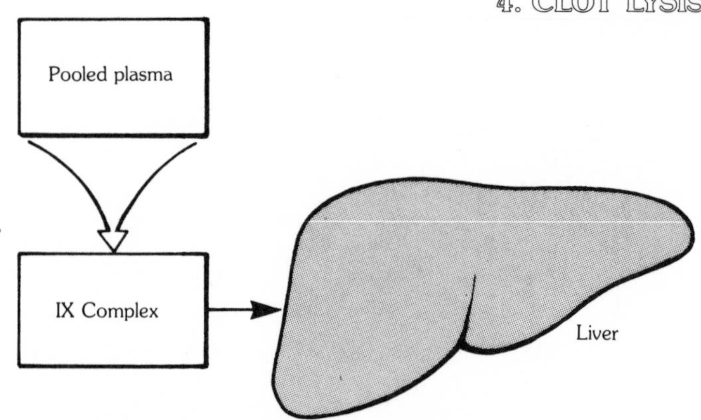

Factor IX complex (Proplex® and Konyne®) is a pooled plasma preparation. It contains substantial quantities of factors II, VII, IX, and X, each vial (approximately 30 ml reconstituted) roughly equivalent to 500 ml of fresh frozen plasma for these four factors. It is **not** treated to inactivate the hepatitis virus(es), and may carry a substantial hepatitis risk by virtue of its multidonor pooled origin.*

Its uses include:

Coumadin overdose Severe liver disease	Severe factor II, VII, IX, or X deficiency
Hemophilia B (Christmas Disease)	Factor IX deficiency
Factor X deficiency	Rare

Recovery rates of the four factors are approximately 50% the expected concentrations based upon contents of the infused concentrate. Factor IX concentrate should be reserved for **severe** bleeding disorders involving (any of) these four factors, and not responsive nor applicable to treatment with fresh frozen plasma and/or vitamin K. Factor IX complex should be used for specific therapy. It is not "vascular glue", and carries a substantial risk of thrombosis, because of the presence of active factors. The necessity for the concentrated administration of any or all of these factors using only a small administered volume (congestive heart failure, infants, etc.) may override other considerations. In DIC, its use should be preceded by heparin administration, if it is used at all, and only upon the advice of a qualified hematologist.

*Exact statistical information regarding the hepatitis risk of this preparation is difficult to document. Many patients critically ill receiving these preparations die from other causes before hepatitis might occur.

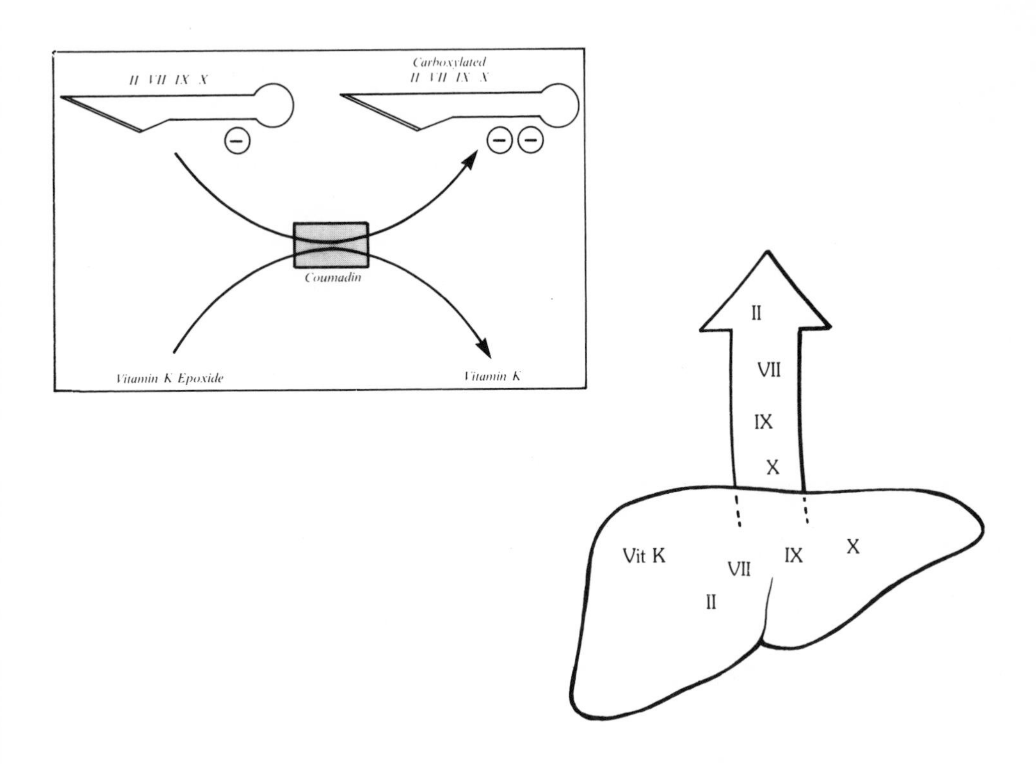

Vitamin K (actually vitamin K_1) is administered to increase the concentrations of the modified factors II, VII, IX, and X. Hepatic function must be adequate to provide the -carboxy glutamic acid modification. If hepatic function is not adequate, vitamin K will have little effect. The dosage is variable, depending upon body size, effect desired, level of coumadin in the plasma, bleeding severity, and prothrombin time prolongation produced by the factor deficiency(ies). Intramuscular or oral dosages of 10-25 mg is usually recommended. Depending upon hepatic function, improvement in the prothrombin time may be seen within hours. The goal is either to normalize the PT (during bleeding), or to improve the PT to approximately 25-30% (if ongoing but lesser coumadin effect is still desired).

---

1. *Vitamin K is used to treat deficiencies of factors ________, ________, ________, and ________.* — ***II, VII, IX, X***
2. *Effective treatment with vitamin K requires nearly normal ________.* — ***hepatic function***
3. *The goal in vitamin K therapy is the normalization of the ________.* — ***PT***

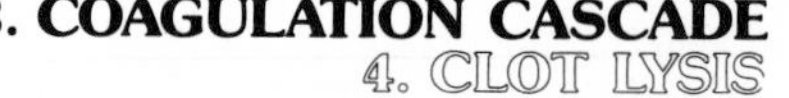

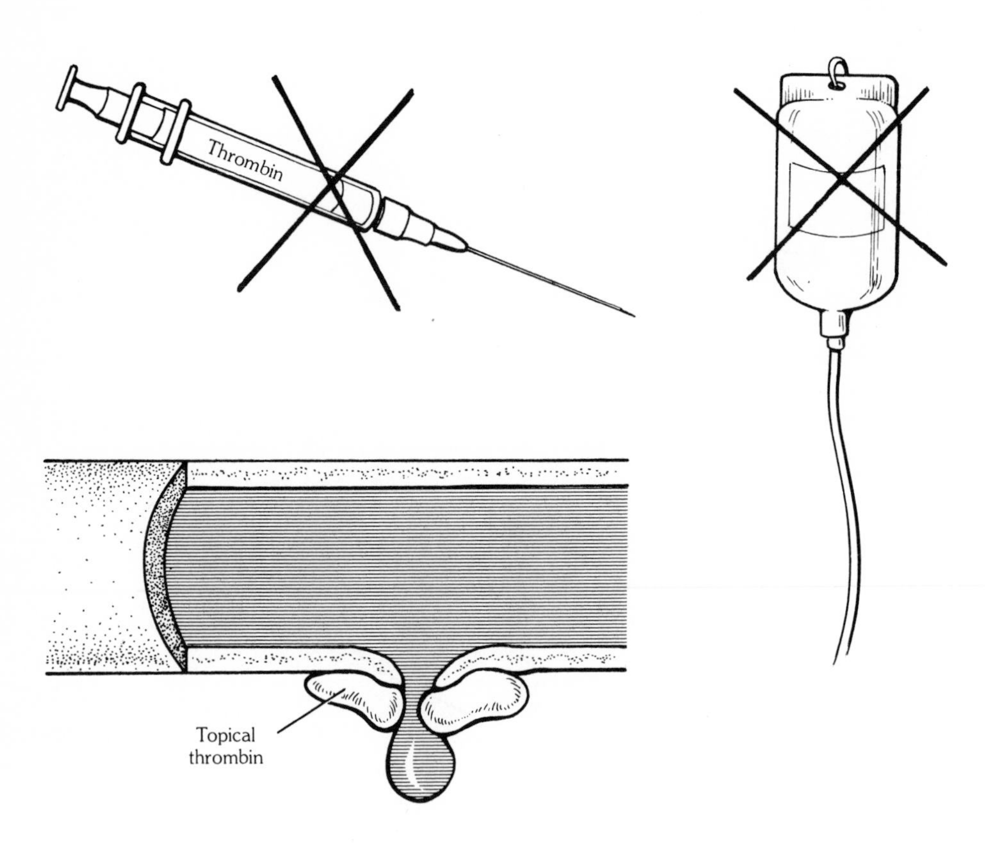

Topical thrombin is a preparation for surface use only, **not for injection**. Its topical use is to provide local fibrin formation. It contains 1,000-10,000 NIH units per vial, each 2 NIH units capable of clotting 1 ml of oxalated human plasma within 15 seconds. (Thus 10,000 NIH units could clot 5,000 ml of oxalated human plasma within 15 seconds—approximately twice the entire adult plasma volume—if injected!)

It is applied as a freshly prepared solution, directly to surgical or traumatic wounds. It also is used orally or via a gastric tube, diluted 10,000 NIH units into milk, in the topical treatment of upper gastrointestinal bleeding.

---

1. *Topical thrombin assists in local __________ formation.* — ***fibrin***
2. *Topical thrombin must __________ be used intravenously.* — ***never***

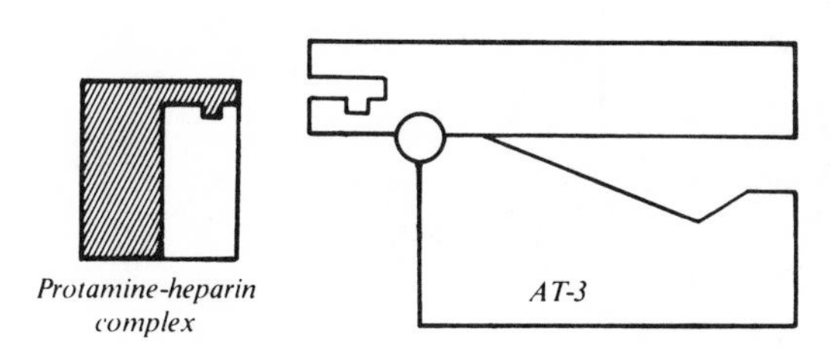

Disorders of **active** factors often involve the increased activity of antithrombin (AT-3), made more avid by heparin. Heparin effect requires antagonism with protamine sulfate. The estimated dose of protamine may be calculated via an ACT-heparin-protamine plot as described in the appendices. The usual initial dose of protamine in the adult is 50-100 mg (5-10 ml reconstituted), given in intravenous increments of no greater than 50 mg per minute. The goal is a normal ACT (the easiest test at the bedside), or a normal thrombin time (the most sensitive laboratory test of heparin effect). If there are other coagulation abnormalities, then the ACT or TT should be as close to the normal values as possible, and other treatment instituted as needed.

Protamine is produced from salmon sperm, so "allergic" responses to its administration are not uncommon. Histamine release may occur, with subsequent vasodilation and hypotension. In addition, protamine may produce myocardial depression via Ca++ binding, the treatment of which is judiciously administered calcium chloride. (Protamine also may produce platelet dysfunction, as previously mentioned.)

---

1. *Heparin inhibition is reversed with ______________.* — ***protamine***
2. *Heparin and protamine require the presence of ______________ for effect.* — ***anti-thrombin***
3. *Protamine may produce ______________, from several etiologies.* — ***hypotension***

1. VASCULAR INTEGRITY
2. PLATELETS
3. COAGULATION CASCADE
4. CLOT LYSIS

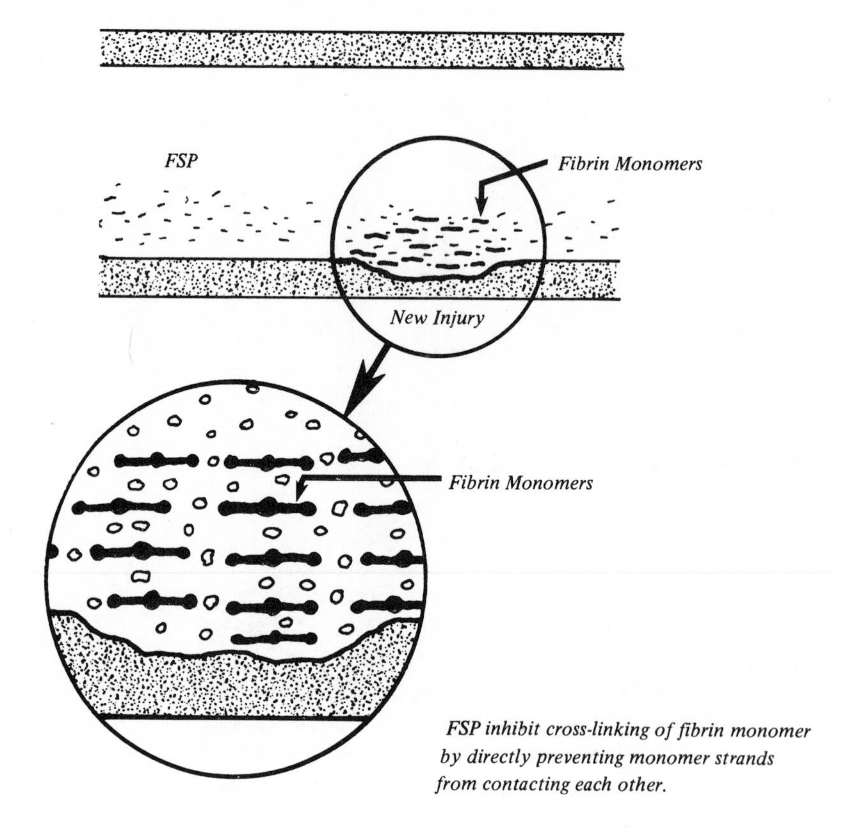

FSP inhibit cross-linking of fibrin monomer by directly preventing monomer strands from contacting each other.

Fibrin split products (FSP) produce **active** factor abnormalities by their action on prevention of fibrin cross-linking, and by completing with thrombin. (They may also produce platelet dysfunction.) The treatment is to find and treat the cause of increased fibrinolysis. Hemodialysis also may offer a beneficial reduction in the concentration of certain FSP fragments.

If snake venoms have produced abnormalities of coagulation by action on factor X, or by thrombin-like effects on fibrinogen, the treatment is heparin, antivenom, debridement of the wound, and treatment of secondary problems.

---

1. *Treatment of FSP inhibition of fibrin cross-linking is to ____________.* — **stop FSP production**
2. *____________ may help reduce FSP concentrations.* — **Hemodialysis**

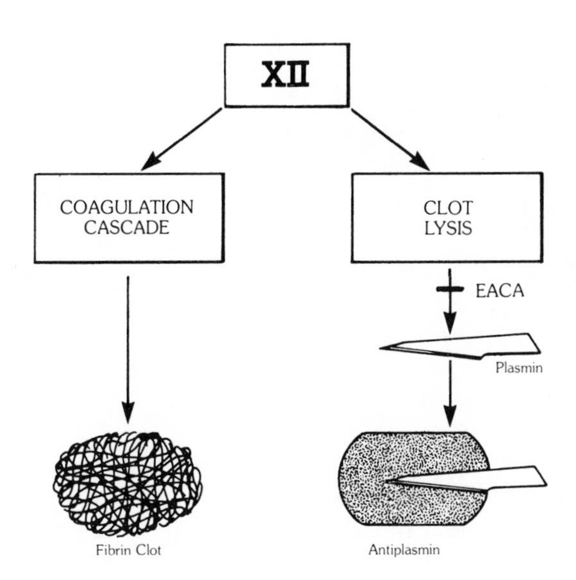

Treatment of disorders of fibrinolysis involves first the determination of whether the increases lysis is secondary to increased clotting, or primary process of increased lysis. In the former circumstance, treatment must be aimed at the clotting process while in the latter, treatment is aimed at the lytic process.

If severe bleeding accompanies the administration of either urokinase or stroptokinase, these drugs must be discontinued. Then, epsilon aminocaproic acid (EACA) may be administered to prevent the transformation of plasminogen activation. EACA has been used experimentally in the adjunctive treatment of hemophilia A and B, in an attempt to minimize fibrin clot degradation, when the amount of fibrin clot being produced is limited by factor VIII or IX deficiencies. In this case, the lytic system is not abnormal, but is being altered anyway. A qualified hematologist should advise in these circumstances, regarding indications, contraindications, and dosage.

---

1. *Treatment of abnormal clot lysis involves finding the ______________.* — ***cause***
2. *If urokinase or streptokinase are in use, ______________ these drugs.* — ***stop***
3. *Attenuation of fibrinolysis is provided by ______________.* — ***EACA***

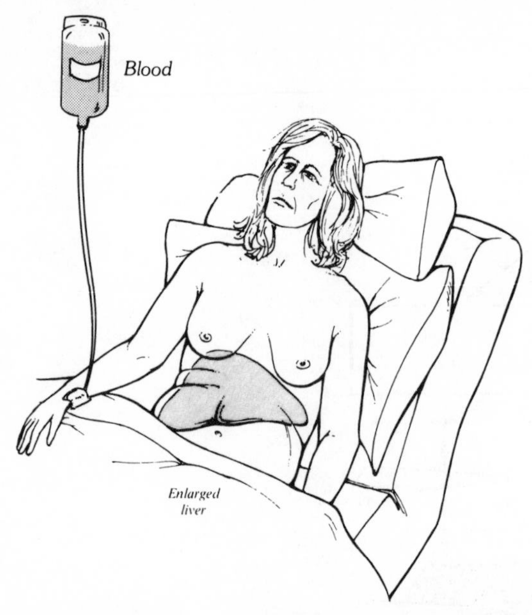

HEPATITIS RISK OF VARIOUS BLOOD PRODUCTS

(Risk varies with donor population, and may be high in some communities, and very low in other.)

1. Risk of Hepatitis from Whole Blood Transfusion

Number of Units	Clinical Hepatitis Incidence
2	2.1%
3-4	1.9%
5-9	2.1%
10 or greater	3.8%

(Grady GF, Bennett AJE: National transfusion hepatitis study. J Amer Med Assoc 220:692, 1972.)

2. Comparative Hepatitis Risk

AHF	3	Platelet unit	1-2
Factor IX Complex	3	Frozen RBCs	1*
Cryoprecipitate	2-3	Albumin	0
Whole Blood	2	Plasma Protein Fraction	0
Packed RBCs	2	Ringer's Lactate Solution	0
FFP unit	2	(*controversial at present)	

3 = **greater** than 1 unit of fresh whole blood
2 = equal to 1 unit of fresh whole blood
1 = **less** than 1 unit of fresh whole blood
0 = virtually zero or zero

COSTS OF VARIOUS BLOOD PRODUCTS

Product	Amount	Approximate Volume	Approximate Cost
"Whole Blood"	1 unit	450 ml	$ 32.- — 40.-
Packed RBCs	1 unit	200 ml	27.- — 38.-
Frozen RBCs	1 unit	200 ml	142.-
Platelets-Regular	6 units	40 ml x 6	162.-/6 u
Platelets-HLA Compatible	6 units	40 ml x 6	202.- — 328.-/6 u
Fresh Frozen Plasma	1 unit	200 ml	27.-
Cryoprecipitate	80-120 factor VIII units	200 ml	12.-/1000 factor VIII units
AHF	100-1000 factor VIII units	25 ml	10¢/unit of VIII
Factor IX Complex	450-500 factor IX units	30 ml	61.-
Plasma Protein Fraction		250 ml	38.-
Albumin 5%		250 ml	42.-
Albumin — "salt poor" 25%		50 ml	45.-
— —			
(Ringer's Lactate Solution)		1000 ml	13.-
— —			
Cross Match Procedure			24.-/unit blood
Blood typing of recipient			16.75

(These are costs to the patient in an average Bay Area medical center blood bank in Spring 1980, provided for comparative information only.)

TREATMENT SUMMARY

Treatment of a bleeding patient has been outlined briefly in the flow sheet at the end of the Chapter on Analysis of a Bleeding Patient, and is summarized in more detail below:

Use blood products judiciously and upon demonstrated need.
Know what substances are provided with each product.
Know the indications, contraindications, and hazards of each product.
Know the hemostasis tests and therapeutic endpoints.

Vascular Integrity

- Prevent further loss by surgical correction or change in blood flow
- Stabilize/normalize the endothelium

Platelets

- Correct quantitative disorders with platelets
- Correct qualitative disorders by stopping drugs or formation of FSP. Correct plasma disorders in von Willebrand's disease, uremia, etc. Administer normal platelets to assist the others
- The goal is a PC 100,000/mm^3, and a normal bleeding time

Coagulation Cascade

- Inactive Factor Disorders
  Hereditary Deficiencies—to normal ACT/aPTT
  —Replace VIII with FFP, cryoprecipitate
  —Replace IX with FFP, Factor IX Complex
  —Replace XI with FFP
  Acquired Deficiencies—to normal ACT/aPTT/PT
  —Replace II, VII, IX, X-vitamin K, FFP, or factor IX Complex
  —Replace V with FFP
  —Replace VIII with WWP, cryoprecipitate
  —Replace I with FFP, cryoprecipitate
- Active Factor Disorders—to normal ACT/aPTT/TT
  Protamine administration for heparin
  Decrease FSP production, and/or remove by dialysis

Clot Lysis

- If DIC—treat as in DIC Chapter
- If produced by urokinase/streptokinase (without concomitant clotting), epsilon aminocaprioc acid (EACA)

If circumstances become uncontrolled, complications appear, or EACA contemplated, consult a hematologist.

We have provided a summary flow sheet again on the next two pages.

SUMMARY
ANALYSIS OF BLEEDING

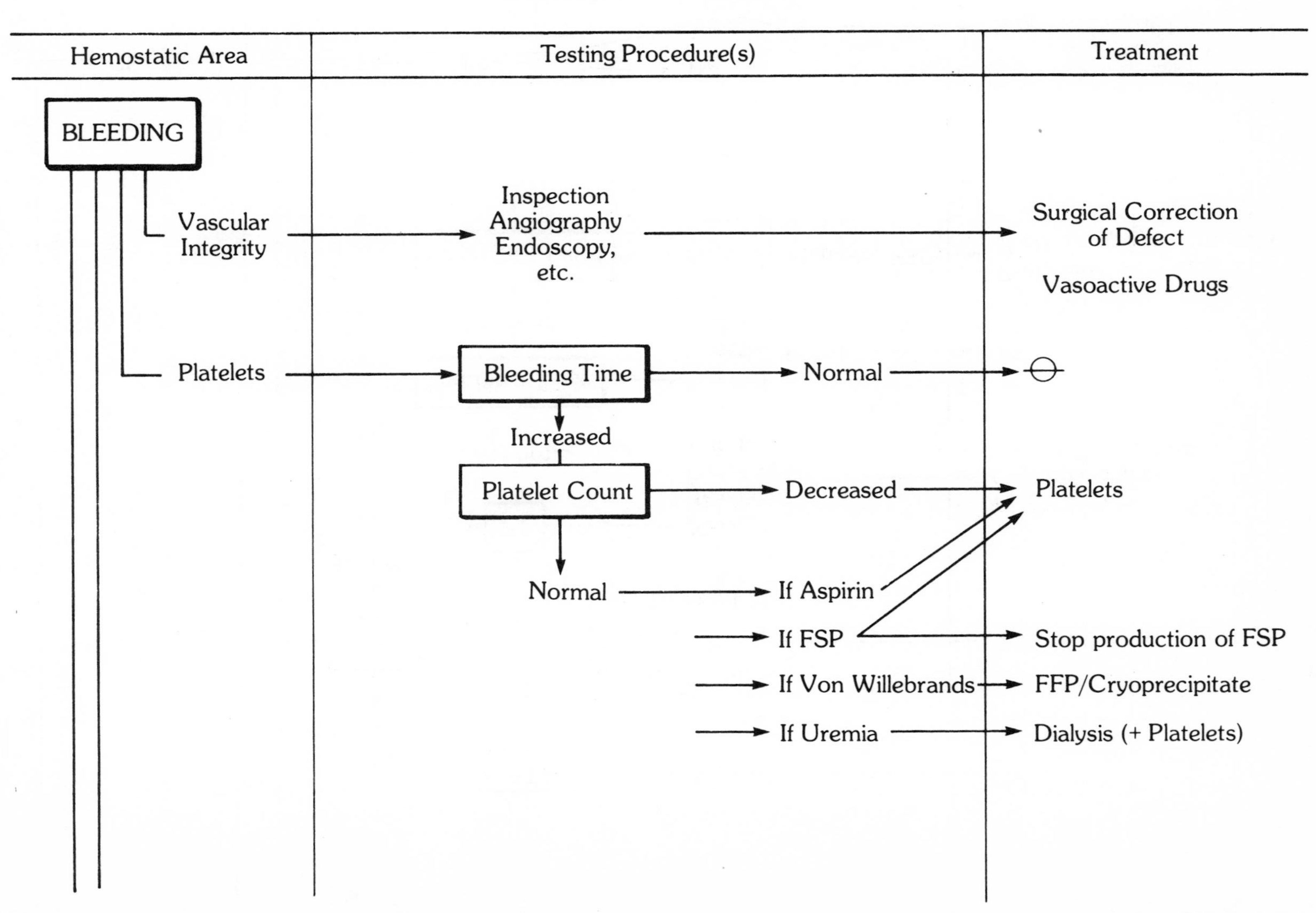

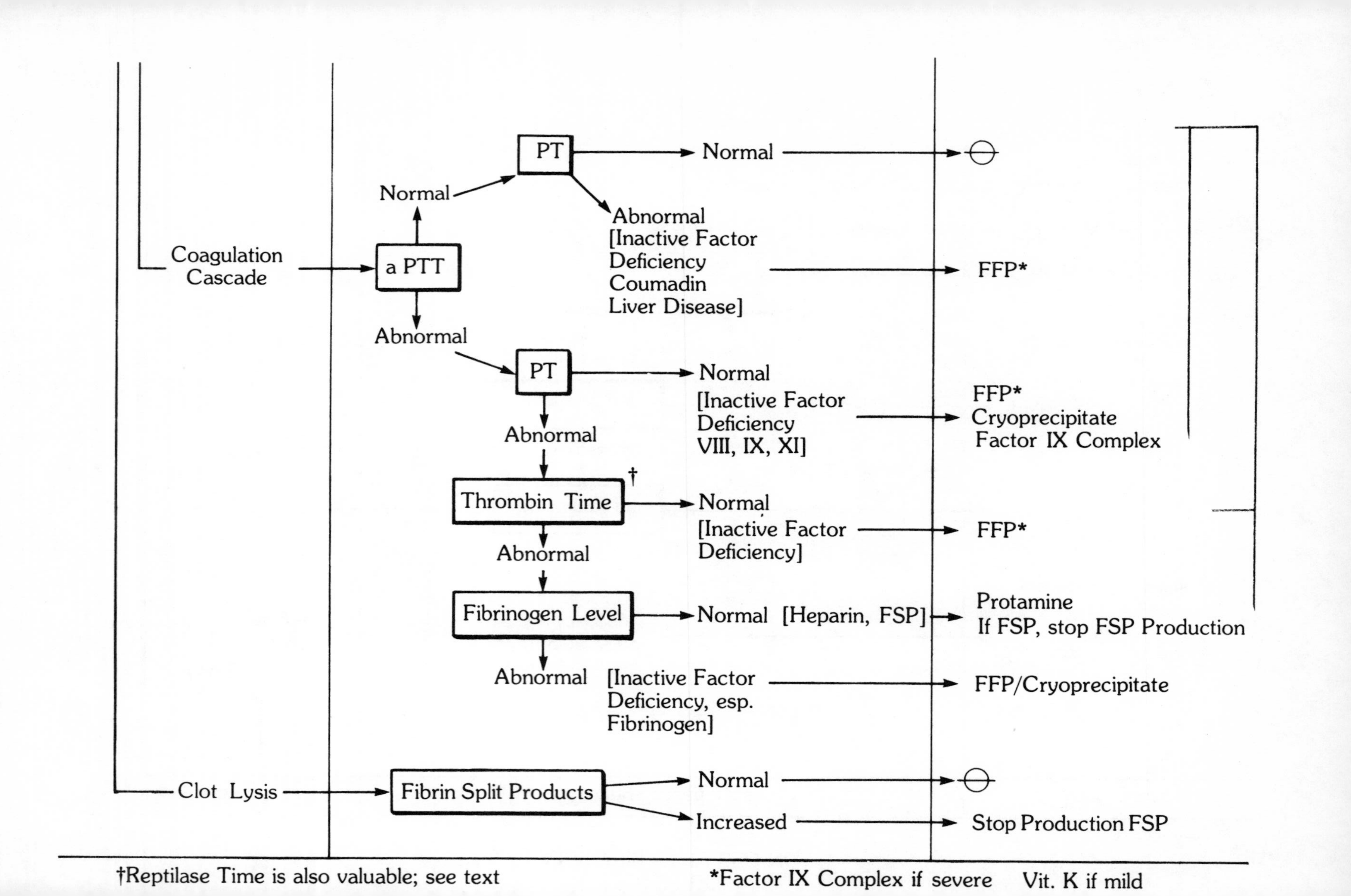

†Reptilase Time is also valuable; see text

*Factor IX Complex if severe Vit. K if mild

Chapter 9

DISORDERS, PREVENTION, AND TREATMENT OF THROMBOSIS

Until now, we have concentrated on those circumstances in which disorders of homostasis produce bleeding. In the other extreme are disorders of hemostasis which are associated with excessive thrombosis.

Each of the first three components of hemostasis — vascular integrity, platelets, and the coagulation cascade — can be the source of unwanted thrombosis. In addition, each of these three components can be modulated or attenuated to minimize or prevent thrombosis. The fourth hemostatic component, clot lysis, is used to treat thrombosis caused by disorders of the first three hemostatic components.

1. VASCULAR INTEGRITY
2. PLATELETS
3. COAGULATION CASCADE
4. CLOT LYSIS

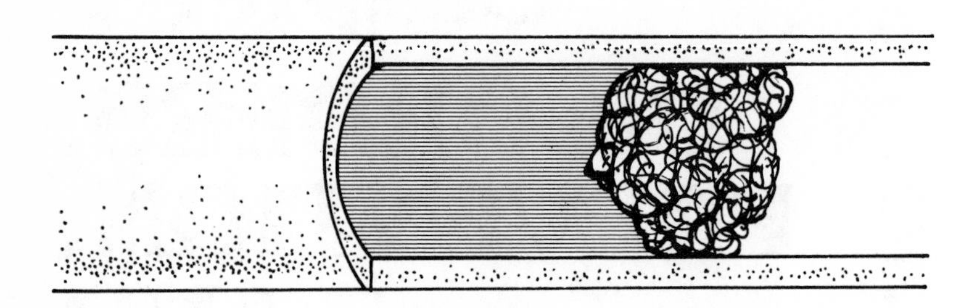

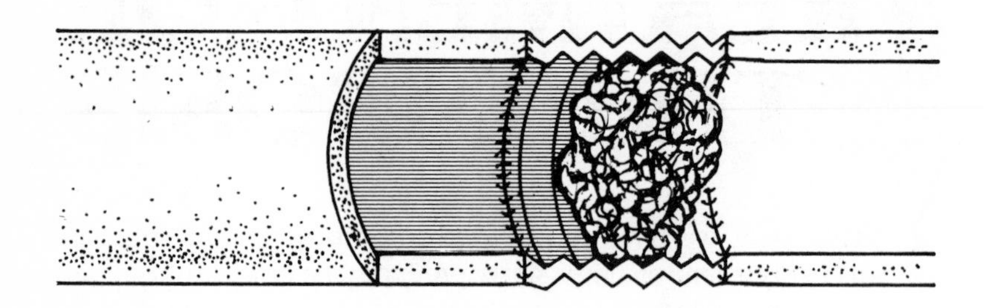

Major disorders of vascular integrity which promote thrombosis are those which involve endothelial injury or endothelial pathology. Atherosclerotic involvement in major blood vessels, abnormal venous structures (wall injury, valve abnormalities, tortuosity, etc.), and circulatory stasis all may predispose to platelet and fibrin deposition.

Artificial intravascular devices (cardiac vascular grafts, shunts and cannulae, etc.) serve as surfaces upon which platelets and fibrin may be deposited. The absence of endothelial prostacyclin (PGI_2) in these artificial surfaces promotes thrombosis even more extensively.

---

1. *Thrombosis is promoted in the presence of ______________ injury.* — ***endothelial***
2. *Thrombosis is promoted by the presence of intravascular ______________ surfaces.* — ***artificial***
3. *Absence of ______________ in artificial grafts promotes thrombosis.* — ***Prostacyclin***

1. VASCULAR INTEGRITY
2. PLATELETS
3. COAGULATION CASCADE
4. CLOT LYSIS

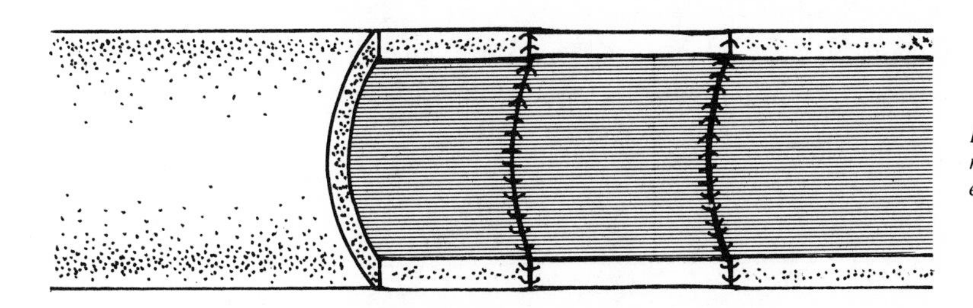

Imitate natural endothelium

The treatment of thrombosis caused by disorders of vascular integrity involves the removal of the inciting pathology, and/or the attenuation of the remainder of the hemostatic system. Thus, alterations in platelet function or in the effectiveness of the coagulation cascade may be necessary.

Development of artificial vascular devices which allow for, or promote, endothelial cell growth on the vascular surface, will minimize exposure of the artificial surface to blood. Prevention of thrombosis is clearly the goal in effective long-term patient management.

---

1. *Treatment of thrombosis caused by disorders of vascular integrity involves __________ of the inciting pathology.* — **removal**
2. *Treatment may involve __________ of the platelet reaction or of fibrin formation.* — **attenuation**
3. *Prevention involves __________ of the endothelial surface.* — **normalization**

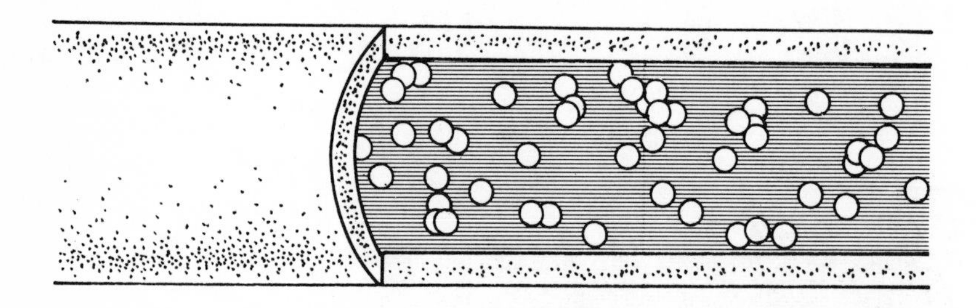

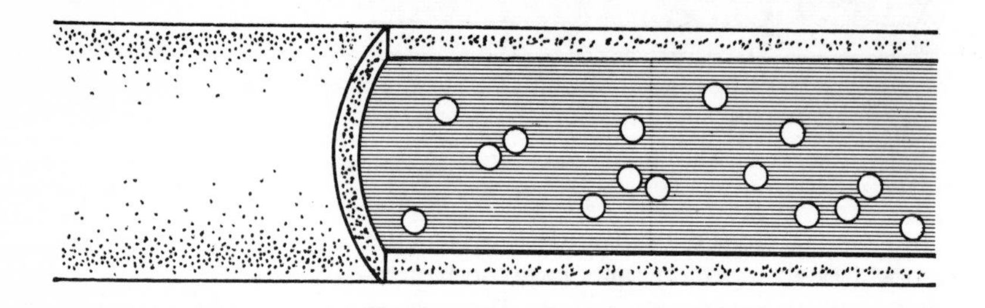

A platelet disorder causing excessive thrombosis is seen in polycythemia vera. In addition to the high number of circulating platelets, these platelets function abnormally. High platelet counts seen occasionally after splenectomy, or after excessive platelet transfusion, normally do not cause thrombosis.

Treatment of excessive platelet numbers is provided by plateletpheresis techniques, hemodilution, and prevention of circulatory statis.

---

1. *Platelets may promote thrombosis if increased, such as in __________.* — ***polycythemia vera***
2. *__________ is used to decrease platelet quantity.* — ***Plateletpheresis***

1. VASCULAR INTEGRITY
2. PLATELETS
3. COAGULATION CASCADE
4. CLOT LYSIS

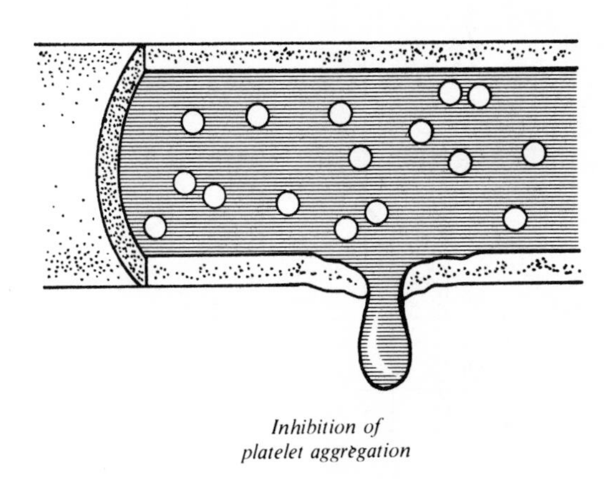

Inhibition of
platelet aggregation

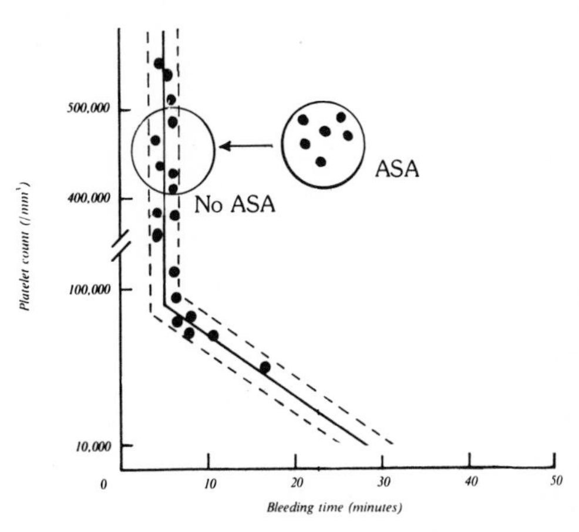

Treatment of excessive platelet aggregation is provided by attenuation of the aggregating capabilities of the platelets. Drugs used clinically, or experimentally, to prevent or minimize platelet aggregation, are summarized below:

Aspirin
Sufinpyrazone
Thromboxane A_2 inhibitors*
Prostacyclin analogs*
Steroids

(*experimental agents presently)

"Anti-platelet" drugs used commonly are:

______________ **aspirin**
______________ **sulfinpyrazone**
______________ **steroids**

1. VASCULAR INTEGRITY
2. PLATELETS
3. COAGULATION CASCADE
4. CLOT LYSIS

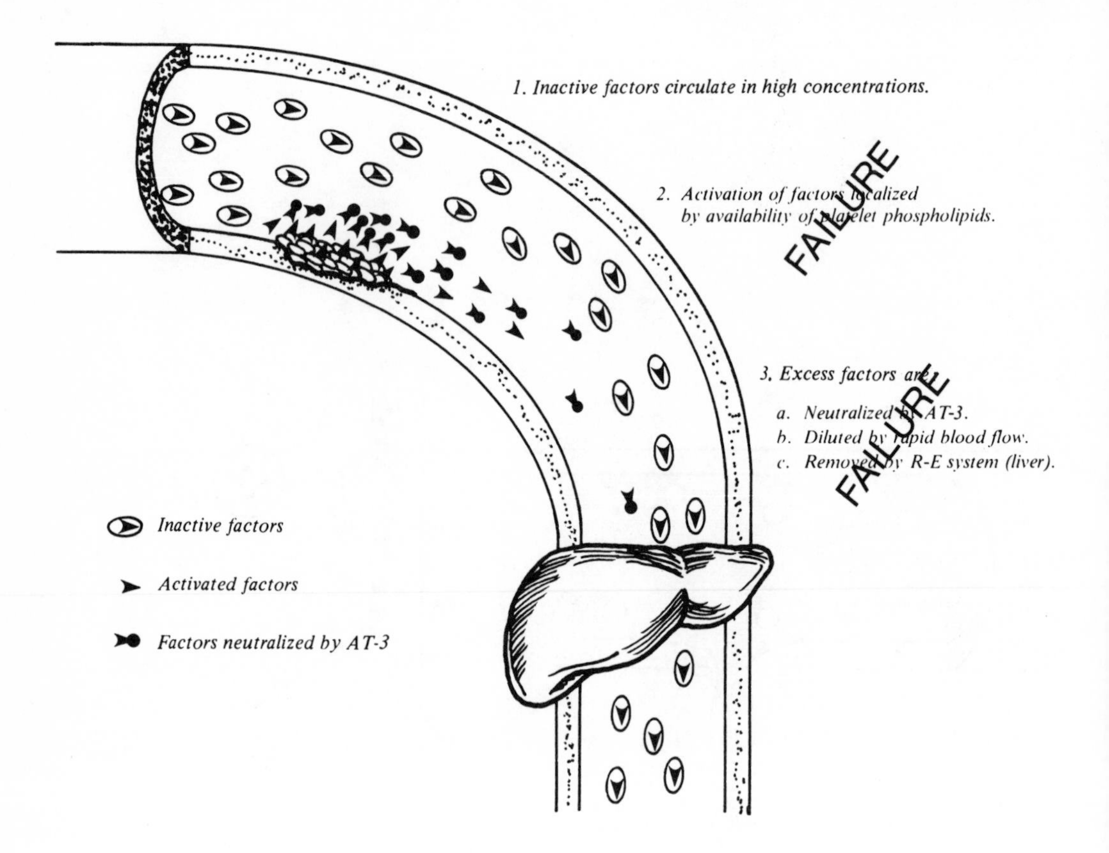

Disorders of the coagulation cascade causing thrombosis are numerous and common. The loss of any of the localizing mechanisms discussed in chapter three, may predispose to fibrin formation, and thus thrombosis. These could include the **failure** of:

Factor Dilution by rapid blood flow	circulatory shock
Factor Removal by the liver	hepatic dysfunction
Lack of activated factor neutralization by antithrombin-3 (At^3)	congenital AT^3 absence acquired AT^3 deficiency

---

1. *Thrombosis may be associated with ineffective __________ of activated serine proteases.* — ***removal***
2. *Thrombosis may be associated with __________.* — ***shock states***
3. *Thrombosis may accompany __________.* — ***hepatic dysfunction***

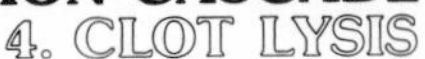

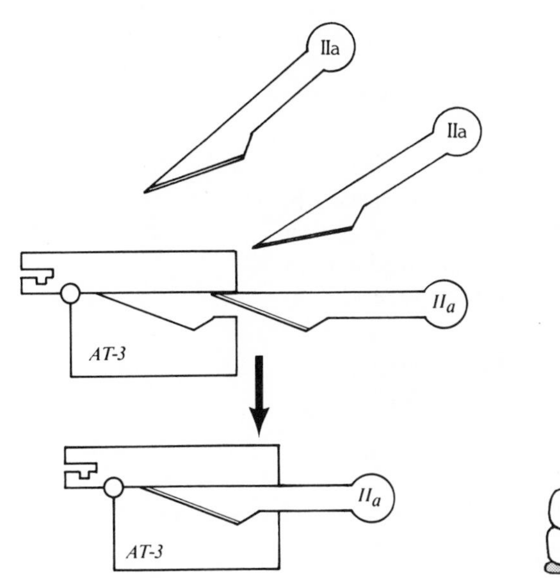

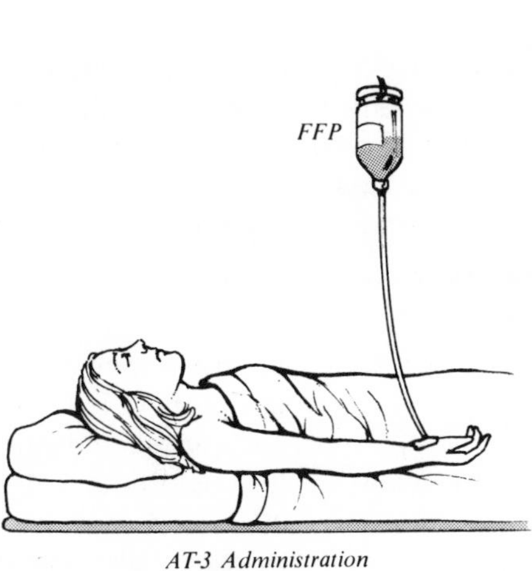

AT-3 Administration

One acquired disorder of an inactive factor which promotes thrombosis is a deficiency of antithrombin-3 (AT-3). A decrease in AT-3 production is reported, although an increase in AT-3 destruction is seen more commonly, such as in DIC. Circulating plasmin destroys AT-3. Levels of AT-3 may be substantially decreased by dilution with crystalloid or bank blood. The treatment for antithrombin deficiency is the administration of antithrombin via fresh frozen plasma. (AT-3 deficiency will make a patient refractory to heparin therapy, since heparin requires AT-3 for its biologic activity.)

---

1. *Fibrin formation may be modulated by ______________ factor levels or effectiveness.* — ***decreasing***
2. *______________ deficiency promotes thrombosis.* — ***antithrombin***
3. *Antithrombin is administered via ______________________.* — ***fresh frozen plasma***

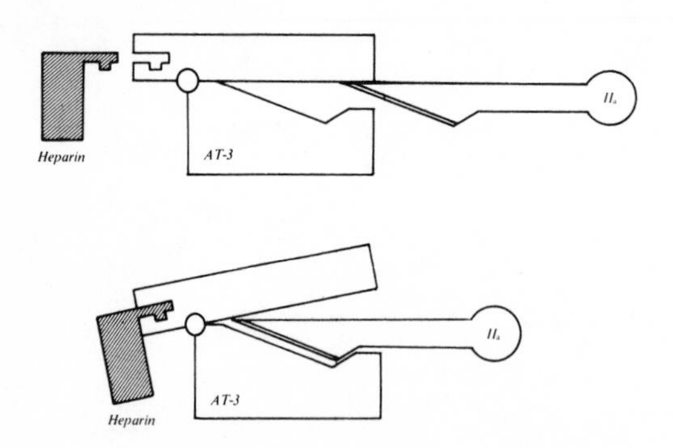

A controlled modulation of **active** factors is accomplished by increasing the effectiveness of antithrombin (AT-3). This can be accomplished by providing heparin to make AT-3 more avid in combining with activated serine proteases (11a, V11a, 1Xa, Xa, and X1a). Thus, fibrin formation is prevented or minimized.

The most commonly recognized goals in heparin therapy are threefold:

"mild"	thrombin time = 2 x normal aPTT or ACT, PT normal ("mini-dose" heparin therapy)
"moderate"	thrombin time = 4 x normal aPTT and ACT = 2-2½ x normal PT essentially normal (pulmonary embolism therapy)
"profound"	thrombin time profoundly prolonged aPTT and ACT = 5-6 x normal (this level is for cardiopulmonary bypass or similar mechanical procedures

The thrombin time (TT) is easily used to provide "fine-tuning" for "low-dose" heparin therapy, and the aPTT or ACT used for "higher dose" heparin therapy. (The actual use of the ACT at the bedside is illustrated in the Appendix.)

Heparin only serves to modulate anti-thrombin's capabilities; **it does not "dissolve" clots.** In fact, heparin-activated At-3 may combine with plasmin to reduce clot lysis.

---

1. *"Low-dose" heparin therapy produces a TT of ______________ normal.* — ***twice***
2. *"Moderate" heparin therapy produces an aPTT approximately ______________ normal.* — ***twice***
3. *"Profound" heparinization produces an aPTT ______________ normal.* — ***5-6 times***

1. VASCULAR INTEGRITY
2. PLATELETS
3. COAGULATION CASCADE
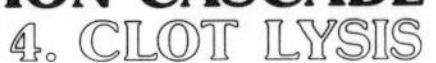

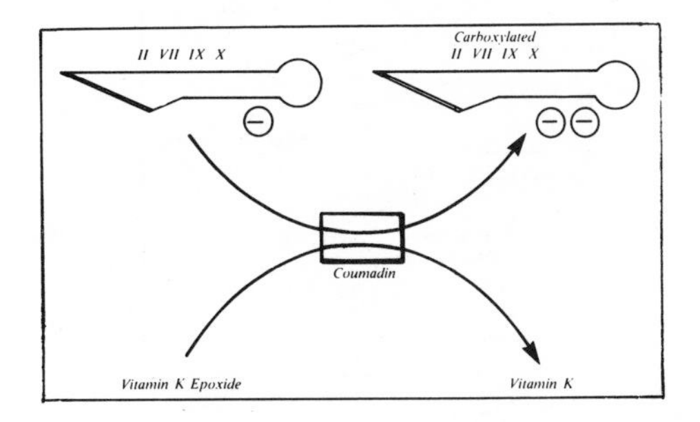

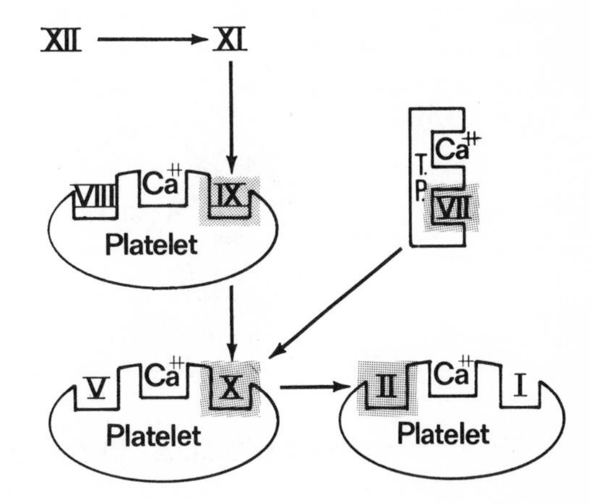

A reduction of inactive factors, to minimize or prevent thrombosis, is often provided in clinical medicine. A controlled reduction of factors II, VII, IX, and X can be produced with coumadin. Since coumadin inhibits the ribosomal modification of factors II, VII, IX, and X, this drug can attenuate selectively the coagulation cascade. A dose of coumadin (often 2.5 - 7.5 mg p.o. each day) necessary to provide a prothrombin time (PT) of approximately 25-30% of normal, is utilized.

---

1. *A reduction of __________ may prevent thrombosis* — ***inactive factors***
2. *Modified factors II, VII, IX, and X are reduced by __________.* — ***coumadin***
3. *Preventative coumadin therapy should provide a PT of __________ of normal.* — ***25-30%***

1. VASCULAR INTEGRITY
2. PLATELETS
3. COAGULATION CASCADE
4. CLOT LYSIS

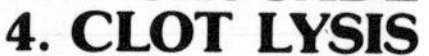

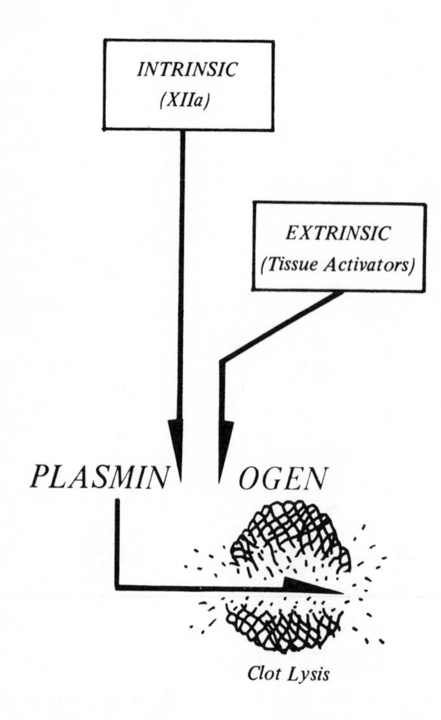

Clot Lysis

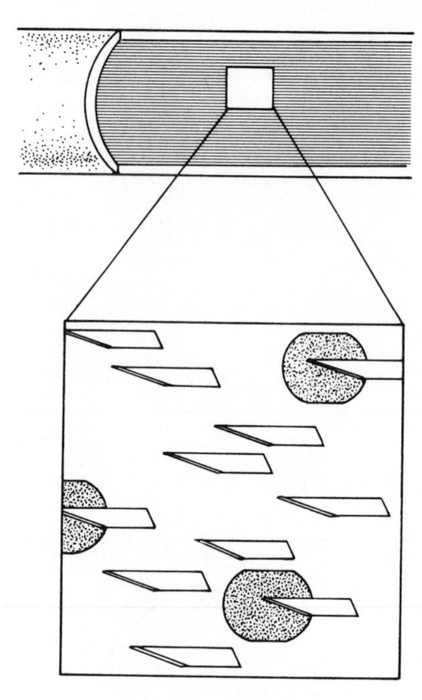

EXCESS PLASMIN

There is no known "natural" abnormality of clot lysis which causes thrombosis.

The use of drugs which enhance the fibrinolytic system is receiving active and enthusiastic investigation. The clinical settings are multiple: acute pulmonary embolism, deep vein thrombosis, dialysis A-V shunt occlusion, and myocardial infarction prevention or treatment. In essence, these drugs serve as plasminogen activators, to allow for the formation of plasmin in substantial concentrations. Their mechanisms of action are slightly different.

Drugs in this category should be used with the advice of a qualified hematologist. The following information is for background and stimulus only. We will discuss only streptokinase and urokinase, even though other agents such as thrombolysin, actase, and various snake venoms are under investigation.

---

1. Fibrinolysis may be improved using ____________ or ____________.

streptokinase
urokinase

2. Three disorders in which thrombolytic agents may be used are: ____________, ____________, and ____________.

pulmonary embolism
deep vein thrombosis
A-V shunt occlusion

1. VASCULAR INTEGRITY
2. PLATELETS
3. COAGULATION CASCADE
4. CLOT LYSIS

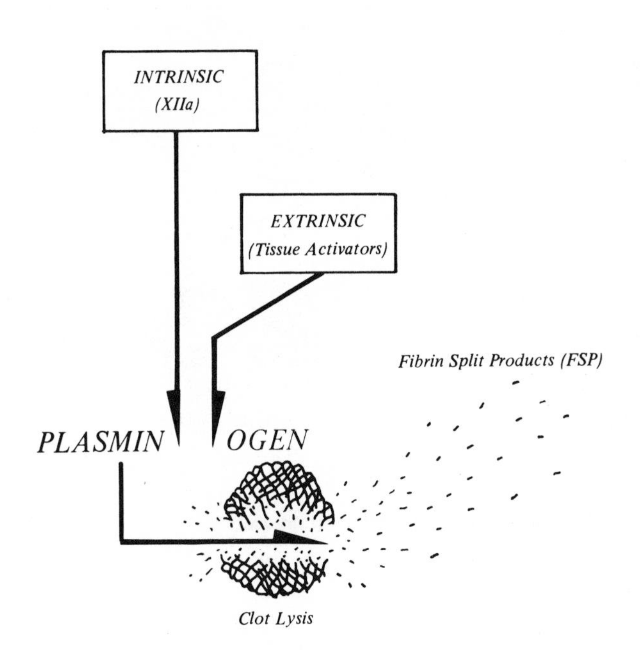

A comparison of streptokinase and urokinase yields the following data.*

	Streptokinase	Urokinase
Source	Group C streptococci	Kidney tissue cultures
Antigenic	yes	no
Pyrogenic	yes	no
Drug Stability	Room Temperature	4° C
Half-Life	First Phase, 18 min Second Phase, 83 min	16 min
Indications presently	Acute Pulmonary Embolism Deep Vein Thrombosis Occluded A-V Cannulae	Acute Pulmonary Embolism
Loading dose	250,000 I.U.	4,400 I.U./kg
Maintenance doses	100,000 U.U./hr.	4,400 I.U./kg/hr
Comments	Antibodies Possible	Expensive

The biodegration and excretion of these two drugs is not fully understood.

(*modified from Sasahara, AA: Drug Therapy, October 1979)

---

1. *Thrombolytic drugs have different ________.* — ***sources***
2. *Streptokinase is ________ and ________.* — ***antigenic***, ***pyrogenic***
3. *Urokinase is ________.* — ***expensive***

1. VASCULAR INTEGRITY
2. PLATELETS
3. COAGULATION CASCADE
4. CLOT LYSIS

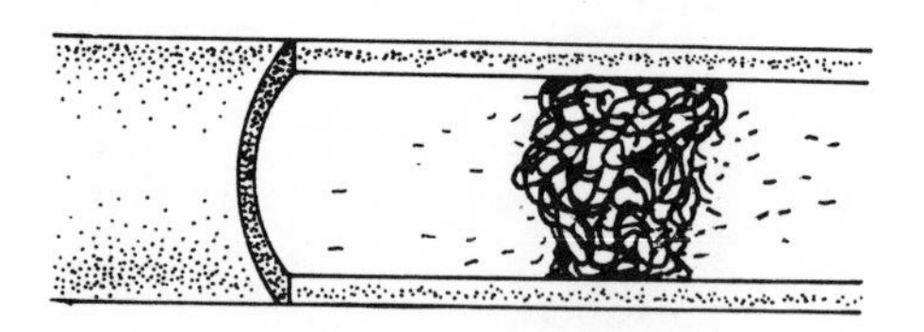

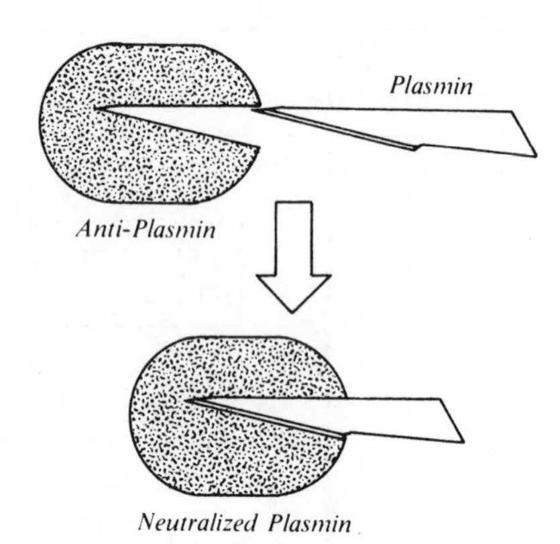

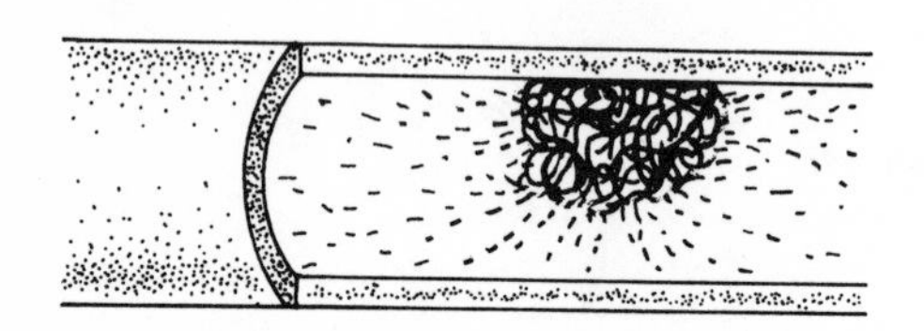

The circumstances* affecting adequate clot lysis with these two drugs include:

- clot location and blood flow to area of clot
- clot duration — preferably less than 7 days old (the younger the better)
- clot size — the smaller the better
- clot plasminogen concentration — the higher the better
- body temperature — no extremes
- ability of fibrinolytic system to be activated — absence of inhibitors or dysfunction of components

Concomitant administration of anticoagulants, platelet inhibitors, and dextran should not occur. The complications of therapy include bleeding, fever, and "allergic" reactions. Overdosage may be treated judiciously with epsilon aminocaproic acid (EACA), after discontinuance of the thrombolytic drug, in conjunction with hematologic consultation.

(*modified from Bell, WR: NEJM 301: 1266-1270, 1979)

---

1. *Clot lysis is affected by many circumstances:* ________, ________ ________, ________.
   location duration size clot plasminogen

2. *Complications of thrombolytic therapy include:* ________, ________, ________.
   bleeding fever "allergic" reaction

3. *Complications from thrombolytic agents may be treated with* ________.
   EACA

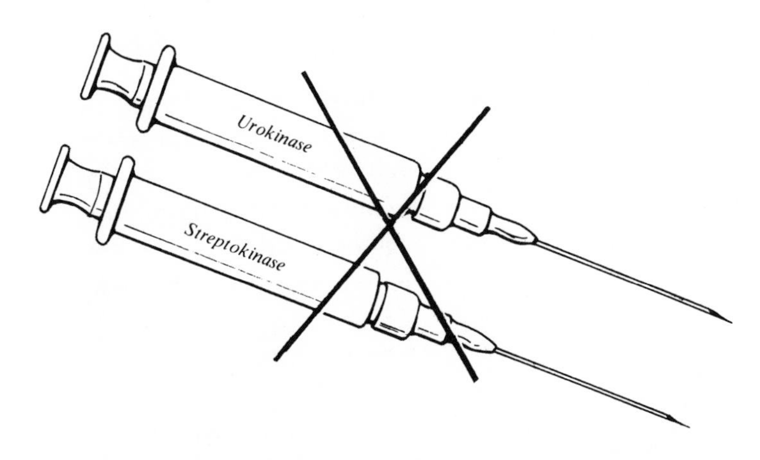

Some patients presently are **not** considered candidates for urokinase or streptokinase therapy, although the list below will undoubtedly undergo revisions during further investigation of these drugs. Contraindications may include:

- Recent surgery, invasive biopsy or drainage, or obstetrical delivery (within 7-10 days?)
- Recent sizable intraarterial invasion (cut-downs, angiograms?)
- Recent CVA, CNS procedure, or CNS neoplasm
- Recent myocardial infarction? (controversial)
- Gastrointestinal bleeding
- Active bleeding or coagulopathy
- Pregnancy
- Pediatric patient?
- Suspicion of presence of intracardiac clot
- Acute/chronic renal or hepatic insufficiency

Those who are candidates for thrombolytic therapy are medicated in such a manner as to produce a prolongation of the thrombin time (TT) 2-5 times normal. The prolongation of the TT is caused by the presence of fibrin split products (FSP). Direct assay of FSP is an alternate monitoring technique.

---

1. Contraindications to thrombolytic therapy may include:
____
____
____
____
____

recent surgery
active bleeding
pregnancy
major CNS disorder
intracardiac clot

2. Thrombolytic therapy should producce a thrombin time ______________ times normal.

2-5

1. VASCULAR INTEGRITY
2. PLATELETS
3. COAGULATION CASCADE
4. CLOT LYSIS

Prevention and treatment of disorders promoting thrombosis are summarized below:

Hemostatic Area	Basic Disorders	Therapy
Vascular Integrity	Endothelial Injury or pathology	Provide an unbroken, normal endothelial surface Promote endothelial growth on artificial surfaces Remove or replace abnormal vessels Attenuate platelet or fibrin function
Platelets	Platelet Aggregation	Reduce platelet number Minimize sludging and stasis Use "antiplatelet" drugs aspirin sulfinpyrazone steroids
Coagulation Cascade	Loss of localizing mechanisms producing increased fibrin formation	Prevent or improve: circulatory shock hepatic dysfunction (enhance clearance of activated serine proteases) Inactive Factors Decrease "production" of II, VII, IX, X withhold Vitamin K Coumadin therapy Active Factors Administer Antithrombin-3 (via FFP) Heparin therapy
Clot Lysis	Need for increased fibrinolysis	Controlled plasmin activation* Streptokinase Urokinase

(*Consultation with a qualified hematologist advised)

Details of Coagulation Testing

This appendix is designed to complement chapter four on coagulation testing. We will not repeat all of the information covered in that chapter, and will concentrate on testing of the coagulation cascade and clot lysis. We will supply the reader with a brief series of steps actually performed in the laboratory, so that details of each laboratory technique may be appreciated.

The reader is reminded of five important points previously stressed:

1. The end point of all tests of the coagulation cascade is the formation of a fibrin clot, sufficiently large enough to be detected by various methods.
2. All laboratory tests are performed on samples in which a calcium chelating agent previously has been added to the collection tube. Thus calcium must be re-added to the plasma in order to perform the tests.
3. Artifacts can be introduced easily into testing systems, if exact technical and collection protocols are not followed precisely.
4. The major difference in initiating and thus testing either the intrinsic or extrinsic pathway is the phospholipid—platelet or tissue—added in the laboratory.
5. Normal values may vary among laboratories. Check with your local coagulation laboratory for accepted local normal values.

Intrinsic Pathway Testing

Remember that the intrinsic pathway is the longest pathway. The names which are longest test this pathway: aPTT (activated partial thromboplastin time), ACT (activated coagulation time), and WBCT (whole blood clotting time).

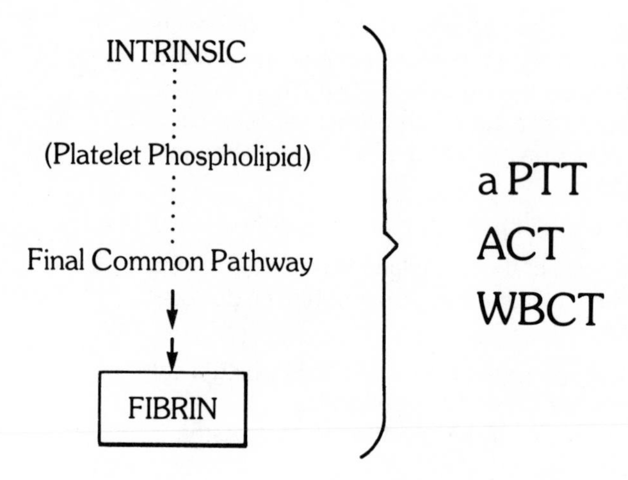

Tests for the Intrinsic Pathway all test the same pathway. All have the same end-point—a fibrin clot. Let us now look at each of these three tests in detail, including a brief summary of the actual method used to perform the tests in the laboratory.

The Activated Partial Thromboplastin Time (aPTT)
(Normal = 26-39 seconds)

Citrated plasma activated by surface activation
- Cephalin (a PF3-like material), or kaolin
- Heat/Agitate
- End product ⟶ clot

INTRINSIC

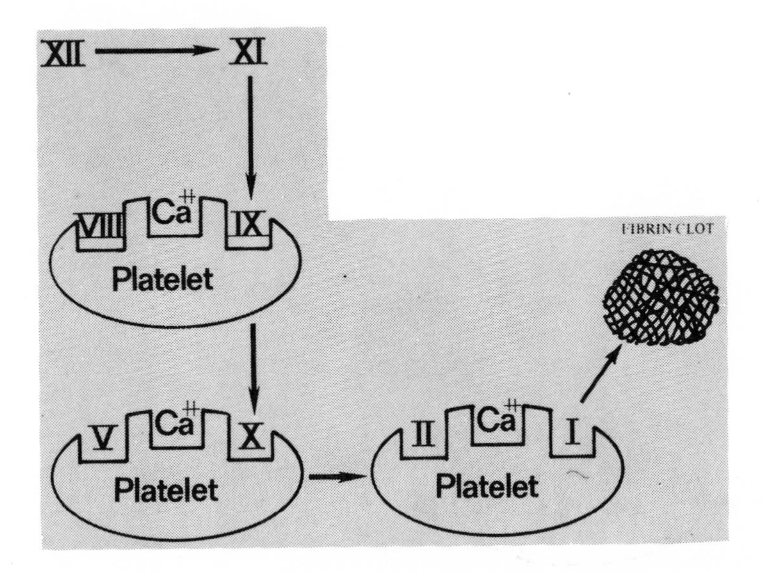

(Specimen is run with a normal control for comparison)

Abnormal: Hemophilia (VIII, IX, or XI deficiency)
Coumadin Therapy
Heparin Therapy
Factor Depletion States
Severe Hepatic Disease

Activated Coagulation Time (ACT)
(Normal by hand 75-90 seconds)
(Normal by Hemochron® 90-120 seconds)

Whole blood specimen added to test tube containing
- celite (diatomaceous earth) for activation
- Heat, agitate or rotate
- End product ⟶ clot

INTRINSIC

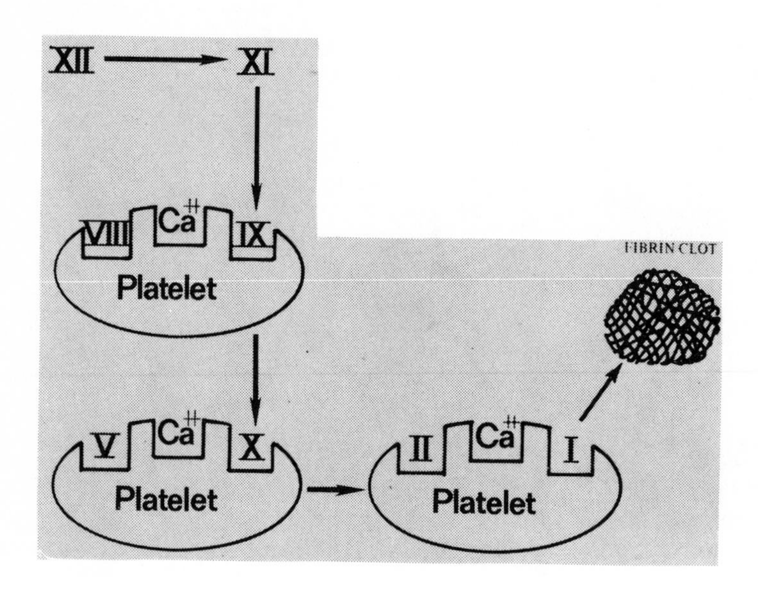

The ACT, activated coagulation time, is nothing more than a simplified aPTT run at the bedside. The information to be derived is exactly the same as that from the aPTT, only with less variability. The endpoint is exactly the same as in the aPTT—formation of a fibrin clot. The endpoint may be visually evaluated, or mechanically determined by a variety of means. A common device presently in use in operating rooms (Hemochron®) measures the endpoint by evaluating the change in magnetic field when a small magnet becomes trapped in the forming fibrin clot. The ACT is the preferred test for intrinsic system testing in the operating room.

Abnormal: Hemophilia (VIII, IX, or XI deficiency)
Coumadin Therapy
Heparin Therapy
Factor Depletion States
Severe Hepatic Disease

Whole Blood Clotting Time (WBCT)
(Also known as the Lee-White WBCT)
(Normal: 2.5-4.25 minutes)

Whole blood is placed in a plain test tube

- Heated
- Tilted periodically
- End product ⟶ clot observed visually

INTRINSIC

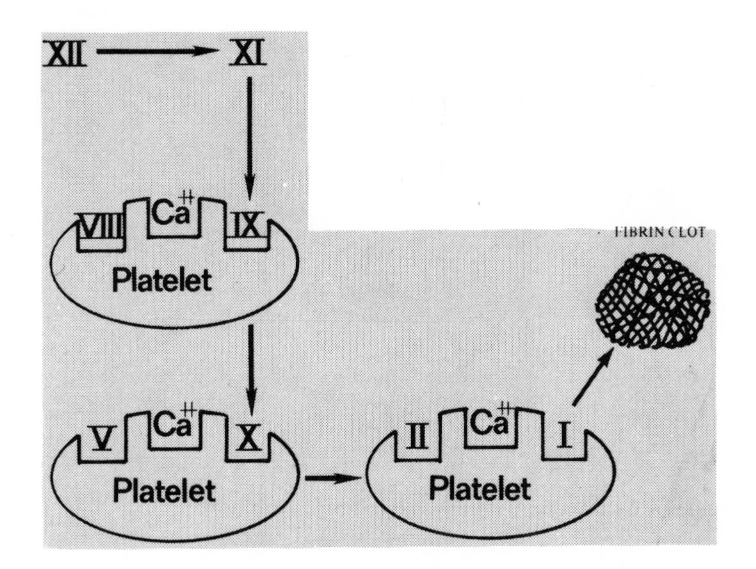

No activating agent is used, as the inside of the test tube serves to activate. The WBCT is far less sensitive than the ACT or aPTT, and has been replaced by the ACT in the operative and ICU settings. (An older modification of the WBCT had used three separate test tubes, but this test is now considered obsolete.)

Abnormal: Hemophilia (VIII, IX, or XI deficiency)
Coumadin Therapy
Heparin Therapy
Factor Depletion States
Severe Hepatic Disease

EXTRINSIC PATHWAY TESTING

Remember that the extrinsic pathway is the shortest pathway. Thus the "shorter names" test this pathway: PT (prothrombin time), and the P & P (prothrombin-proconvertin time).

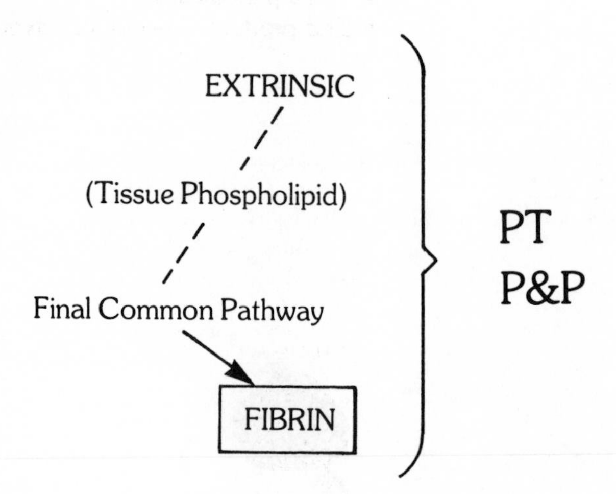

Tests for the extrinsic pathway test the final common pathway as well. We will look at a modification of the PT, called the P & P, which helps separate coagulation factor deficiencies from thrombin inhibitors in extrinsic pathway testing.

Prothrombin Time (PT)
(Normal: Approximately 11 seconds; also reported as 60%)

To Citrated plasma, add:
- Calcium
- Platelets
- Tissue phospholipid
- Heat
- End product → clot

EXTRINSIC

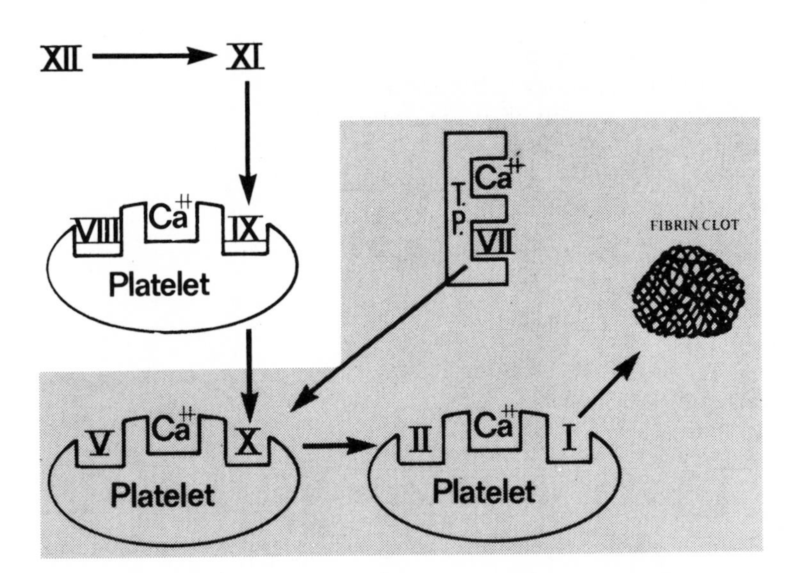

The PT, prothrombin time ("the test with the shorter name tests the shorter pathway") serves to evaluate the extrinsic pathway. In addition, of course, it also tests the final common pathway, since the end product of the test is, again, a fibrin clot. Results are reported in seconds, along with a control specimen. These two values may be compared as a "percent" figure taken from a **non-linear** calibration curve. Normal values will vary, but are generally greater than 60%.

Abnormal: Coumadin Therapy
Heparin Therapy
Factor Depletion States
Severe Hepatic Disease

There is a clever manipulation of the PT. If the PT is abnormal, there is usually one of two common problems occurring:

1. Heparin effect (acting via AT-3)
2. Extrinsic factor deficiencies (VII, X, V, II, and I)

How might these two categories be differentiated from each other? Remember that only approximately 10% of the normal concentrations of each of the coagulation factors is required for normal coagulation. If the specimen with an abnormal PT secondary to heparin was diluted 1:10 and another PT performed, any heparin effect would be diluted, and the PT normalized. This manipulation is called the **P & P, prothrombin-proconvertin time**. (Some minor additions are required as detailed on the next page.)

A summary of the comparison between the PT and the P & P is as follows:

PT	P & P	Problem
normal	normal	normal extrinsic system
prolonged	normal or much nearer to normal	heparin effect
prolonged	equally prolonged	deficiency of factor VII, X, II (most likely VII). (If aPTT is normal, VII is the problem.)

Prothrombin-Proconvertin Time (P & P)
(Normal: Approximately 11 seconds, also reported as 60%)

To Citrated plasma, add:
- Calcium
- Platelets
- Tissue phospholipid
- Proaccelerin (V)
- Fibrinogen (I)
- Dilute specimen with normal saline
- Heat
- End product → clot

EXTRINSIC

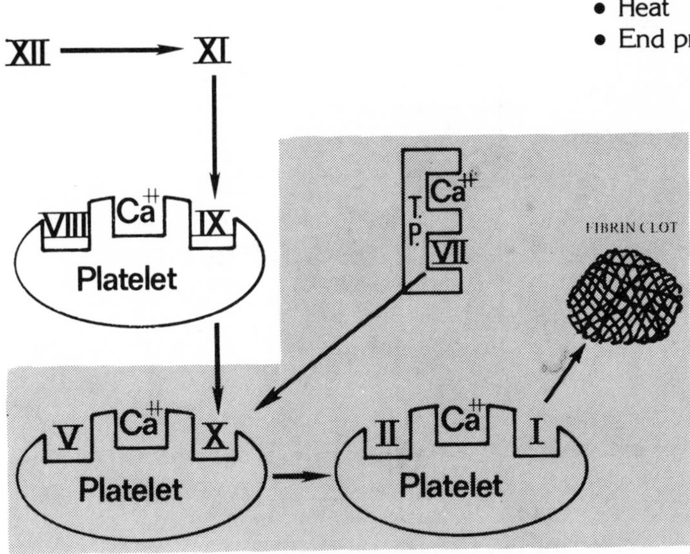

The Prothrombin-Proconvertin Time (P & P) is just a modified PT. It is diluted to minimize the effects of heparin (the heparin concentration is thus greatly reduced). Fibrinogen (I) is added so that a firm clot can be obtained (counteracting the dilutional effects on fibrinogen). Proaccelerin (V) is added to remove abnormalities caused by this labile cofactor. Thus, the P & P measured deficiencies of factor VII, and to some extent II and X.

Abnormal: Factor VII Deficiency
Coumadin Therapy
Hepatic Disease
Factor II, X Deficiency
Very High Heparin Concentrations

Testing of the Final Stage in the Final Common Pathway

The end product in the final common pathway is a fibrin clot. Fibrin is produced by the action of thrombin on fibrinogen. Thus an evaluation of the formation of fibrin will tell a great deal about the amount or type of fibrinogen. In addition, the presence of thrombin inhibitors or inhibitors of fibrin cross-linking will be evident.

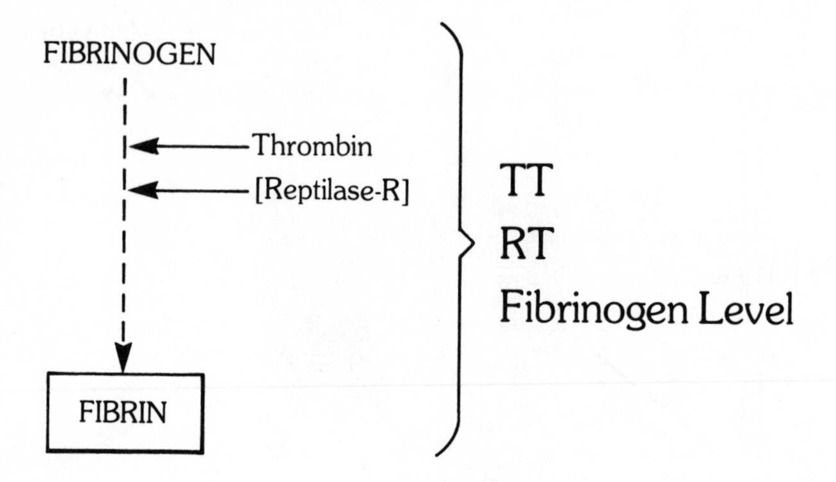

We will thus look at the thrombin time (TT), reptilase time (RT), and fibrinogen level, as three tests to evaluate this final stage in the final common pathway.

Thrombin Time (TT)
(Normal: Approximately 15 seconds)

To Citrated plasma, add:
- Thrombin
- Heat
- End product ⟶ clot

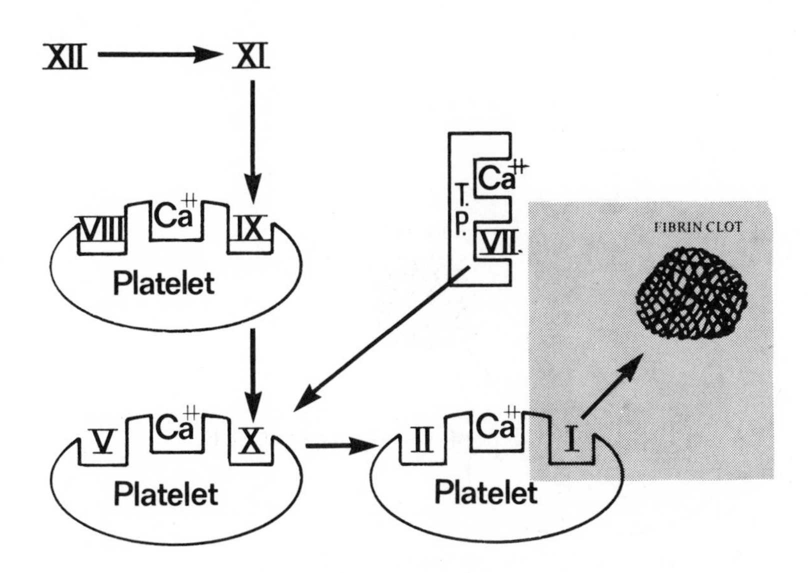

This test measures the last stage of the final common pathway, since thrombin is already added in the performance of the test. The end product of the test is a fibrin clot. (Enough thrombin is added so that a normal plasma specimen will clot in 15-35 seconds.) Each specimen will be run with a control for comparison.

Abnormal: Low fibrinogen level (200 mg%)
An abnormal type of fibrinogen
Presence of a thrombin inhibitor
(such as heparin-activated anti-thrombin (AT-3), or fibrin split products)

Reptilase Time (RT)
(Normal: 14-21 seconds)

To Citrated plasma, add:
- Reptilase-R
- Heat
- End product ⟶ clot

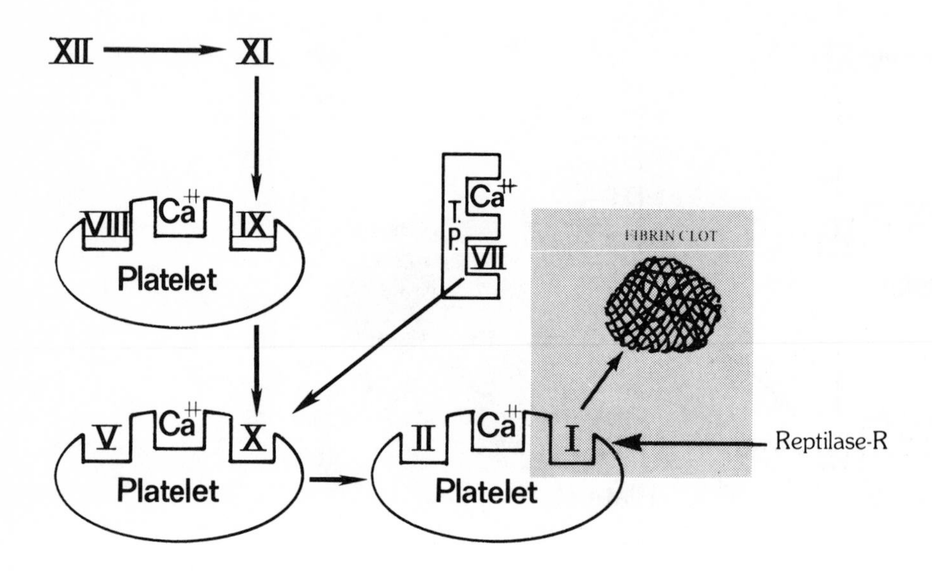

The reptilase time is a modification of the thrombin time. Like thrombin, Reptilase-R is an enzyme capable of cleaving fibrinogen, however it splits off only firbinopeptides A and AP. These fragments are able to cross-link in the presence of fibrin split products, explaining the minimal effect of FSP on the reptilase time. Reptilase-R does **not** split fibrin (and is thus free of fibrinolytic activity).

In the presence of heparin, thrombin is inhibited, via antithrombin. However, heparin does **not** affect Reptilase-R's ability to cleave fibrinogen. Thus a comparison of the thrombin time and reptilase time will assist in evaluating the presence of thrombin inhibitors such as heparin.

Thrombin Time	Reptilase Time	Problem
Prolonged	Equally Prolonged	Low Fibrinogen
Prolonged	Strongly Prolonged	Dysfibrinogenemia
Prolonged	Normal	Heparin Presence
Prolonged	Slightly Prolonged	Fibrin(ogen) Split Products

Fibrinogen Level
(Normal: 160-350 mg%)

To Citrated Plasma, add:
- Thrombin in excess
- Heat
- End product ⟶ clot

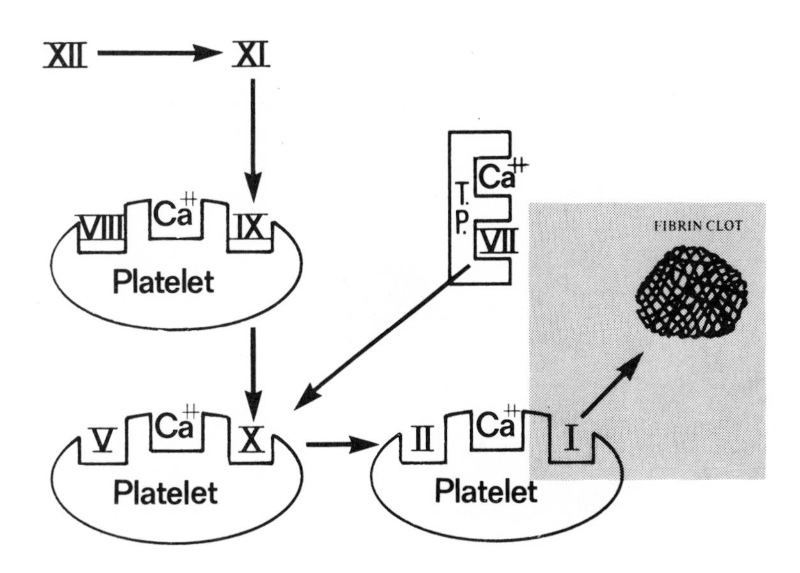

The fibrinogen level is another test used to evaluate the last stage in the final common pathway. In essence, it is a thrombin time performed with an excess of thrombin. The excess thrombin is used to "overpower" any thrombin inhibitors (such as heparin-activated antithrombin). Controls are run using samples containing known concentrations of fibrinogen.

Abnormal: Low fibrinogen concentration (<160 mg%)
An abnormal type of fibrinogen

Fibrin Split Products (FSP) by Latex Testing

(Normal: 10 micrograms/ml)

To patient serum **after** clot has formed:

- Serially dilute specimen samples
- Add latex suspension
- Mix and spread
- Observe for clumping

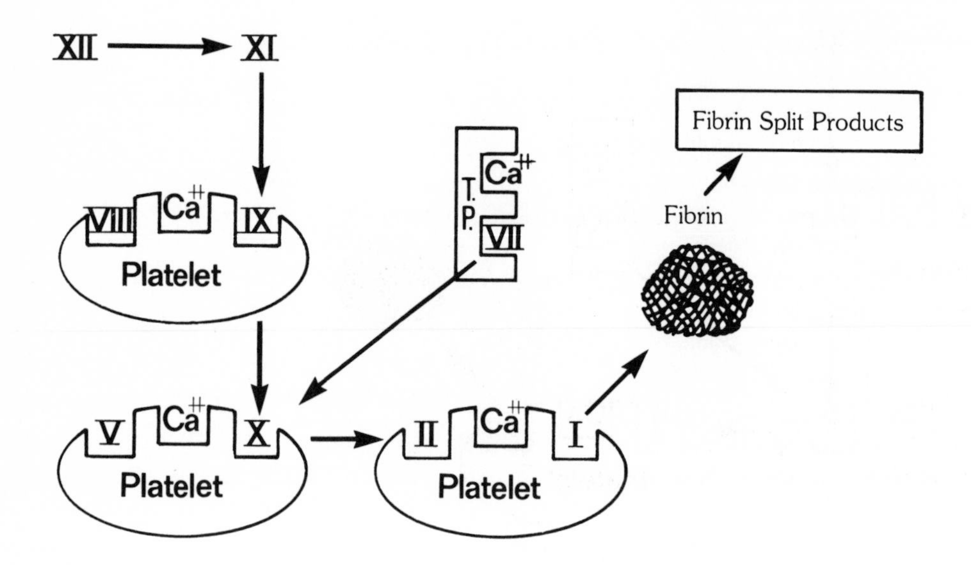

Degradation products of fibrin or fibrinogen will cause macroscopic agglutination (clumping) when combined with certain latex particles. These particles have been previously coated with antisera to the D and E fibrin fragments. (There are details in the testing procedure which are necessary, but will not be discussed in detail here, such as adding thrombin to the collection tube, and the use of epsilon amino caproic acid during collection to inhibit post-collection fibrinolysis.) Human fibrinogen standards, as positive controls, and negative serum controls are also used.

Abnormal: Active Fibrinolysis, including DIC

False negative: Patient with depleted fibrinogen and/or depleted fibrin (consumption)

Hemostatic Abnormalities Which May Occur Specifically After Surgery Involving Cardiopulmonary Bypass—A Summary

Vascular Integrity

- Surgical holes
- Hypertension—arterial or venous
- Intimal vascular damage from atherosclerosis
- Inflammatory process (endocarditis, vasculitis)

Platelets

- Quantitative disorder from sequestration, dilution, or destruction
- Qualitative disorders
  - Drugs—ASA, dextran, aminoglycosides, or protamine
  - Effects of fibrin split products
  - Storage defects in transfused platelets
  - Presence of uremic plasma

Coagulation Cascade

- Hypothermia (decreased enzymatic reaction rates)
- Inactive factor deficiencies
  - Dilution, destruction, consumption (V, VIII, I, AT-3)
  - Coumadin therapy, Hepatic dysfunction, Dilution } (II, VII, IX, X)
- Active factor deficiencies
  - Heparin effect (II, VII, IX, X, XI)
  - Inhibition by fibrin split products

Clot Lysis

- DIC with increased fibrinolysis, secondary to inadequate heparinization, deficiency of AT-3, circulating tissue phospholipids, sepsis, etc.
- Fibrinolysis secondary to streptokinase therapy
- Hemolytic anemia secondary to transfusion reaction

(Combinations of any of the above)

PRODUCTS CONTAINING ASPIRIN
(Alphabetical Order)

PRODUCT	MANUFACTURER
	A
ACA Caps & No. 2	Scrip
ACD	Philips Roxane
Acetabar*	Philips Roxane
Acetasem*	Philips Roxane
Acetonyl	Upjohn
Aidant	Noyes
Aidant c Dovers powder*	Noyes
Aidant c gelsemium	Noyes
Alka Seltzer	Miles
Allylgesic*	Elder
Allylgesic c ergotamine*	Elder
Alprine*	Ulmer
Aluprin	Lemmon
Amsodyne*	Elder
Amytal c ASA*	Lilly
Anacin	Whitehall
Anexsia c codeine	Massengill
Anexsia-D*	Massengill
Anodynos	Buffington
Ansemco No. 1 & 2	Massengill
APAC*	N Amer Pharm
Apamead*	Spencer Mead
APC	Various manufacturers
APC c codeine*	Various manufacturers
APC c Demerol	Winthrop
APC c gelsemium*	Sutliff & Case
Aphodyne	Gold Leaf
Aphophen*	Gold Leaf
Arthra-Zene caps	Xttrium
ASA	Lilly
ASA compound	Lilly
ASA compound c codeine	Lilly
Asalco No. 1 & 2	Jenkins
Ascaphen	Schlicksup
Ascaphen compound	Schlicksup
As-csa-phen	Ulmer
Ascodeen-30*	Burroughs Wellcome
Ascription	Rorer
Ascriptin c codeine*	Rorer
Aspadine tab*	N Amer Pharm
Aspergum	Pharmaco
Asphac-G*	Central

Asphac-G c codeine	Central
Asphencaf	Cole
Asphyte	Cowley
Aspirbar	Lannett
Aspir-C	Jenkins
Aspireze	Stanlabs
Aspirin (USP)	Various manufacturers
Aspirin aluminum	Abbott
Aspirin children's	Abbott
Aspirin compound c Dover's powder*	Fellows
Aspirin-Pb tab*	American Drug
Aspirin-secobarbital Supprettes No. 1 & 2 & 3 & 4*	Webster
Aspirin Supprettes	Webster
Aspirjen Jr Tabs	Jenkins
Aspirocal*	McNeil
Aspir-phen	Spencer-Mead & Robinson
Aspodyne	Blue Line
Aspodyne c codeine*	Blue Line
Axotal*	Warren-Teed
B	
Babylove	Amer Pharm
Ban-O-Pain	Daniels
Bayer	Glenbrook
Bayer children's	Glenbrook
Bayer timed-release	Glenbrook
Brogesix*	Brothers
Bufabar*	Philips Roxane
Buff-A	Mayrand
Buffacetin	Kay & Bowman
Buff-a-Comp*	Mayrand
Buffadyne	Lemmon
Buffadyne A-S Tab*	Lemmon
Buffadyne c barbiturates	Lemmon
Bufferin	Bristol-Meyers
Bufferin arthritis strength	Bristol-Meyers
Buffinol	Otis Clapp
C	
Calurin	Dorsey
Cama Inlay	Dorsey
Capron	Bryant-Vitarine
Causalin*	Amfre-Grant
Cephalgesic*	Smith, Miller & Patch
Cheracol caps	Upjohn
Cirin	Zemmer
Clistanal*	McNeil
Codasa tab*	Stayner

Codempiral No. 2 & 3	Burroughs Wellcome
Codesal No. 1 & 2	Durst
Coldate	Elder
Colrex	Rowell
Colrex compound*	Rowell
Cogesprin	Bristol-Meyers
Congesprin	Bristol-Meyers
Cope	Glenbrook
Coralsone modified*	Zemmer
Cordex*	Upjohn
Cordex forte*	Upjohn
Cordex buffered*	Upjohn
Cordex forte buffered*	Upjohn
Coricidin	Schering
Coricidin "D"	Schering
Coricidin Demilets	Schering
Coricidin Medilets	Schering
Co-ryd	Daniels
Counter Pain	Squibb
Covangesic	Mallinekrodt
D	
Darvon c ASA*	Lilly
Darvon-N c ASA*	Lilly
Darvon compound 32 & 65*	Lilly
Darvo-Tran*	Lilly
Dasikon	Beecham-Massengill
Dasin caps*	Beecham-Massengill
Dasin-CS*	Beecham-Massengill
Dasin ¼ strength*	Beecham-Massengill
Decagesic*	Merck, Sharp & Dome
Delenar*	Schering
Derfort*	Cole
Derfule*	Cole
Dolcin	Dolcin
Dolene compound 65*	Lederle
Dolor	Geriatric Pharm
Doloral*	Wolly
Dorodol*	Durst
Drinacet*	Philips-Roxane
Dristan Tab	Whitehall
Drocogesic No. 3*	Century Lab
Duopac*	Spencer-Mead
Duradyne	Durst
Duragesic	Meyer
E	
Ecotrin	Smith, Kline & French

Empiral*	Burroughs Wellcome
Empirin	Burroughs Wellcome
Empirin	Burroughs Wellcome
Empirin compound c codeine	Burroughs Wellcome
Emprazil	Burroughs Wellcome
Emprazil-C*	Burroughs Wellcome
Epragen*	Lilly
Equagesic*	Wyeth
Excedrin	Bristol-Meyers
Excedrin PM	Bristol-Meyers
F	
Fiorinal*	Sandoz
Fiorinal c coden No. 1 & 2 & 3*	Sandoz
Fizrin	Glenbrook
Formasal caps & tabs	First Texas
4-Way cold tabs	Bristol-Meyers
G	
Gelsodyne*	Blue Line
Grillodyne*	Fellows Med
H	
Hasamal CT*	Arnar-Stone
Henasphen	Drug Products
Histadyl & ASA compound	Lilly
Hypan	Lemmon
I	
I-PAC*	Spender-Mead
K	
Kryl*	Ayerst
L	
Liquiprin	Thayer
Lumasprin c hyoscyamus*	Rorer
M	
Marnal tab & cap	N Amer Pharm
Measurin	Breon
Medadent*	Upjohn
Medaprin*	Upjohn
Midol	Glenbrook
Multihist & APC caps†	Dorsey
N	
Nembudeine ¼ & ½ & 1*	Abbott
Nembu-Gesic*	Abbott
Nipirin*	Elder
Norgesic*	Riker
Novahistine c APC	Dow Chemical
Novrad c ASA*	Lilly

	O
Opacedrin	Elder
Opasal	Elder
	P
Paadon*	Rorer
Pabirin	Dorsey
PAC compound tab*	Upjohn
PAC compound c codeine*	Upjohn
PAC c Cyclopal	Upjohn
Palgesic*	Pan Amer
PC-65*	Caribe Chemical
Pedidyne	Lemmon
Pentagesic	Kremers-Urban
Pentagill	Beecham-Massengill
Percobarb*	Endo
Percobarb-Demi*	Endo
Percodan*	Endo
Percodan-Demi	Endo
Persistin	Fisons
Phac tab*	Cole
Phenaphen*	Robins
Phenaphen c codeine	Robins
Phencasal	Elder
Phencaset improved	Elder
Phenergan compound tabs*	Wyeth
Phenodyne	Blue Line
Pheno-Formasal*	First Texas
Phensal	Dow Chemical
Pirseal	Fellows-Testagar
Polygesic CT*	Amar-Stone
Ponodyne	Fellows-Testagar
Predisal*	Mallard
Prolaire-B*	Stuart
Pyrasal	Philips-Roxane
Pyrhist Cold	Daniels
Pyrroxate	Upjohn
Pyrroxate c codeine*	Upjohn
	R
Rhinex	Lemmon
Robaxisal*	Robins
Robaxisal-PH*	Robins
Ryd	Daniels
	S
Sal-Aceto	Fellows-Testagar
Sal-Fayne	Kenton
Salibar Jr*	Jenkins

Salipral*	Kenyon
Sarogesic*	Saron
Sedagesic*	Kay
Sedalgesic*	Table Rock
Semaldyne*	Beecham-Massengill
Sigmagen*	Schering
Sine-Off	Menley & James
Spirin Buffered	Schlicksup
Stanback	Stanback
Stero-Darvon c ASA*	Lilly
St. Joseph	Plough
St. Joseph for Children	Plough
Supac	Mission
Super-Anahist	Warner-Lambert
Synalgos*	Ives
Synalgos-DC*	Ives
Synirin*	Poythress
T	
Tetrex-APC c Bristamin*	Bristol
Thephorin-AC†	Roche
Toloxidyne	Durst
Trancogesic*	Winthrop
Trancoprin*	Winthrop
Triaminicin	Dorsey
Trigesic	Squibb
Triocin	Commerce
V	
Vanquish	Glenbrook
Z	
Zactirin*	Wyeth
Zactirin compound*	Wyeth

Unlisted products identified in 5 community pharmacies:

BiAct cold tabs	Sauter Labs
Defencin	Grove Labs
Haysma	Haysma Co
Monacet	Rexall
Quiet World	Whitehall Labs
Saleto	Mallard Inc
Sine-Aid	Johnson & Johnson
Soltice cold tabs	Chatlem Drug & Chemical Co

*On prescription only. †Discontinued.

(Reproduced by Permission. Leist ER, Banwell JG: Products Containing Aspirin, New England Journal of Medicine: 291: 710-712, 1974.)

Treatment of Hemophilia-A

The level or activity of factor VIII is related to the severity of clinical manifestations by the relationships below:

Efficacy of Hemostasis	VIII level (% of normal)
Normal	>50
Bleeding with major trauma	25-50
Severe bleeding after minor trauma or surgery	5-25
Spontaneous bleeding, hemarthroses	1-5
Crippling bleeding disorder	<1

The various available sources for factor VIII treatment may produce the following recipient factor VIII levels:

Source	Level (% of normal)
Fresh whole blood	4-6
Fresh frozen plasma	15-20
Cryoprecipitate	60-80
Lyophilized human AHG	60-80
Lyophilized animal AHG	≈ 150

The basic method by which the amount of factor VIII required can be calculated is:

$$\frac{\text{Patient Wgt (kg)} \times \text{Desired rise in VIII (\%)}}{K} = \text{total units factor VIII required}$$

where K = 2 for fresh frozen plasma
K = 1.5 for human AHG or cryoprecipitate
K = 1.0 for animal AHG

Example 1: A 70 kg patient with a factor VIII level of 3%, scheduled for surgery, and needing treatment to produce a 90% level, using cryoprecipitate:

$$\frac{70 \times (90 - 3)}{1.5} = \frac{70 \times (87)}{1.5} = 4060 \text{ factor VIII units}$$

This amount of factor VIII would produce a normal level, and would require the factor VIII from approximately 45 donors (at approximately 90 units per donor).

Example 2: The same patient requires treatment to a factor VIII level of 50%, and is not expected to receive any bank blood, dilutional IV solutions, nor major surgery:

$$\frac{70 \times (50 - 3)}{1.5} = \frac{70 \times 47}{1.5} = 2193 \text{ factor VIII units}$$

This represents enough factor VIII from approximately 24 donors.

Thus treatment requires knowledge of the patient's present factor VIII level, a proposed new level appropriate to the clinical circumstances, and the type of agent available for treatment, in a patient of known or closely estimated weight.

An alternate method is to estimate an initial dose, and maintenance dose based upon calculated plasma volume (PV), and clinical circumstances. Plasma volume is calculated as:

$$PV = \text{Patient wgt (kg)} \times 70 \text{ ml blood/kg} \times \left(\frac{100 - HCt(\%)}{100}\right)$$

After calculating plasma volume, the schedule is as follows:

	Initial dose	Maintenance dose
Major Surgery (preop)	1 PV	½ PV q 8 hr × 3 ½ PV q 12 hr × 16 ¼ PV q 12 hr × 16
Hemorrhage		
Major	1PV	½ PV q 8 hr × 3 ½ PV q 12 hr × 8
Minor	½ PV	½ PV q 12

1 PV = 1 unit of factor VIII for each ml of plasma volume

Example: A 70 kg patient scheduled for surgery with a hematocrit of 32% would receive factor VIII preoperatively as below:

$$70 \times 70 \times \left(\frac{100 - 32}{100}\right) = 3332 \text{ ml PV}$$

$$= 3332 \text{ factor VIII units}$$

This second method is less precise than the first, and only guesses at the patient's starting level and goal level.

Treatment of Hemophilia-B

The level or activity of factor IX is related to the severity of clinical manifestations by the same relationship as factor VIII, detailed in the previous appendix. The goal in therapy is to produce a level at least 50 percent of normal, during bleeding, or higher if continued losses, dilution, or consumption are anticipated. The two materials most available for treatment are fresh frozen plasma, and factor IX complex (Proplex®, Konyne®). The administered volume of FFP required is often prohibitively high. The formula for factor IX replacement is:

$$\frac{\text{Patient wgt (kg)} \times \text{Desired rise in factor IX (\%)}}{K} = \text{total units of factor IX needed}$$

where K = 1.2 for factor IX complex

Example: A 70 kg patient with known Christmas Disease (Hemophilia-B) and a factor IX level of 6%, scheduled for emergency surgery, requires treatment to the 70% level:

$$\textbf{Total units of factor IX} = \frac{70 \times (70 - 6)}{1.2}$$

Total units of factor IX = 3733 factor IX units via factor IX complex

The blood bank will determine the volume of factor IX complex necessary for use. Factor IX levels may not rise to the expected level—the kinetics are not well understood. A hematologist should be consulted.

Use of the ACT to Guide Heparin and Protamine Therapy

The ACT measures the effectiveness of the intrinsic and final common pathways. The action of heparin (and antagonism by protamine) on antithrombin, allows for modulation of these two pathways. It should be remembered that the thrombin time (TT) is a sensitive indicator of heparin effect, but the TT is not readily performed at the bedside (O.R., I.C.U., etc.). The ACT serves as a readily available, easy to perform test for heparin effect, but slightly less sensitive, and of course altered by many other disorders (factor V, VIII, and I deficiencies especially). The ACT may be performed by hand or by mechanical means (Hemochron®). The technique of heparin or protamine dose control is as follows:

1. Perform a control ACT (no heparin, etc.). Barring other problems, the ACT should be normal (90-120 seconds). Plot at point A.
2. Administer the dose of heparin estimated to double the control ACT, ≈1.5 mg/kg. Perform an ACT, plot as point B.
3. Administer any additional heparin estimated to place the ACT at a desired level (i.e. at 450-500 for cardiopulmonary bypass). This is estimated from the slope of the A-B line, i.e. 4 mg/kg total. Thus 2.5 mg/kg more is needed. Another ACT, plot as point C.
4. There is now a 3 point dose-response curve, along which **this patient, at this temperature,** roughly will track.
5. To achieve a **higher** ACT, the goal is projected from the A-B-C line, and the difference of heparin in mg/kg required to achieve this goal is read off the heparin scale. (To go to an ACT of 600 it would require an effective 6 mg/kg of heparin, thus 2 mg/kg more would be needed.)
6. To achieve a **lower** ACT, either time will provide a degradation of heparin, or protamine can be used to antagonize heparin's effect. If the ACT at point C is desired reduced to 200 seconds, this point would be at ≈1.5 mg/kg of protamine effect, and the **difference** 5.2 - 1.5 = 3.7 mg/kg of protamine would be given.
7. Thus the patient can be moved up or down the **individual** dose-response curve by giving the **difference** of the heparin or protamine dose required to move between two points.

Use of the ACT to Guide Heparin and Protamine Therapy

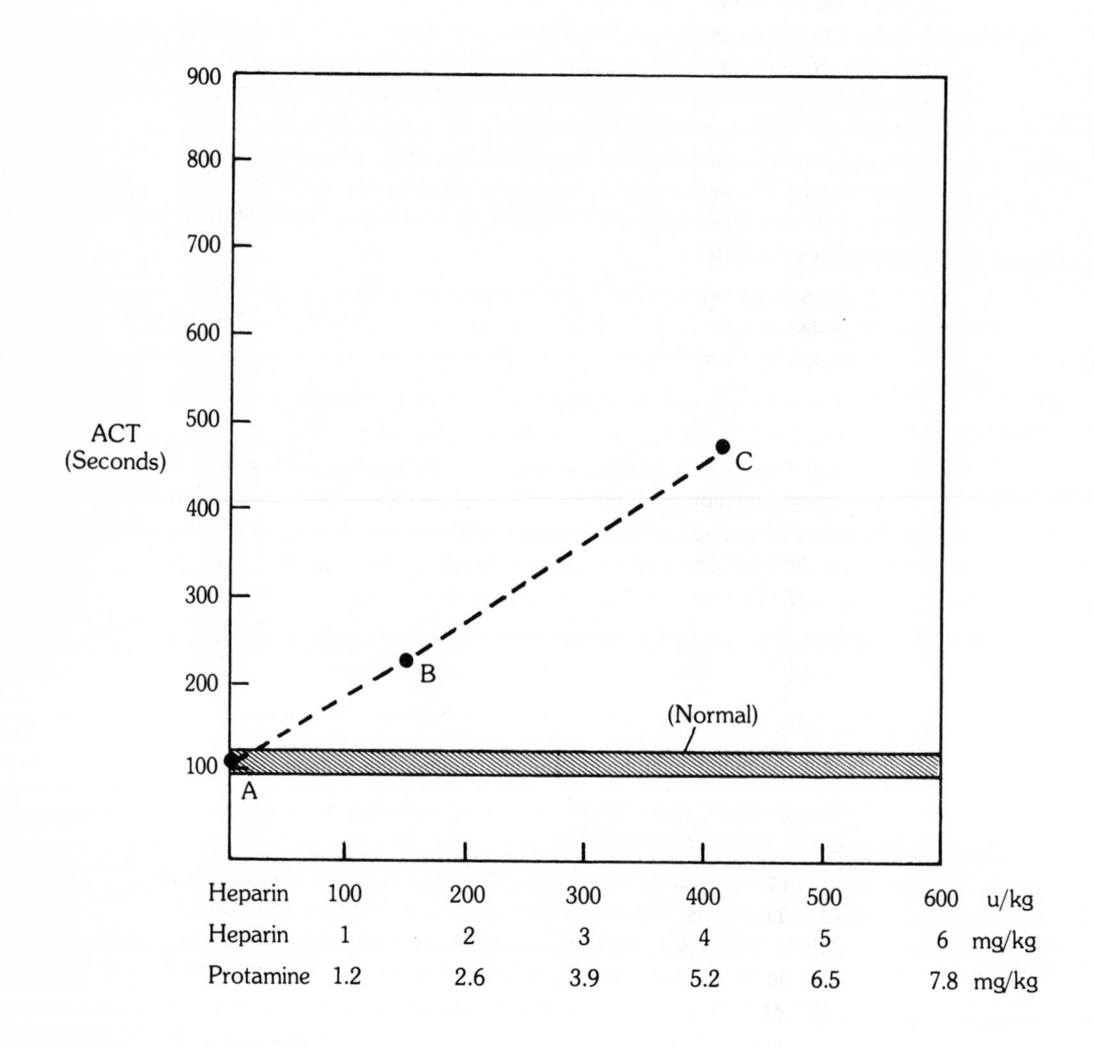

SUPPORTIVE READING

The sources listed below are compiled from a reference collection of over 800 articles. They are listed by subject, roughly in chronological order, and represent those articles which the authors believe provide the most informative supporting data.

GENERAL INFORMATION

1. Biggs R (Ed): Human Blood Coagulation, Haemostasis, and Thrombosis, 2nd edition. Blackwell (Lippincott), Oxford (Philadelphia) 1976 (An encyclopedic tome; excellent source book; not light nor quick reading)
2. Hirsch J, Brain EA: Hemostasis and Thrombosis — A Conceptual Approach. Churchill-Livingstone, New York 1979 (A small illustrated book with information on inherited and acquired disorders, medical conditions associated with coagulopathies, and thrombotic complications)
3. Ellison N: Coagulation Evaluation and Management, in Ream AK, Fogdall RP (eds) *Acute Cardiovascular Management: Anesthesia and Intensive Care.* Lippincott, Philadelphia (In Press) (an up-to-date chapter of direct clinical use)

LABORATORY INFORMATION

4. Harker LA: Hemostasis Manual. University of Washington, Seattle 1970. (some basics plus laboratory information)
5. Scully RE, McNeely BU, Galdabini JJ: Normal Reference Laboratory Values. New Eng J Med 302:37-48, 1980.

PLATELETS

General

6. Deykin D: Emerging Concepts of Platelet Function, New Eng J Med 290:144-151, 1974.
7. Weiss HJ: Platelet Physiology and Abnormalities of Platelet Function. New Eng J Med 293:531-541, 1975; 293:580-588, 1975.
8. Barrer MJ, Ellison N: Platelet Function. Anesthesiology 46:202-211, 1977.
9. Harker LA, Slichter SJ: The Bleeding Time as a Screening Test for Evaluation of Platelet Function. New Eng J Med 287:155-159, 1972.
10. Stuart MJ, Murphy S, Oski FA, et al: Platelet Function in Recipients of Platelets from Donors Ingesting Aspirin. New Eng J Med 287-1105-1109, 1972.
11. Harker LA, Slichter SJ: Platelet and Fibrinogen Consumption in Man. New Eng J Med 287:999-1005, 1972.
12. Handin RI, Valeri CR: Hemostatic Effectiveness of Platelets Stored at 22°C. New Eng J Med 285:538-543, 1974.
13. Needleman P, Kaley G: Cardiac and Coronary Prostaglandin Synthesis and Function. New Eng J Med 298:1122-1128, 1978.
14. Moncada S, Vane JR: Arachidonic Acid Metabolites and the Interactions between Platelets and Blood-Vessel walls. New Eng J Med 300:1142-1147, 1979.
15. Stuart MJ, Gerrard JM, White JG: Effect of Cholesterol on Production of Thromboxane B_2 by Platelets in Vitro. New Eng J Med 302:6-10, 1980.
16. McGiff JC: Thromboxane and Prostacyclin: Implications for Function and Disease of the Vasculature. Advances in Internal Medicine 25:199-216, 1980.
17. Kelton JG, Neame PB, Gauldie J, et al: Elevated Platelet-associated IgG in the Thrombocytopenia of Septicemia. New Eng J Med 300:760-764, 1979.
18. Green LM, Seroppian E, Handin RI: Platelet Activation during Exercise-induced Myocardial Ischemia. New Eng J Med 302:193-197, 1980.
19. Weiss HJ: Platelets and Ischemic Heart Disease (editorial). 302:225-226, 1980.

Platelet Abnormalities

20. Weily HS, Steele PP, Davis H, et al: Platelet Survival in Patients with Substitute Heart Valves. New Eng J Med 290:534-539, 1974.
21. Beurling-Harbury C, Galvan CA: Acquired Decrease in Platelet Secretory ADP Associated with Increased Postoperative Bleeding in Postcardiopulmonary Bypass Patients and in Patients with Severe Valvular Heart Disease. Blood 52:13-23, 1978.
22. Bachmann F, McKenna R, Cole ER, et al: The Hemostatic Mechanism After Open-Heart Surgery. I. Studies on Plasma Coagulation Factors and Fibrinolysis in 512 Patients After Extracorporeal Circulation. J Thorac Cardiovasc Surg 70:76-85, 1975.
23. McKenna R, Bachmann F, Whittaker B, et al: The Hemostatic Mechanism After Open-Heart Surgery. II. Frequency of Abnormal Platelet Functions During and After Extracorporeal Circulation. J Thorac Cardiovasc Surg 70:298-308, 1975.
24. Bick RL: Alterations of Hemostasis Associated with Cardiopulmonary Bypass: Pathophysiology, Prevention, Diagnosis, and Management. Seminars in Thrombosis and Hemostasis 3:59-82, 1976.
25. Lichtenfeld KM, Schiffer CA, Helrich M: Platelet Aggregation During and After General Anesthesia and Surgery. Anesth Analg 58:293-296, 1979.
26. Lum LG, Tubergen DG, Corash L, et al: Splenectomy in the Management of the Thrombocytopenia of the Wiskott-Aldrich Syndrome. New Eng J Med 302:892-896, 1980.
27. Hoar PF, Stone JG, Wicks AE, et al: Thrombogenesis Associated with Swan-Ganz Catheters. Anesthesiology 48:445-447, 1978.
28. Richman KA, Kin YL, Marshall BE: Thrombocytopenia and Altered Platelet Kinetics Associated with Prolonged Pulmonary-artery Catheterization in the Dog. Anesthesiology 53:101-105, 1980.

Platelets and Drugs

29. Folts JD, Crowell, EB, Rowe GG: Platelet Aggregation in Partially Obstructed Vessels and its Elimination with Aspirin. Circulation 54:365-370, 1976.
30. Bedford RF, Ashford TP: Aspirin Pretreatment Prevents Post-Cannulation Radial-Artery Thrombosis. Anesthesiology 51:176-178, 1979.
31. Pantely GA, Goodnight SH, Rahimtoola SH, et al: Failure of Antiplatelet and Anticoagulant Therapy to Improve Potency of Grafts After Coronary-Artery Bypass. New Eng J Med 301:962-966, 1979.
32. Marcus AJ: How Useful is Antiplatelet Therapy? Drug Therapy (Hosp) 53-62, October 1979.
33. Anturane Reinfarction Trial Research Group — S. Sherry, Chrm. Sulfinpyrazone in the Prevention of Sudden Death After Myocardial Infarction. New Eng J Med 302:250-256, 1980.

Von Willebrand's Disease and Factor VIII

34. Zimmerman TS, Abildgaard CF, Meyer D: The Factor VIII Abnormality in Severe Von Willebrand's Disease. New Eng J Med 301:1307-1310, 1979.
35. Ruggeri ZM, Pareti FI, Mannucci PM, et al: Heightened Interaction between Platelets and Factor VIII/Von Willebrand Factor in New Subtype at Von Willebrand's Disease. New Eng J Med 302:1047-1051, 1980.
36. Mandalaki T, Louizou C, Dimitriadou C, et al: Variations in Factor VIII During the Menstrual Cycle in Normal Women. New Eng J Med 302:1093-1094, 1980.
37. Lusher JM, Shapiro SS, Palascak JE, et al: Efficacy of Prothrombin-Complex Concentrates in Hemophiliacs with Antibodies to Factor VIII. New Eng J Med 303:421-425, 1980.

COAGULATION CASCADE

Heparin and Protamine

38. Rosenberg RD: Actions and Interactions of Antithrombin and Heparin. New Eng J Med 292:146-151, 1975.

39. Rosenberg RD, Rosenberg JS: The Anticoagulant Function of Heparin. Drug Therapy (Hosp) 87-95, September 1979.
40. Bull BS, Huse WM, Braver FS, et al: Heparin Therapy During Extracorporeal Circulation II. The use of a dose-response curve to individualize heparin and protamine dosage. J Thorac Cardiovasc Surg 69:685-689, 1975.
41. Bull BS, Korpman RA, Huse WM, et al: Heparin Therapy During Extracorporeal Circulation I. Problems inherent in existing heparin protocols. J Thorac Cardiovasc Surg 69:674-684, 1975.
42. Bull MH, Muse WM, Bull BS: Evaluation of Tests Used to Monitor Heparin Therapy During Extracorporeal Circulation. Anesthesiology 43:346-353, 1975.
43. Guffin AV, Dunbar RW, Kaplan JA, et al: Successful Use of a Reduced Dose of Protamine After Cardiopulmonary Bypass. Anesth Analg 55:110-113, 1976.
44. Salzman EW, Deykin D, Shapiro RM, et al: Management of Heparin Therapy. Controlled Prospective Trial. New Eng J Med 292:1046-1050, 1975.
45. Simon TL: The Rationale for Continuous Heparin Infusion. Drug Therapy (Hosp) 17-25, November 1978.
46. Estes JW: Heparin in Clinical Practice. Drug Therapy (Hosp) 69-80, September 1979.
47. Palermo LM, Andrews RW, Ellison N; Avoidance of Heparin Contamination in Coagulation Studies Drawn from Indwelling Lines. Anesth Analg 59:222-224, 1980.

Coumadin and Vitamin K

48. Koch-Weser J, Sellers EM: Drug Interactions with Coumadin Anticoagulants. New Eng J Med 285:487-498, 1971; 285:547-558, 1971.
49. Suttie JW: How Coumarin Anticoagulants Work. Drug Therapy (Hosp) 117-125, September, 1979.
50. Gallop PM, Lian JB, Mauschka PV: Carboxylated Calcium — Binding Proteins and Vitamin K. New Eng J Med 302:1460-1466, 1980.
51. Furie B: Using Oral Anticoagulants Effectively. Drug Therapy (Hosp) 108-112, September, 1979.

TREATMENT

52. Myhre BA (Ed): Blood Component Therapy — A Physician's Handbook. American Association of Blood Banks, 1975.
53. Miller RD, Robbins TO, Tong MJ, et al: Coagulation Defects Associated with Massive Blood Transfusions. Ann Surg 174:794-801, 1971.
54. Miller RD: Complications of Massive Blood Transfusions. Anesthesiology 39:82-93, 1973.
55. Allen JG: The Case for the Single Transfusion (Editorial). New Eng J Med 287:984-985, 1972.
56. Ellison N: Diagnosis and Management of Bleeding Disorders. Anesthesiology 47:171-180, 1977.
57. Grady GF: Transfusions and Hepatitis: Update in '78 (Editorial). New Eng J Med 298:1413-1415, 1978.
58. Tabor E, Hoofnagle JH, Smallwood LA, et al: Studies of Donors Who Transmit Post-transfusion Hepatitis. Transfusion 19:725-731, 1979.

THROMBOEMBOLISM AND FIBRINOLYSIS

59. Pechet L: Fibrinolysis. New Eng J Med 273:966-973, 1965.
60. Sherry S: Fibrinolysis and Afibrinogenemia. Anesthesiology 27:465-474, 1966.
61. Evarts CM: Thromboembolic Disease: Prophylaxis and Treatment. Crit Care Med 4:62-66, 1976.
62. McKee PA: The Prevention of Thromboembolism (Editorial). Drug Therapy (Hosp) 25-27, September 1979.
63. Moroz LA, Sniderman AD, Marpole DGF: Leukocyte — Plasma Interaction in Fibrinolysis. A New Dimension in the Action of Urokinase. New Eng J Med 301:1100-1104, 1979.

64. Bell WR, Meek AG: Guidelines for the Use of Thrombolytic Agents. New Eng J Med 301:1266-1270, 1979.
65. Sasahara AA, Ho DD, Sharma GVRK: When and How to Use Fibrinolytic Agents. Drug Therapy (Hosp) 67-84, October 1979.
66. European Cooperative Study Group: Streptokinase in Acute Myocardial Infarction. New Eng J Med 301:797-802, 1979.
67. Sullivan JM: Streptokinase and Myocardial Infarction (Editorial). New Eng J Med 301:836-837, 1979.

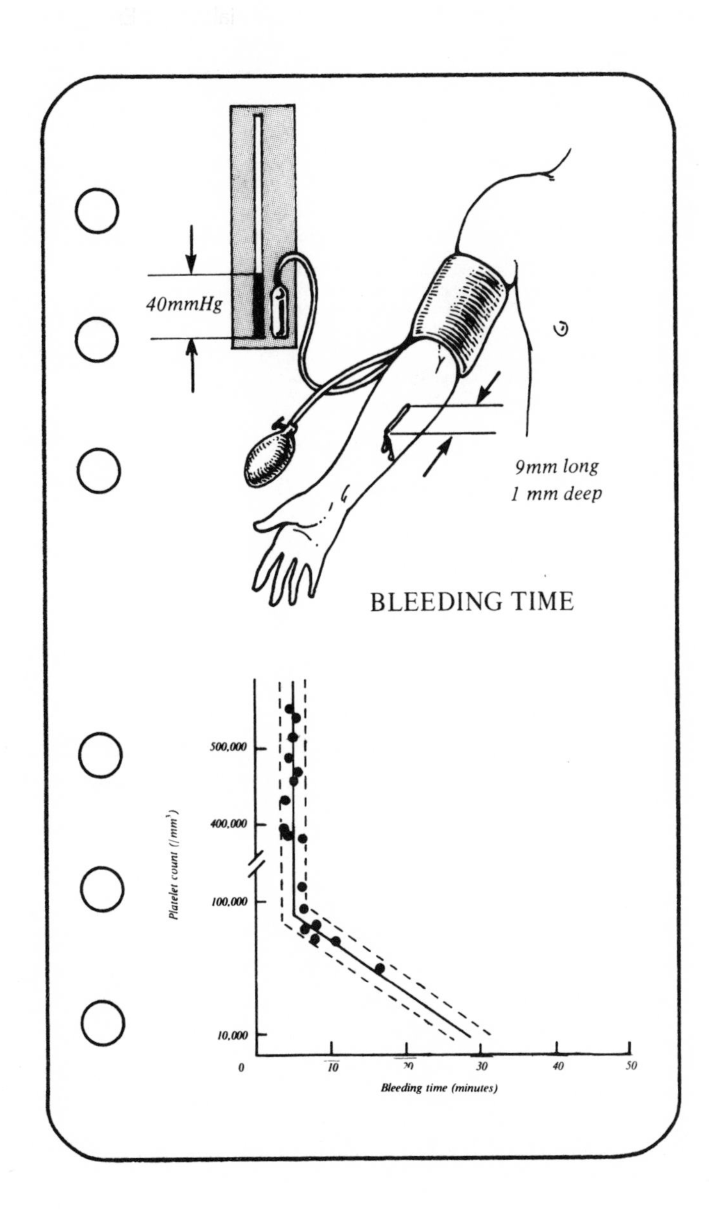
40mmHg
9mm long
1 mm deep
BLEEDING TIME
500,000
400,000
100,000
10,000
Platelet count (/mm³)
0
10
30
40
50
Bleeding time (minutes)

In order to avoid confusion, an international committee* established a standard nomenclature assigning Roman Numerals to the clotting factors. They were numbered in the order of discovery. Active factors were indicated by the subscript "a".

Roman Numeral	Protein Coagulation Factor
I	Fibrinogen
II	Prothrombin
III	Platelet Factor 3 (thromboplastin)
IV	Calcium
V	Labile Factor (proaccelerin)
VI	(Not Assigned)
VII	Stable Factor—Proconvertin
VIII	Antihemophiliac Factor A (AHF)
IX	Antihemophiliac Factor B, Christmas Factor
X	Stuart-Prower Factor
XI	Antihemophiliac Factor C
XII	Hageman Factor
XIII	Fibrin Stabilizing Factor

Note: Factor III is a phospholipid in the platelet surface membrane. Factor IV is the calcium ion.

(*Biggs—Second Edition, p. 15.)

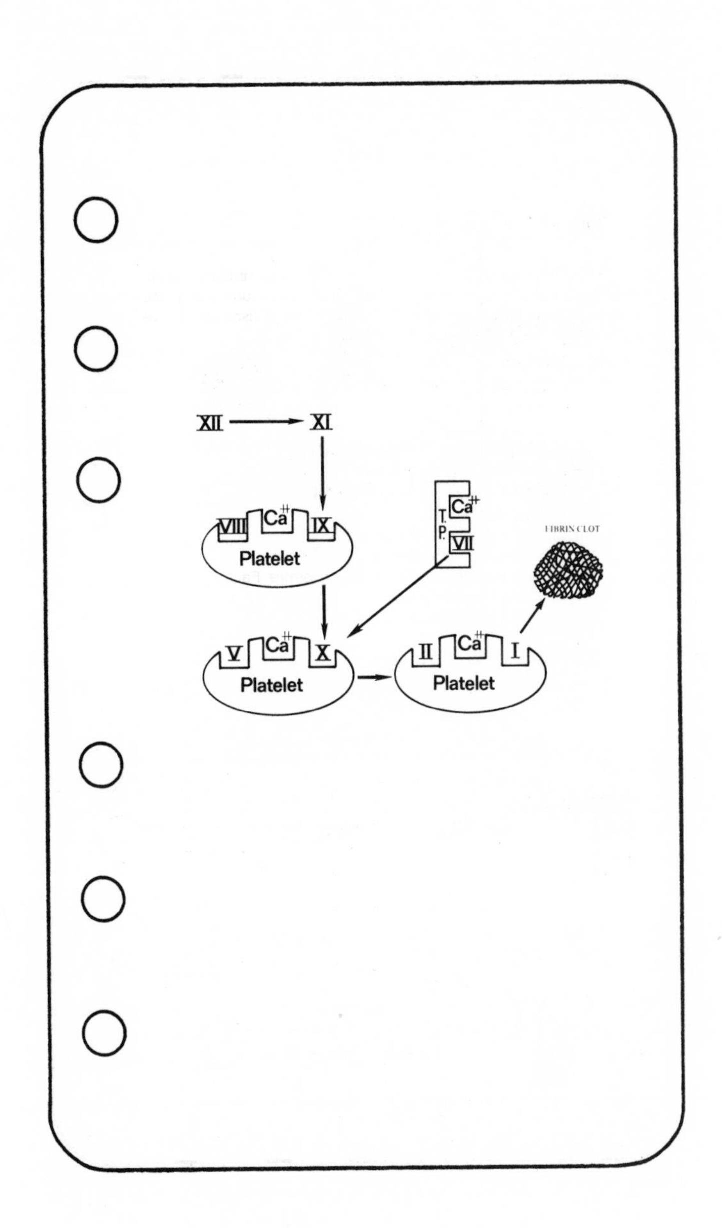
XII
XI
VIII
Ca++
IX
Platelet
T.
P.
Ca++
VII
FIBRIN CLOT
V
Ca++
X
Platelet
II
Ca++
I
Platelet

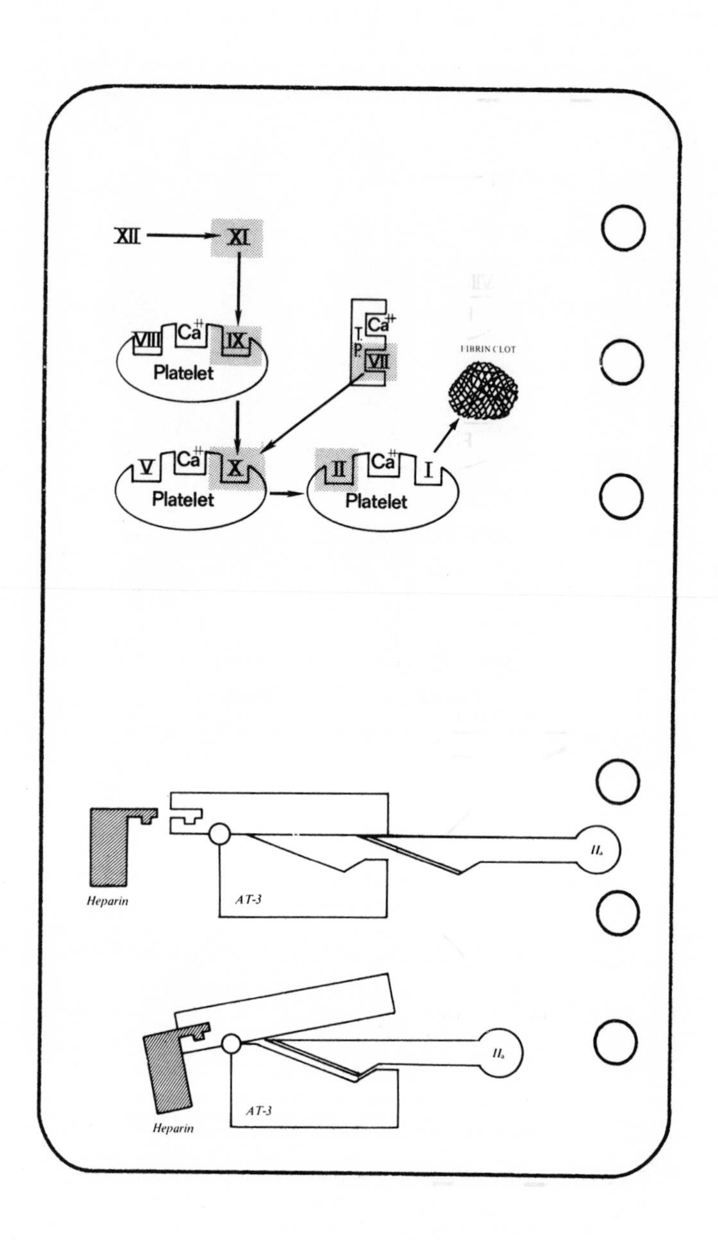
XII
XI
VIII
Ca++
IX
Platelet
T.
P.
Ca++
VII
FIBRIN CLOT
V
Ca++
X
Platelet
II
Ca++
I
Platelet
Heparin
AT-3
IIa
Heparin
AT-3
IIa

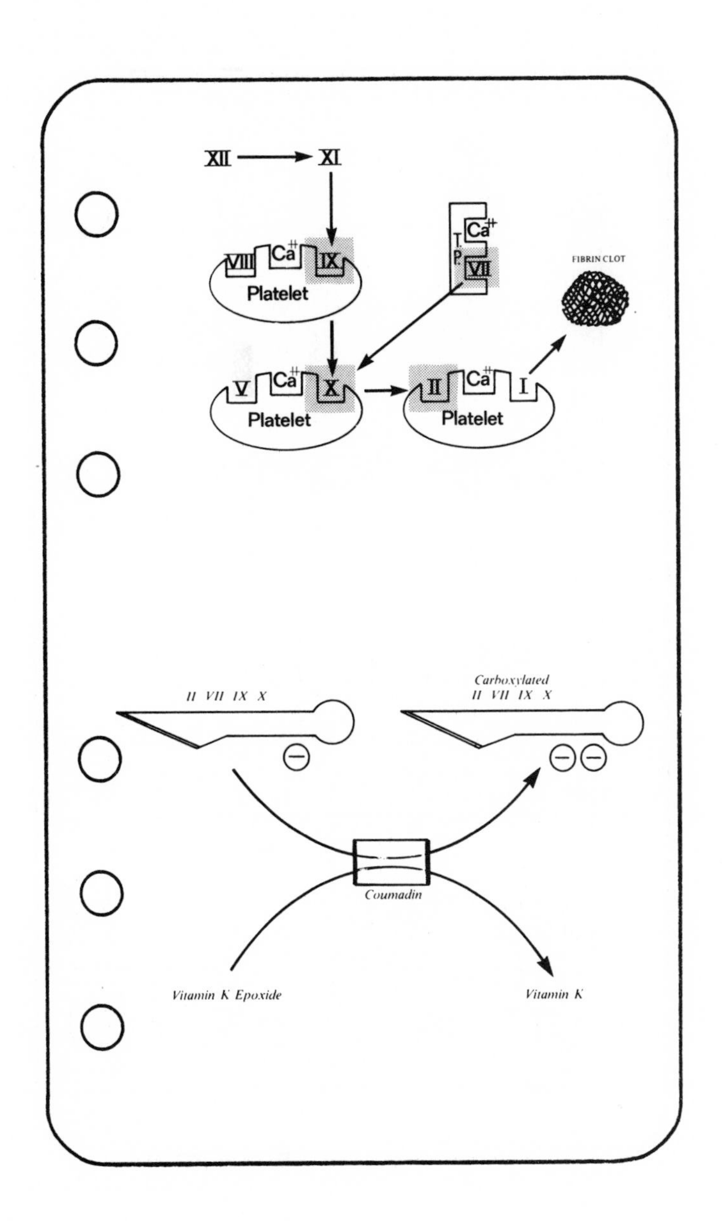
XII
XI
VIII
Ca++
IX
Platelet
T.
P.
Ca++
VII
FIBRIN CLOT
V
Ca++
X
Platelet
II
Ca++
I
Platelet
II VII IX X
Carboxylated
II VII IX X
Coumadin
Vitamin K Epoxide
Vitamin K

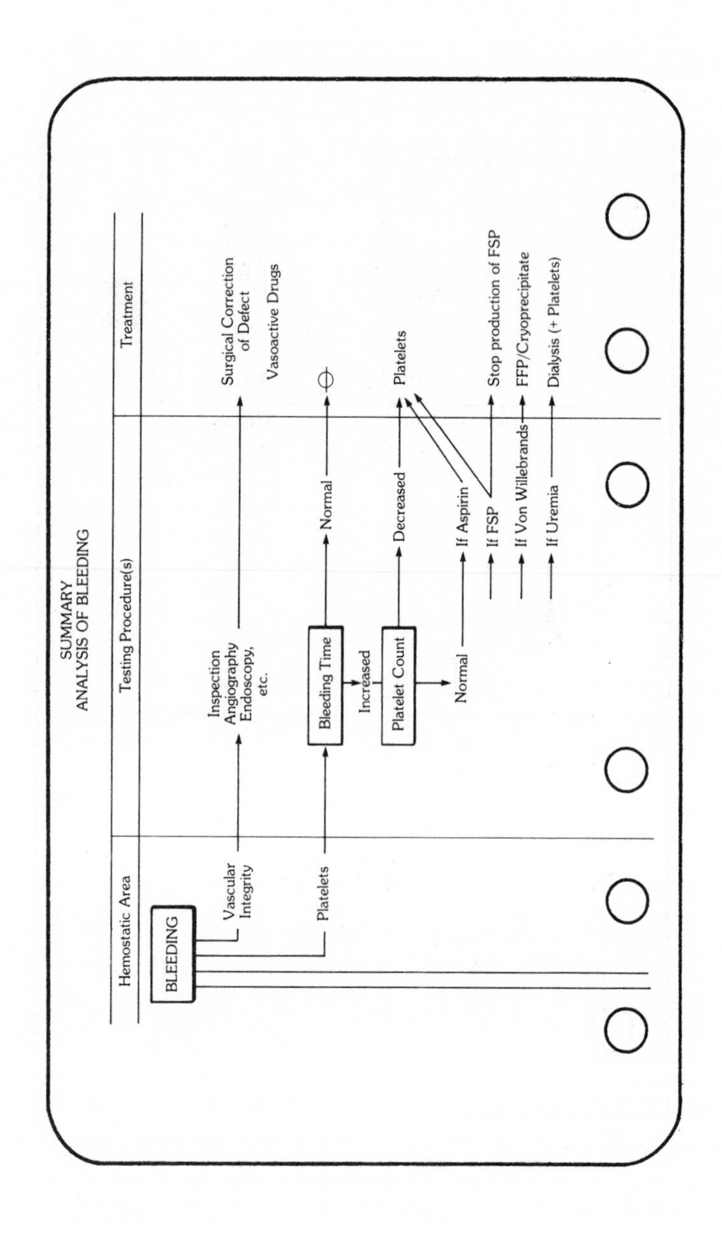
SUMMARY
ANALYSIS OF BLEEDING
Hemostatic Area
Testing Procedure(s)
Treatment
BLEEDING
Vascular Integrity
Platelets
Inspection
Angiography
Endoscopy,
etc.
Surgical Correction of Defect
Vasoactive Drugs
Bleeding Time
Normal
Increased
Platelet Count
Decreased
Platelets
Normal
If Aspirin
If FSP
If Von Willebrands
If Uremia
Stop production of FSP
FFP/Cryoprecipitate
Dialysis (+ Platelets)

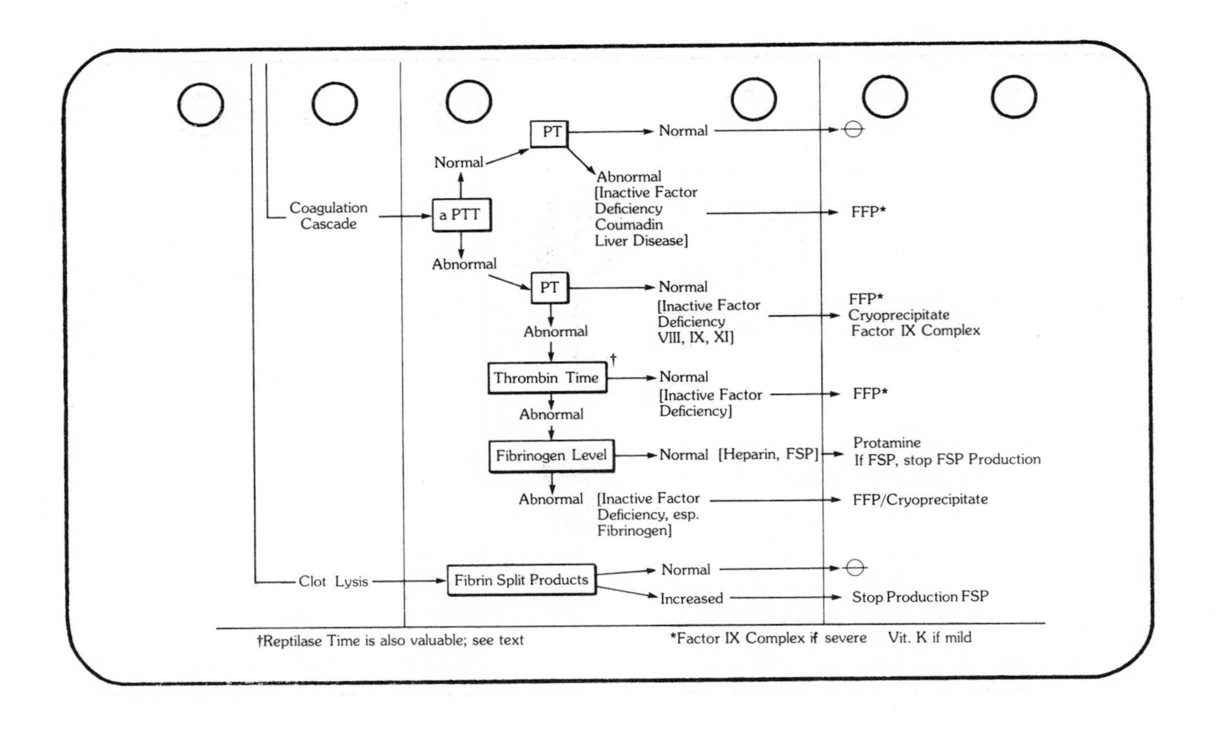
Coagulation Cascade
a PTT
Normal
Abnormal
PT
Normal
Abnormal [Inactive Factor Deficiency Coumadin Liver Disease]
FFP*
PT
Normal [Inactive Factor Deficiency VIII, IX, XI]
FFP* Cryoprecipitate Factor IX Complex
Abnormal
Thrombin Time†
Normal [Inactive Factor Deficiency]
FFP*
Abnormal
Fibrinogen Level
Normal [Heparin, FSP]
Protamine If FSP, stop FSP Production
Abnormal [Inactive Factor Deficiency, esp. Fibrinogen]
FFP/Cryoprecipitate
Clot Lysis
Fibrin Split Products
Normal
Increased
Stop Production FSP
†Reptilase Time is also valuable; see text
*Factor IX Complex if severe Vit. K if mild

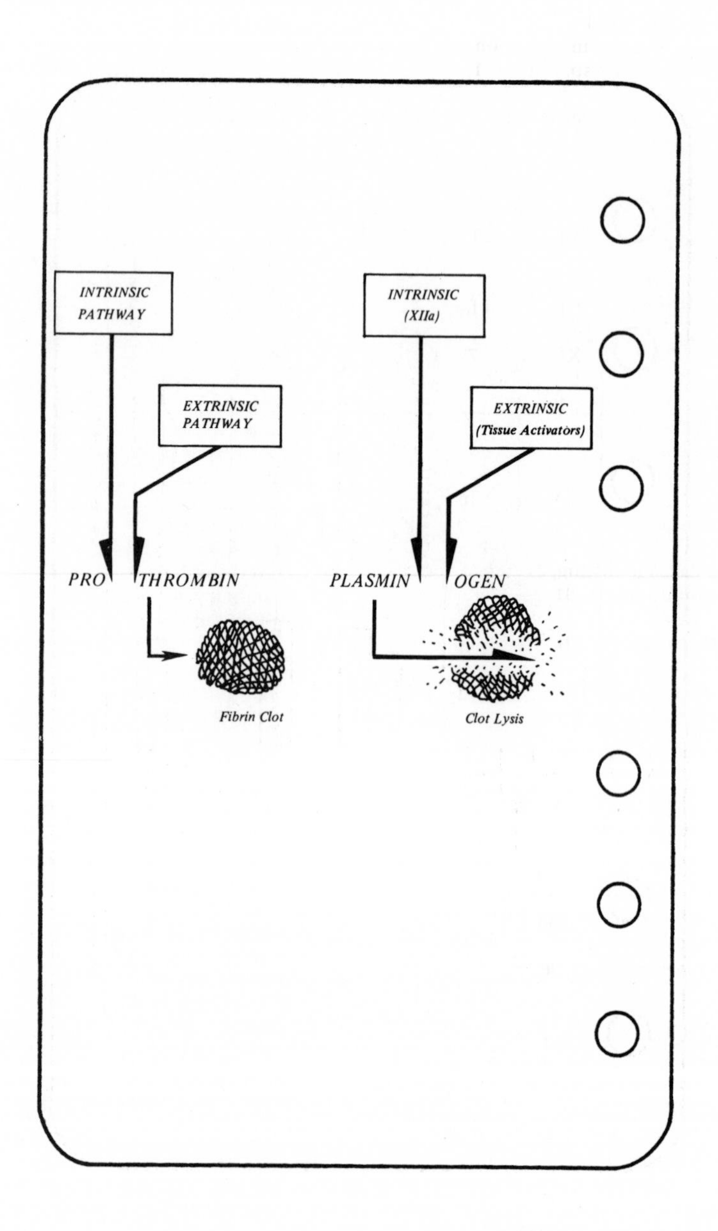
INTRINSIC PATHWAY
EXTRINSIC PATHWAY
PRO THROMBIN
Fibrin Clot
INTRINSIC (XIIa)
EXTRINSIC (Tissue Activators)
PLASMIN OGEN
Clot Lysis

Index